Reprint from ADDICTIVE DISEASES:
An International Journal,
Volume II, Numbers 1 and 2, 1975

Perinatal Addiction

Proceedings of a conference sponsored by
the National Institute on Drug Abuse and Vanderbilt University,
Nashville, Tennessee, September 1974

Editor: Raymond D. Harbison

Vanderbilt University School of Medicine
Nashville, Tennessee

S P Books Division of
SPECTRUM PUBLICATIONS, INC.

New York

Distributed by Halsted Press
A Division of John Wiley & Sons

New York   Toronto   London   Sydney

SPECTRUM PUBLICATIONS, INC.
86-19 Sancho Street, Holliswood, N.Y. 11423

Distributed solely by the Halsted Press division of John Wiley & Sons, Inc., New York

Library of Congress Cataloging in Publication Data
Main entry under title:

Perinatal addiction.

    (Sociomedical science series)
    "Reprint from Addictive diseases: an international journal, volume II, numbers 1 and 2, 1975."
    1. Drug withdrawal symptoms—Congresses. 2. Drugs and infants—Congresses. 3. Drugs and women—Congresses. 4. Narcotic habit—Congresses. I. Harbison, Raymond D. II. National Institute on Drug Abuse. III. Vanderbilt University, Nashville. IV. Addictive diseases. [DNLM: 1. Drug addiction—Congresses. 2. Maternal-fetal exchange—Drug effects—Congresses. 3. Fetus—Drug effects—Congresses. WQ210 P441 1974]

RJ506.N3P47 1975   618.3'2   75-29065

ISBN 0-470-35148-9

CONTENTS

PREFACE—*WILLIAM POLLIN*

OVERVIEW OF THE PERINATAL NARCOTIC ADDICTION
CONFERENCE AND FUTURE RESEARCH GOALS IN
DEVELOPMENTAL PHARMACOLOGY OF ABUSED DRUGS
—*RAYMOND D. HARBISON, MONIQUE C. BRAUDE* 1

EPIDEMIOLOGY

USE OF LEGAL SUBSTANCE WITHIN THE GENERAL
POPULATION: THE SEX AND AGE VARIABLES
—*CARL D. CHAMBERS, MICHAEL S. GRIFFEY* 7

CURRENT CONCEPTS IN THE MANAGEMENT OF
THE PREGNANT OPIATE ADDICT
—*JAMES F. CONNAUGHTON, JR., LORETTA P.
FINNEGAN, JACOB SCHUT, JOHN P. EMICH* 21

PRENATAL DRUG EXPOSURE

METABOLIC CAPABILITIES OF THE HUMAN FETUS:
DRUG BIOTRANSFORMATION
—*M.R. JUCHAU* 37

DRUGS OF ABUSE: TERATOGENIC AND MUTAGENIC
CONSIDERATIONS
—*MICHAEL A. EVANS, MICHEL W. STEVENS, BERNARDO
MANTILLA-PLATA, RAYMOND D. HARBISON* 45

CYTOGENETIC RISKS TO THE OFFSPRING OF
PREGNANT ADDICTS
—*CYRIL A.L. ABRAMS* 63

THE FETAL ALCOHOL SYNDROME
—*KENNETH LYONS JONES* 79

HEAT-STABLE ALKALINE PHOSPHATASE IN
METHADONE-MAINTAINED PREGNANCIES
—*RITA G. HARPER, GEORGE SOLISH,*
    ELLEN FEINGOLD, MYRON SOKAL 89

CLINICAL OBSERVATIONS ON METHADONE-MAINTAINED
PREGNANCIES
—*ROY C. DAVIS, JOHN N. CHAPPEL, ALFONSO*
    MEJIA-ZELAYA, JOHN MADDEN 101

NEONATAL CONSIDERATIONS

NEONATAL ABSTINENCE SYNDROME:
RECOGNITION AND DIAGNOSIS
—*MURDINA M. DESMOND, GERALDINE S. WILSON* 113

BIOMEDICAL APPLICATIONS OF VAPOR PHASE ANALYSIS
—*EUGENE HEATH, J. THROCK WATSON* 123

NEONATAL ABSTINENCE SYNDROME:
ASSESSMENT AND MANAGEMENT
—*LORETTA P. FINNEGAN, REUBEN E. KRON,*
    JAMES F. CONNAUGHTON, JR., JOHN P. EMICH 141

ACUTE MANAGEMENT OF NEONATAL ADDICTION
—*CARL ZELSON* 159

DISPOSITION OF METHADONE AND ITS RELATIONSHIP
TO SEVERITY OF WITHDRAWAL IN THE NEWBORN
—*TOVE ROSEN, CHARLES E. PIPPENGER* 169

PHENOBARBITAL DISPOSITION IN THE NEONATE
—*L.K. GARRETTSON* 179

A STUDY OF FACTORS THAT INFLUENCE THE SEVERITY
OF NEONATAL NARCOTIC WITHDRAWAL
—*ENRIQUE M. OSTREA, CLEOFE J. CHAVEZ,*
    MILTON E. STRAUSS 187

DRUG IMPEDIMENTS TO MOTHERING BEHAVIOR
—*H.P. COPPOLILLO* 201

ADDICTIVE DISEASES: AN INTERNATIONAL JOURNAL VOLUME 2, NO. 2, 1975

CONTENTS

GENERAL DISCUSSION 209

**SPECIAL CONSIDERATIONS OF ADDICTIVE
DRUG EFFECTS ON THE NEONATE**

NEUROLOGICAL ASPECTS OF PERINATAL NARCOTIC
ADDICTION AND METHADONE TREATMENT
  —*MIRYAM DAVIS, BETTY SHANKS* 213

NEONATAL ADDICTION: A TWO-YEAR STUDY
  —*ANN LODGE, CYRIL M. RAMER, MARILYN M. MARCUS* ... 227

THE ASSESSMENT OF BEHAVIORAL CHANGE IN INFANTS
UNDERGOING NARCOTIC WITHDRAWAL: COMPARATIVE
DATA FROM CLINICAL AND OBJECTIVE METHODS
  —*REUBEN E. KRON, STUART L. KAPLAN, LORETTA P.
  FINNEGAN, MITCHELL LITT, MARIANNE D. PHOENIX* 257

PERINATAL NARCOTIC ADDICTION IN MICE:
SENSITIZATION TO MORPHINE STIMULATION
  —*LUIS SHUSTER, G.W. WEBSTER, G. YU* 277

SYMPATHO-ADRENAL DEVELOPMENT IN
PERINATALLY ADDICTED RATS
  —*THEODORE A. SLOTKIN, THOMAS R. ANDERSON* 293

SOME EFFECTS OF PRENATAL EXPOSURE TO
D-AMPHETAMINE SULFATE AND PHENOBARBITAL
ON DEVELOPMENTAL NEUROCHEMISTRY AND
ON BEHAVIOR
  —*JOHN W. ZEMP, LAWRENCE D. MIDDAUGH* 307

SOMATIC GROWTH EFFECTS ON PERINATAL ADDICTION
  —*GERALDINE S. WILSON* 333

DIFFERENTIAL EFFECTS OF HEROIN AND METHADONE
ON BIRTH WEIGHTS
  —*STEPHEN R. KANDALL, SUSAN ALBIN, EVAN DREYER,*
  MARCIA COMSTOCK, JOYCE LOWINSON 347

EFFECT OF HEROIN ON PERINATAL RESPIRATION
  —*LEONARD GLASS, HUGH E. EVANS,*
  B.K. RAJEGOWDA, ERIC J. KAHN 357

MORPHINE ADMINISTRATION TO PREGNANT RABBITS:
EFFECT ON FETAL GROWTH AND LUNG DEVELOPMENT
  —*DIETRICH W. ROLOFF, WILLIAM F. HOWATT,*
  WILLIAM P. KANTO, JR., ROBERT C. BORER 369

GENERAL DISCUSSION 381

SUBJECT INDEX 385

PREFACE

With a marked increase in addiction in recent years has come a similarly large increase in the number of infants born of addicted mothers. There is now a slim but growing volume of knowledge on how to better treat both the mothers and the newborn so as to minimize health hazards to these children. As multiple drug use becomes increasingly common we can expect new complications to arise in the management of the pregnant drug abuser and of her offspring. This monograph represents an initial attempt to bring together some of the latest insights into the problem of perinatal addiction from both a basic and an applied research perspective. It is our hope that as knowledge increases, this monograph will be succeeded by others so as to encourage a more sophisticated approach to the public health management of children born of drug-abusing mothers and to foster the basic research that must serve as the ultimate foundation for better health care.

William Pollin
National Institute on Drug Abuse

Addictive Diseases: an International Journal 2 (1): 1-5 (1975)

Overview of the Perinatal Narcotic Addiction Conference and Future Research Goals in Developmental Pharmacology of Abused Drugs

RAYMOND D. HARBISON
Department of Pharmacology
Division of Pediatric Clinical Pharmacology
Vanderbilt Medical Center
Nashville, Tennessee

MONIQUE C. BRAUDE
National Institute on Drug Abuse
Division of Research
Biomedical Research Branch
Washington, D.C.

We have recently learned that commonly used therapeutic agents can produce extraordinary responses in developing organisms. The sedative hypnotic drug thalidomide produced the most dramatic example of a drug-induced change during perinatal development. Since this acknowledgment of the first drug-induced change during in utero development, we have recognized that a diverse array of pharmacologically active compounds can affect perinatal growth and development. Despite these facts, relatively few guidelines have been determined objectively for clinicians who must treat women of the child-bearing ages, pregnant women, the newborn, and young children. The major concerns are treatment efficacy, compliance, safety, dosage, and adverse effects.

Approximately 4 million females and 4 million males under the age of 35 regularly use phenobarbital, amphetamine, major and minor tranquilizers, and alcohol. In addition, combinations of these as well as with other drugs are frequently used. The use of drug combinations increases the possibility of adverse reactions.

Thus, a large number of females and males are exposed to drugs, both intentionally—for therapeutic purposes—as well as for self-medication purposes during the reproductive years. The hazard of this exposure to the unborn child, the potential for drug-induced mutations and the possible drug-induced adverse effects during neonatal growth and development and subsequent postnatal development are of major concern and constitute the subject of this conference.

Drug-induced human developmental anomalies have been documented by a number of the participants in this conference (Jones, Glass, Kandall, Abrams, and Connaughton). These anomalies range from the fetal alcohol syndrome to physiological dysfunctions, biochemical abnormalities, and an increased perinatal mortality. Also, additional drug-induced biochemical and behavioral defects have been documented in animal models (Slotkin, Shuster, Roloff, and Zemp). Increased susceptibility of newborn animals to methadone-induced toxicity was also demonstrated (Evans). Despite the wide variety of pharmacologically diverse compounds used and abused during the reproductive ages, we have only limited information on the developmental pharmacology-toxicology of a few of these drugs. Human studies document that drug-induced changes are produced in the fetus and newborn, and animal studies suggest additional drug-induced changes are possible but not yet recognized in the human population.

Medical management of the pregnant addict and subsequently the management of her addicted offspring was a major theme of the conference and a top-priority area. Low-dose methadone maintenance plus intense psychosocial support is best for treatment of the pregnant addict and her offspring and least compromises the newborn's physiological functions. Methods for objective assessment of withdrawal severity have been presented (Finnegan). Objective, semiquantitative clinical methods involving the assessment of sucking behavior, the adaptive behavior of the addicted infant, and the subsequent effects of pharmacological treatment on these parameters were also described (Kron). These represent important achievements. In the past, answers to major pharmacological questions were obtained solely by therapeutic empiricism with its attendant risks. These newly described objective measures will help refine pharmacologic treatment of the addict newborn. Development of a new body of fundamental pharmacologic and toxicologic information applicable to the developing human is the necessary route to establishing a rational basis for the use of drugs in this special patient population.

Effects of narcotic drugs on long-term somatic growth and subsequent behavioral development have long been discussed and were refocused at this conference (Wilson and Desmond). The consequences of the reported drug-induced low birth weights, reduced body lengths, and reduced head circumferences are not yet known.

As sophisticated, sensitive analytical pharmacological techniques have become available for analysis of drugs in small samples of biological fluids, we now urgently need pharmacokinetic data to correlate blood drug levels with efficacy in the treatment of neonatal withdrawal. For instance, Garrettson reported that the plasma half life of phenobarbital is prolonged in the newborn and that drugs should be administered with caution to the newborn because detoxification systems are developing at this time (Juchau). Also, additional studies are urgently needed to describe placental transfer of narcotics and their subsequent disposition in the offspring (Rosen). Drug dosage regimens cannot be established for treatment of the pregnant addict or her addicted offspring unless we have some knowledge of the pharmacokinetics of these drugs, specifically in this special addict patient population. The treatment of the newborn addicted syndrome was discussed at length following Zelson's and Ostrea's presentation. There was no consensus between the conference participants regarding the best pharmacological treatment of this withdrawal syndrome. Prospective efficacy studies for pharmacological treatment of the neonatal withdrawal syndrome are urgently needed.

Finally, the long-term effects produced by exposure in utero to narcotics is unknown. A great deal of discussion during the conference was directed to the presence or absence of tremors and seizures in the infants born of addicted mothers. Again, no consensus was reached, but future studies should look more specifically for this and other definite signs of central nervous system changes. The mother-infant relationship might be impaired, thereby producing permanent predispositional changes in adult behavior. This might lead to a vicious cycle of propagated drug abuse (Coppolillo). Long-term longitudinal follow-up studies are urgently needed.

Based on the proceedings of this conference, it is clear that to design appropriate studies in this area of perinatal drug addiction requires a cooperative multidisciplinary effort involving the disciplines of obstetrics, pediatrics, genetics, toxicology, developmental biochemistry, and basic pharmacology. The persons involved in this multidisciplinary activity must be concerned not only with acquiring data, but with transmitting this information to the clinician responsible for treatment of this special patient population. Programs for training pediatric clinical pharmacologists and developmental pharmacologists should be sponsored.

From what was learned here, we have tried to outline the gaps that exist in our basic information of the developmental pharmacology of abused drugs in the various areas covered by the conference. The following need special attention:

A. Factors affecting drug transfer to embryo and fetus
　　1. Physicochemical
　　　　a. solubility
　　　　b. molecular size
　　　　c. binding
　　　　d. ionization

    2. Physiological
        a. gestational age and placental maturation
        b. transplacental transfer
        c. blood flow
        d. placental dysfunction
    3. Placental metabolism
        a. detoxification and bioactivation
        b. therapeutic significance
    4. Comparative pharmacology
        a. development of suitable animal models for transfer study
  B. Toxicological effects of transplacental passage of drugs
      1. Teratogenetic
      2. Cytogenetic
      3. Mutagenic
      4. Carcinogenic
  C. In utero drug disposition
      1. Relative drug disposition in fetus and maternal organism
      2. Accumulation of drugs of abuse in specialized tissues, such as brain, adrenals, etc.
      3. Fetal drug metabolism
      4. Fetal drug distribution and excretion (pharmacokinetics)
  D. Postnatal drug action and disposition
      1. Drug metabolism, distribution, and excretion in newborn
      2. Changing volume of distribution and influence on drug levels
      3. Development of blood-brain barrier
      4. Pharmacologic reactivity
      5. Drug-induced changes on production, distribution, metabolism, and excretion of endogenous materials during normal development
        a. hormones
        b. steroids
        c. phospholipids
  E. Toxicology
      1. Drug-induced long-term effects on behavioral development and somatic growth
      2. Drug-drug interactions
      3. Malnutrition-drug and disease-drug interactions
      4. Development of micromethodology for drug analysis

In summary, this conference strongly emphasized the need for supporting both basic and clinical developmental pharmacology studies in the drug abuse area. Exposure of the pregnant patient and newborn to abused drugs is a significant public health problem. The hazards of this exposure for future generations must be assessed and the subsequent treatment of drug-induced adverse effects programatically planned. The highest priority should be given to filling the gaps in the knowledge outlined above and to training qualified persons to ensure a continuous flow of information essential for rational decision-making.

Addictive Diseases: an International Journal 2 (1): 7-19 (1975)

Use of Legal Substances Within the General Population: The Sex and Age Variables

CARL D. CHAMBERS
MICHAEL S. GRIFFEY
Department of Epidemiology and Public Health
University of Miami School of Medicine
Miami, Florida

As requested by your conference chairmen, we have prepared a presentation which my colleagues and I believe both dramatizes the extent of substance use in this country and characterizes those most likely to be involved. The numbers which will be presented have been derived from more than 30,000 face-to-face interviews conducted within the general populations of 16 states and the District of Columbia and are projected to the nation as a whole. As far as we know, our data base is the largest in this country. Even so, we acknowledge and caution you to remember that our numbers are statistical projections which, although they are highly reliable problem indicators, are not to be confused with the precision of a full census.

We would also like to point out that the most dysfunctional people were *excluded* from our surveys and our subsequent projections. Our survey data are based on household residents and therefore do *not* include persons who are residents of institutions, e.g., mental hospitals, nursing homes, jails or penitentiaries, etc., and do not include those persons who do not have a permanent residence, e.g., skid-row alcoholics, migrant workers, etc.

For ease of presentation, we have elected to array our data by drug or drug class describing the prevalence of use and characterizing the users by sex and age cohorts. Because of time limitations, we have restricted the presentation to the extent of current regular use of six prescription drugs and classes—the barbiturates, non-barbiturate sedatives, minor tranquilizers, antidepressants, amphetamines, and the non-narcotic analgesics—and alcohol. We have elected not to present data on users of illicit drugs partly because of space limitations and partly because these drugs are not available to everyone.

BARBITURATES

The barbiturates were first synthesized and introduced into medicine in Germany in 1903. Since that time, more than 2,000 different barbiturates have been compounded, yet fewer than a dozen of these account for the bulk of current use. The barbiturates most commonly prescribed include amobarbital (Amytal), pentobarbital (Nembutal), phenobarbital (Luminal), secobarbital (Seconal, Tuinal), and butabarbital (Butisol, Fiorinal). In 1970 some $31,779,000 were spent on the barbiturates, with prescriptions from general practitioners accounting for 38% and internists accounting for 19% of this total.

Our survey data indicate that the use of barbiturates is widespread throughout the general population. For purposes of describing the extent of this use, we have projected our survey data for the total population above age 13 with the following results:

In excess of 24 million people (some 16% of everyone over the age of 13) have taken one or more of the barbiturates.

As many as 9 million people have probably used these drugs within the past six months. We project, therefore, that about one of every three people who have ever taken a barbiturate has done so recently.

Probably as many as 4.5 million people use one of these prescription sedatives on a regular basis.

4,500,000 Regular Users of Barbiturates			
Males	14-17	3%	135,000
	18-24	6%	270,000
	25-34	4%	180,000
	35 +	29%	1,305,000
Females	14-17	4%	180,000
	18-24	6%	270,000
	25-34	7%	315,000
	35 +	41%	1,845,000

Our data suggest that no more than 85% of the regular users of barbiturates obtain *all* of these barbiturates with their own legal prescription.

Our data further suggest that no more than 75% of the regular users of barbiturates take them exactly as they were prescribed.

Over one-third of all the regular users of barbiturates are concurrently using one or more of the other prescription psychoactive medications—usually a non-barbiturate sedative or one of the minor tranquilizers.

About 50% of all regular users of barbiturates are also regular users of alcohol and 10% can be considered as heavy drinkers.

Women in the general child-bearing age cohort (18-34) represent 12% of the total population. Women within this age group represent 13% of that population which regularly use barbiturates. Our data would suggest therefore, that women of general child-bearing age are proportionately represented in the regular use of these drugs.

NON-BARBITURATE SEDATIVES

The more commonly prescribed non-barbiturate sedatives include: Doriden, Valmid, Placidyl, Noludar, Quaalude and Sopor.

In 1970 some $22 million were spent on the non-barbiturate sedatives, with prescriptions from general practitioners accounting for 30 percent and those from internists accounting for 14 percent of this total.

Our survey data indicate that the use of the non-barbiturate sedatives is less extensive than the use of the barbiturates. Projections from our surveys lead us to conclude the following:

We believe some 4.5 million people (some 3% of everyone over the age of 13) have taken a non-barbiturate sedative at some time during their lives.

We further believe that over a million of these people have used these drugs within the past six months, or about one of every nine people who have ever used these drugs has done so recently.

Probably as many as 350,000 people are regular users of these drugs.

Based on our total survey data, we believe only some 70% of the regular users of the non-barbiturate sedatives obtain *all* of these drugs with their own legal prescription. In addition, only about 70% of all these regular users take them exactly as they were prescribed.

One can expect over one-third of all the regular users of the non-barbiturate sedatives to also use another of the prescription psychoactive medications. This concurrent regular use most frequently involves the barbiturates and/or the minor tranquilizers.

Some 70% of the regular users of non-barbiturate sedatives are also regular users of alcohol, but less than 10% are heavy drinkers.

350,000 Regular Users of Non-Barbiturate Sedatives			
Males	14-17	4%	14,000
	18-24	10%	35,000
	25-34	7%	24,500
	35 +	33%	115,500
Females	14-17	8%	28,000
	18-24	5%	17,500
	25-34	7%	24,500
	35 +	26%	91,000

Women in the general child-bearing age cohort (18-34) represent 12% of the total population. Women within this age group represent 12% of that population which regularly use the non-barbiturate sedatives. Our data would suggest therefore, that women of general child-bearing age are proportionately represented in the regular use of these drugs.

MINOR TRANQUILIZERS

The minor tranquilizers refer to a group of anxiolytic sedatives that were introduced into medical practice during the 1950's. They are designated as minor tranquilizers. effective in the reduction of anxiety and tension, as opposed to the major tranquilizers, which are antipsychotic drugs employed in the treatment of severe mental disorders. Librium, Valium, Miltown and Equanil are the most widely prescribed of the minor tranquilizers.

In 1970 some $357,300,000 were spent on these minor tranquilizers, with prescriptions from general practitioners accounting for 32% and prescriptions from internists accounting for 17% of the total.

Our survey data indicate the use of the minor tranquilizers to be more extensive than the use of any other group of prescription psychoactive medications. Projections from our surveys suggest the followingest the following:

More than 20 million people (some 18% of everyone over the age of 13) have at some time used one of the prescription minor tranquilizers.

More than 13.5 million people can be considered as *recent* users of these drugs, having used them within the last six months.

Probably as many as 5 million people are regular users of minor tranquilizers.

5,000,000 Regular Users of Minor Tranquilizers			
Males	14-17	1%	50,000
	18-24	3%	150,000
	25-34	5%	250,000
	35 +	23%	1,150,000
Females	14-17	2%	100,000
	18-24	6%	300,000
	25-34	9%	450,000
	35 +	51%	2,550,000

Based on our total survey data, our conclusion is that 90% of all regular users of minor tranquilizers obtain *all* of these drugs with their own legal prescription but that only about 70% take them exactly as they were prescribed.

Only about 15% of those who regularly use these drugs concurrently use other prescription psychoactive drugs on a regular basis. If another drug is used concurrently, it is usually one of the sedatives.

Only about 40% of the regular users of minor tranquilizers are also regular users of alcohol and about 15% are heavy drinkers.

Women in the general child-bearing age cohort (18-34) represent 12% of the total population. Women within this age group represent 15% of that population which regularly use the minor tranquilizers. Our data would suggest therefore, that women of general child-bearing age are overrepresented in the regular use of these drugs.

ANTIDEPRESSANTS

The introduction of antidepressants some fifteen years ago has greatly facilitated the management of a wide variety of depressive states. Generally known as mood elevators, these drugs have chemical structures quite different from those of the amphetamines and have largely replaced them in the treatment of depression.

In 1970 some $57 million were spent on antidepressants, with prescriptions from general practitioners accounting for 16% of the total, internists accounting for 10% of the total, and psychiatrists accounting for almost 60% of the total. The most widely prescribed of the antidepressants are Elavil, Tofranil, and Sinequan.

The use of antidepressants is the least prevalent of all the prescribed psychoactive medications. Projections from our surveys suggest the following involvements:

Only some 3 million people (less than 2% of everyone over the age of 13) have ever used one of these antidepressants.

About a million people can be considered as *recent* users of these drugs, having used them within the past six months. This does suggest, however, that one of every three people who have *ever* used them has done so recently.

Probably 500,000 people are *regular* users of the antidepressants.

500,000 Regular Users of Antidepressants			
Males	14-17	1%	5,000
	18-24	3%	15,000
	25-34	6%	30,000
	35 +	27%	135,000
Females	14-17	2%	10,000
	18-24	8%	40,000
	25-34	11%	55,000
	35 +	42%	210,000

We believe most regular users of antidepressants (over 85%) obtain *all* of these drugs with their own legal prescription but that as many as 20% do *not* take the drugs as they are prescribed.

One can expect half of those who regularly use antidepressants to concurrently use other prescription psychoactive drugs on a regular basis, usually sedatives or minor tranquilizers.

Only about 20% of the regular users of antidepressants are regular alcohol users, and less than 10% can be considered as heavy drinkers.

Women in the general child-bearing age cohort (18-34) represent 12% of the total population. Women within this age group represent 19% of that population which regularly use antidepressants. Our data would suggest therefore, that women of general child-bearing age are significantly overrepresented in the regular use of these drugs.

AMPHETAMINES

We have limited our inquiry into the use of prescription stimulants to amphetamines and amphetamine base stimulants and hunger suppressants.

Amphetamines were initially synthesized during the latter part of the Nineteenth century, but were not used extensively in medical practice until the 1930s.

In 1970 some $85 million were spent on the amphetamines and amphetamine base stimulants and hunger suppressants. Prescriptions from general practitioners accounted for 62% of this total and internists accounted for an additional 11%.

The amphetamines are frequently used, both clinically and illicitly, in conjunction or in alternation with a variety of depressant drugs such as sedatives, alcohol, or heroin. Amphetamines also reportedly prolong, intensify, or otherwise alter the effects of other stimulants, sedatives, analgesics and hallucinogenic drugs.

The amphetamines are typically misused for their energizing and euphorigenic properties. Self-medication has been common in groups such as housewives, students, truck drivers, and factory workers. Although recent controls placed on these drugs have curtailed their availability, we have every reason to believe that those persons who used and misused them in the past will either continue to seek them out or will seek out other non-amphetamine stimulants.

Pep Pills

For the purposes of our surveys, pep pills were defined as those prescription amphetamines which are taken for their energizing effects. We have encountered only two drugs with any regularity, *Benzedrine* and *Dexedrine.*

Our survey data indicate the admitted use of amphetamines specifically for their energizing effects has involved some six million people (almost 4% of everyone above the age of 13). We are projecting some 1.5 million people as recent users and some 750,000 people as being current regular users.

750,000 Regular Users of Amphetamine "Pep Pills"			
Males	14-17	9%	67,500
	18-24	36%	270,000
	25-34	2%	15,000
	35 +	12%	90,000
Females	14-17	10%	75,000
	18-24	11%	82,500
	25-34	3%	22,500
	35 +	17%	127,500

The availablility of amphetamine pep pills during the period of our surveys (1973-1974) from other than strictly legal sources was quite high. We found only some 30% of the regular users of these drugs obtained *all* of their drugs with their own legal prescription. Even among those who did obtain their drugs with a legal prescription, only a third of them took these drugs as they had been prescribed.

At least one-fourth of those who regularly use amphetamines for their stimulating effect can be expected to also be regularly using minor tranquilizers. Indicating the popularity of these drugs among drug abusers, we have noted that about one-half of the regular users of amphetamine pep pills are also regular users of illegal drugs, usually marijuana.

Our data indicate almost all regular users of amphetamine pep pills are also drinkers with about half of them being heavy drinkers.

Women in the general child-bearing age cohort (18-34) represent 12% of the total population. Women within this age group represent 14% of that population which regularly use the "pep pills." Our data would suggest, therefore, that women of general child-bearing age are *overrepresented* in the regular use of these drugs.

Diet Pills

Diet pills most often consist of an amphetamine in combination with a central nervous system depressant. When combined this way, the stimulant acts to reduce appetite, and the depressant serves to counteract any overstimulation which might otherwise occur.

The use of amphetamine-containing diet pills appears to be closely related to their ability to create a sense of well-being. As such, they may be useful when taken for short periods of time. However, their long-term effectiveness in weight control has been properly questioned.

Our survey data indicate the use of amphetamines ostensibly for their hunger suppressant effects has involved some 12 million people (some 8% of everyone above the age of 13). We are projecting some 3 million people as recent users and more than 1.5 million as current regular users.

1,500,000 Regular Users of Amphetamine "Diet Pills"			
Males	14-17	2%	30,000
	18-24	7%	105,000
	25-34	5%	75,000
	35 +	8%	120,000
Females	14-17	6%	90,000
	18-24	21%	315,000
	25-34	17%	255,000
	35 +	34%	510,000

Our data suggest that only about 70% of all regular users of amphetamine "diet pills" obtain *all* of their drugs with their own legal prescription, and only about 70% of those who do, take them exactly as they were prescribed.

Persons who regularly use the amphetamine base "diet pills" do not normally use any other prescription psychoactive drug on a regular basis.

About one-half of all regular users of amphetamine "diet pills" can be expected to be heavy users of alcohol.

Women in the general child-bearing age cohort (18-34) represent 12% of the total population. Women within this age group represent 38% of that population which regularly use "diet pills." Our data would suggest, therefore, that women of general child-bearing age are greatly *overrepresented* in the regular use of these drugs.

NON-NARCOTIC ANALGESICS

In our surveys we have attempted to assess the extent to which people are involved in the management of pain with the prescription non-narcotic analgesics. The two drugs we encounter most frequently are propoxyphene (Darvon) and Pentazocine (Talwin). In 1970 some $98.5 million were spent on the prescription non-narcotic analgesics, with prescriptions from general practitioners accounting for 58% and internists accounting for 14% of this total.

Not unexpectedly, our survey data indicate the use of these drugs to be widespread throughout the general population. For purposes of describing the extent of this use, we have projected our survey data for the total population above age 13 with the following results:

In excess of 36 million people (some 24% of everyone over the age of 13) has taken one or more of the non-narcotic analgesics.

As many as 12 million people have probably used these drugs within the past six months. We project, therefore, that about one of every three people who have ever used these drugs has done so recently.

Probably as many as 3,750,000 people use one of these prescription non-narcotic analgesics on a regular basis.

Our data suggest that no more than 70% of the regular users of non-narcotic analgesics obtain *all* of these drugs with their own legal prescription.

Our data further suggest that no more than 75% of these regular users take them exactly as they are prescribed.

Only about 15% of all the regular users of these drugs are concurrently using one or more of the prescription psychoactive medications—usually a sedative or minor tranquilizer.

About 50% of all regular users of non-narcotic analgesics are also regular users of alcohol, and some 10% can be considered as heavy drinkers.

Women in the general child-bearing age cohort (18-34) represent 12% of the total population. Women within this age group represent 27% of that popu-

3, 750, 000 Regular Users of Prescription Non-Narcotic Analgesics			
Males	14-17	4%	150, 000
	18-24	9%	337, 500
	25-34	6%	225, 000
	35 +	18%	675, 000
Females	14-17	6%	225, 000
	18-24	13%	487, 500
	25-34	14%	525, 000
	35 +	30%	1, 725, 000

lation which regularly use non-narcotic analgesics. Our data would suggest, therefore, that women of general child-bearing age are greatly overrepresented in the regular use of these drugs.

The surveys have clearly established the extensive utilization of the barbiturate sedatives, minor tranquilizers, and non-narcotic analgesics. As many as 24 million people have at some time relied on these sedatives; 20 million have sought to tranquilize themselves against the effects of anxiety, stress, or tension; and 36 million have sought to relieve pain with the prescription non-narcotic analgesics. The surveys have suggested that as many as 4.5 million people regularly use these sedatives, 5 million people regularly use the minor tranquilizers and 3,750,000 people regularly use these analgesics.

We might also point out that probably as many as a million people use one of the nonprescription (OTC) sleeping medications every week; as many as 500,000 people use a nonpescription (OTC) stimulant every week; and as many as 500,000 people use a nonprescription (OTC) tranquilizer every week.

ALCOHOL

While roughly one-third of America's population above the age of 13 claim abstinence—that is, no drinking in the year preceding their interview—we project that the remaining two-thirds (68% or more than 100 million persons) drank *some* alcohol last year. Almost half of these are "*regular drinkers*"; that is, they drink alcohol *at least* once a month.

Our data indicate there are some 18 million people who can be considered *heavy drinkers*—persons who typically drink every day and often consume five or six drinks at each setting or several drinks during the day.

Women in the general child-bearing age cohort (18-34) represent 12% of

18,000,000 Heavy Users of Alcohol			
Males	14-17	8%	1,440,000
	18-24	30%	5,400,000
	25-34	28%	5,040,000
	35 +	11%	1,980,000
Females	14-17	2%	360,000
	18-24	9%	1,620,000
	25-34	9%	1,620,000
	35 +	3%	540,000

the total population. Women within this age group represent 18% of that population which are heavy users of alcohol. Our data would suggest, therefore, that women of general child-bearing age are overrepresented in the regular use of these drugs.

The prevalence of heavy drinking is noticeably higher among *minority groups* and persons in the *lower socioeconomic classes*. According to our survey data, almost half of the heavy drinkers surveyed are employed as either skilled, semi-skilled, or unskilled workers.

SUMMARY

We have attempted to describbbe the dimensions of the extent to which people in our society have come to rely on chemicals to assist the management of their lives. In addition, we have attempted to characterize those who regularly cope with themselves, others, and their life situation through the use of drugs. Projecting from data obtained from more than 30,000 interviews, we believe the numbers of people who are currently or regularly coping chemically to be as follows:

Barbiturate Users 4,500,000
Non-Barbiturate Sedative Users 350,000
Minor Tranquilizer Users 5,000,000
Antidepressant Users 500,000
Amphetamine "Pep Pill" Users 750,000
Amphetamine "Diet Pill" Users 1,500,000

Over-the-Counter Sleep Inducers 1,000,000
Over-the-Counter Stimulants 500,000
Over-the-Counter Tranquilizers 500,000

Regular Drinkers 50,000,000
Heavy Drinkers 18,000,000

When we control for persons who use more than one substance on a regular basis we find the following:

There are some 12 million people who regularly use one or more of these legal drugs but who do not drink enough to be considered heavy drinkers.

There are some 15 million heavy drinkers who are not regular users of the other drugs.

There are some 3 million people who are both regular users of these drugs and heavy drinkers.

In attempting to characterize those who habitually respond to boredom, loneliness, frustration, and stress by turning to alcohol or psychoactive medications, we have determined the following *generalizations*:

Women tend to cope with "medications" while men cope with alcohol.

Whites tend to cope with "medications" while blacks cope with alcohol.

Persons over age 35 tend to cope with "medications"; persons under age 35 cope with alcohol.

Middle and upper socioeconomic groups tend to cope with "medications," while the lower groups cope with alcohol.

Housewives, sales workers, clerks and other white-collar workers tend to cope with "medications," while skilled, semiskilled and unskilled workers cope with alcohol.

Among those coping with "medications," younger persons and men are more likely to use stimulants, and older persons and women are more likely to use sedating and tranquilizing drugs.

Although the use of illicit drugs was not the subject of our presentation here, we would like to make a brief comment relative to the regular use of these drugs among women of child-bearing age.

Women in the general child-bearing age cohort (18-34) represent 12% of the total population, and this same group comprises 19% of all current and regular users of marijuana, 25% of all regular social/recreational users of heroin, 12% of all current and regular users of LSD and 18% of all regular social/recreational users of cocaine. Our data do suggest, therefore, that women within the child-bearing ages are at least proportionately represented and normally overrepresented among current and regular users of illicit drugs.

Note:

Reprint request should be addressed to Dr. Carl D. Chambers, Department of Epidemiology and Public Health, University of Miami School of Medicine, Miami, Florida 33124.

Addictive Diseases: an International Journal 2 (1): 21-35 (1975)

Current Concepts in the Management of the Pregnant Opiate Addict

JAMES F. CONNAUGHTON, JR.
Department of Obstetrics and Gynecology
University of Pennsylvania School of Medicine and
Philadelphia General Hospital
Philadelphia, Pennsylvania

LORETTA P. FINNEGAN
Department of Pediatrics
University of Pennsylvania School of Medicine and
Philadelphia General Hospital
Philadelphia, Pennsylvania

JACOB SCHUT
Department of Psychiatry
University of Pennsylvania School of Medicine and
West Philadelphia Mental Health Consortium
Philadelphia, Pennsylvania

JOHN P. EMICH
Department of Obstetrics and Gynecology
University of Pennsylvania School of Medicine and
Philadelphia General Hospital
Philadelphia, Pennsylvania

INTRODUCTION

In 1969, the increasing concern with the problem of drug-dependent pregnant women and the resultant passively drug-dependent newborn prompted the opening of a special prenatal clinic at the Philadelphia General Hospital. Prior to that year, little work had been done in this field, and published data were largely limited to retrospective studies describing the horrors of narcotics addiction combined with pregnancy (Krause, S.O., Murray, P.M., Holmes, J.B., and Burch, R.E., 1958; Sussman, S., 1963; Perlmutter, J.F., 1967; Stern, R., 1966; Stone, M.L., Salerno, L.J., Green, M., and Zelson, C., 1971). Since that time, numerous programs addressing themselves to the care of the pregnant drug-dependent woman have flourished throughout the United States, and a substantial number of studies have been published (Harper, R.G., Sia, C.G., and Blenman, S., 1973; Newman, R.G., 1973; Scott, N.R., and Ryan, J.J., 1973; Blinick, G., Wallach, R.C., and Jerez, E., 1969; Davis, R.C., and Chappel, J.N., 1973).

This report addresses itself to the evaluation of a comprehensive approach in the care of 206 pregnant addicts and their infants. This type of approach employed at the Philadelphia General Hospital has decreased the complication rate substantially. The literature has been reviewed in an attempt to isolate pertinent findings so that future work can be directed toward maximum improvement of methods now being used to manage these difficult cases.

One of the most difficult problems in analyzing data obtained from these patients is defining a control group. In most of the previously published studies, the control group is composed of non-treated addicted patients. Along with the comparison of previously published data, this manuscript will compare a group of pregnant women addicted to heroin and treated with methadone maintenance and/or detoxification with a group of randomly selected non-addicted pregnant women from the same socioeconomic level treated in the outpatient clinics and delivered at Philadelphia General Hospital.

BACKGROUND

In reviewing the literature, an attempt must be made to limit the number of parameters reported by each author and thereby significantly compare the results. The obstetrical complication most consistently reported and probably most significant is pre-eclampsia. The neonatal complications are low birth weight with its subsequent sequelae and the neonatal withdrawal syndrome.

Table I lists the early studies prior to published data on "treated" patients (Krause, S.O., Murray, P.M., Holmes, J.B., and Burch, R.E., 1958; Sussman, S., 1963; Perlmutter, J.F., 1967; Stern, R., 1966; Stone, M.L., Salerno, L.J., Green, M., and Zelson, C., 1971). All are retrospective studies with varying numbers of drug-dependent mothers. It was noted then, as it is now, that low birth weight is the most significant factor influencing perinatal mortality and morbidity. All of the authors reported an extremely high incidence of low birth weight and, in these reports, pre-eclampsia was present in a large number of mothers.

In 1969, Blinick [Blinick, G., Wallach, R.C., and Jerez, E. (Table II)] from the Beth Israel Hospital in New York reported the first data on "treated" patients obtained through a combined approach with the Dole-Nyswander Methadone Program. For the first time, pregnant patients were given comprehensive

TABLE I
Early Literature Statistics

INVESTIGATORS	YEAR REPORTED	NO. OF PATIENTS	TOXEMIA	LBW
Krause et al.	1958	18	10%	39%
Sussman	1963	22	--	50%
Perlmutter	1967	22	--	56.5%
Stern	1966	66	15%	18.5%
Stone et al.	1971	382	11%	49%

LBW = low birth weight

care in an effort to treat the medical problems of pregnancy as well as the problems of addiction. A high percentage of patients in the Blinick study returned to the use of heroin; however, maternal complications were reduced to 7%. The incidence of low birth weight, however, remained high (34%).

Since the work of Blinick et al. (Blinick, G., Wallach, R.C., and Jerez, E., 1969), there have been a series of reports dealing with the various methods of treatment of pregnant drug-dependent women and the successes of each. Table II lists the largest series and the results.

It is interesting to note that even with the use of methadone in various doses, the incidence of low birth weight was not significantly reduced, but as in Blinick's study, prenatal care apparently reduced the incidence of pre-eclampsia to negligible levels, comparable to that in a non-addicted population.

The most comprehensive study is that of Davis and Chappel in which a large number of patients were studied and six different groups analyzed [(Table III), Davis, R.C., and Chappel, J.N., 1973]. In their report, there is a minimal reduction in the incidence of low birth weight no matter how intense the therapy. (In Groups 3, 4 and 5, besides methadone maintenance and intensive prenatal care, the patient had superior counseling with psychological support.)

PHILADELPHIA GENERAL HOSPITAL STUDY
MATERIALS AND METHODS

Two hundred and six drug-dependent pregnant patients were studied. All were delivered at Philadelphia General Hospital between 1969 and 1973. The patients are divided into three groups: *Group A*—patients who received no counseling and delivered while still actively using heroin ("street addicts on heroin"); *Group B*—patients who were admitted to the Family Center Program

TABLE II
Recent Literature Statistics

AUTHORS	TYPE OF TREATMENT	TOTAL PATIENTS	LBW INCIDENCE	PRE-ECLAMPSIA	INCIDENCE OF INFANT WITHDRAWAL
Harper	11>60 mg.				
	26<60 mg.	37	15/37 (40%)	12/37 (5.4%)	95%
Newman	100>40 mg.				
	20<40 mg.	120	N.R. (- %)	3/120 (2.0%)	79%
Scott	Mean dose 60 mg.	24	11/24 (46%)	0.24 (0%)	58%
Blinick	Detox- Maint--dosage*	100	34/100 (34%)	3/100 (3.0%)	N.R.**

*Patients were detoxified or maintained on methadone but no dosages were given in this report.

**Not reported.

LBW = low birth weight

24

TABLE III
Treatment of 155 Pregnant Drug-Dependent Women Illinois Drug-Treatment
Program, Chicago

GROUPS	INCIDENCE	LBW
1. Heroin Withdrawal (N=14)	3/11*	27%
2. Outpatient Methadone (N=40)	7/22*	31%
3. Outpatient Methadone-Psychiatric Therapy (N=11)	2/11	18%
4. Outpatient Methadone-Para-Professional Counseling (N=37)	10/37	29%
5. Outpatient Methadone (N=38)**	10/35*	28%
6. Unregistered Heroin Addict (N=15)	5/14*	35%

*Some patients were lost to the program and delivery statistics are unknown.

**Affiliated with Chicago Lying-In Interagency Program

LBW = low birth weight

for drug-dependent mothers but received minimal (less than four clinic visits) prenatal care and counseling for this addiction; *Group C*—patients who were admitted to the Family Center Program and who received intensive counseling with methadone maintenance or detoxification as well as "adequate" prenatal care (four or more visits to prenatal clinic).

The daily dose of methadone given to each patient varied from 5 to 120 mg. Nearly 70% of the patients received less than 50 mg daily (Table IV). Also included for comparison are two groups labeled *D* and *E*. These are randomly selected non-drug-dependent pregnant patients who delivered at Philadelphia General Hospital between 1969 and 1973. Group D patients had no prenatal care, and Group E had more than four prenatal visits.

The method of management of each patient in the Family Center Program is one of intensive prenatal care as well as psychosocial counseling for the patient's drug-dependent state. On the patient's initial visit, the history is obtained and physical examination performed. The patient is admitted to the hospital and subsequently has a chest X-ray, urinalysis and blood tests including complete blood count, serology for syphilis, blood type and an SMA-12. A urine specimen is sent to the toxicology laboratory in order to substantiate her claim to

TABLE IV
Methadone Dosage in 137 Patients
Family Center Program
Philadelphia General Hospital
January 1969 to December 1973

METHADONE DOSAGE IN MGS.	% OF PATIENTS ON VARIOUS DOSAGES OF METHADONE	
5-10	13.1	Low Dose
11-20	21.2	
21-30	11.7	
31-40	8.8	
41-50	13.9	68.6
51-60	13.1	
61-70	7.3	High Dose
71-80	5.8	
81-90	2.2	
91-100	1.5	31.4
101-110	0.7	
111-120	0.7	

heroin addiction. Analysis for heroin, quinine, barbiturates, amphetamines and cocaine is accomplished by thin layer chromatography.

Initial prenatal education is provided, including abortion option in early pregnancy. Discussions are held regarding the relationship of heroin addiction to the serious complications of pregnancy and, if the patient is not already receiving therapy for her addiction, a psychiatrist and a counselor from the Family Center Program interview her and begin treatment with methadone, providing drug-dependence is proven by withdrawal symptomatology and subsequently by urine toxicology. The patient's husband or consort is likewise admitted to the program, and a public health nurse along with the social worker is assigned to the family. After about four days of hospitalization, during which time laboratory tests are accomplished and methadone dosage stabilized, the patient is discharged and given her methadone on an outpatient basis to be followed in a special prenatal clinic by the same physician throughout her pregnancy.

During the hospital stay, the neonatologist meets with the expectant mother and explains potential neonatal problems of withdrawal, the nursery management of the neonate, and the need for follow-up neonatal care in the special pediatric clinic. During the subsequent prenatal visits, classes by the nurse educator are conducted in nutrition, fetal maternal changes, process of labor, delivery and anesthesia.

When the patient presents herself to the hospital in labor, she is managed with minimal regard to her methadone dependence. Physicians in charge of the labor floor are aware of her drug usage, however, and an effort is made to start conduction anesthesia as early as possible to avoid use of narcotic analgesics. A record is made of when the last dose of methadone was taken and, if necessary, methadone is given to the patient for analgesia and prevention of withdrawal symptoms.

RESULTS

Data collected on all Family Center Program patients include demographic, social, medical (obstetrical), laboratory, and neonatal parameters. In this paper, only the significant medical and neonatal parameters are reported.

Overall figures for obstetrical and medical complications are given in Table V so that all five groups may be evaluated against one another. The maternal statistics are of interest in that the obstetrical complications show a definite

TABLE V
Obstetrical Complications by Groups
Philadelphia General Hospital
1969-1973

GROUPS	No. Patients	Ave. No. Prenatal Visits	Obstetrical Complications %	Incidence of LBW %
A	56	0	35.7	48.2
B	58	1.8	17.2	43.1
C	92	7.3	23.9	22.8
D*	50	0	34.0	16.0
E**	50	8.7	20.0	18.0

*Non-clinic control

**Clinic control

LBW = low birth weight

TABLE VI
Other Major Obstetrical Complications (Groups A-E)
Philadelphia General Hospital
1961-1973

GROUPS	No. of Patients	Ave. No. Prenatal Visits	Overall Obstetrical Complications %	Pre-eclampsia %	PROM* %	Abruptio Placenta %	Amnionitis %	Postpartum Hemorrhage %
A	56	0	35.7	10.7	10.7	3.6	1.8	3.6
B	58	1.8	17.2	1.7	6.9	0	0	0
C	92	7.3	23.9	6.5	4.3	1.1	1.1	2.2
D**	50	0	34.0	10.0	4.0	4.0	2.0	0
E***	50	8.7	20.0	5.0	2.0	0	0	0

*Premature rupture of membranes>20 hours

**Non-clinic control

***Clinic control

trend downward in Groups B and C compared to Group A, with the obstetrical complications present in 35.7% of non-clinic addicts, as compared to 17.2% and 23.9% in groups with prenatal care.

An interesting comparison is that of Group A (addicts with no prenatal care) with Group D (non-addicts without prenatal care) showing 35.7% and 34% incidence of obstetrical complications, respectively, and Groups C and E (addict and non-addict patients with more than four prenatal visits) evidencing 23% and 20% incidence of obstetrical complications.

The incidence of low birth weight infants is remarkable and extremely significant. In Group A, 48.2% of the patients delivered infants weighing less than 5½ pounds, whereas in Group C the incidence was 22%. The fact that the non-clinic, non-addicted patients (Group D) only had a 16% incidence of low birth weight infants is most impressive, since this is the first time that it has been possible to implicate narcotics *per se* for obstetrical complications rather than the lack of prenatal care. A comparison of the two non-clinic groups (addict—A; and non-addict—D) reveals values that are statistically significant (P 0.0005). The difference in incidence of low birth weight in the clinic groups (addict—C; and non-addict—E) is not significant.

Patients on methadone with good prenatal care and counseling are comparable to non-addict patients with prenatal care. One may postulate the irregularity with which a "street" addict receives her supply, which in turn causes withdrawal symptoms, causing uterine irritability and, hence, increased incidence of premature labor with subsequent birth of light-weight infants.

Other major obstetrical complications observed in each group (A-E) are listed in Table VI. The incidence of pre-eclampsia, abruptio placenta and amnionitis is greater in both non-clinic groups (A, D), addict and non-addict, but this increase is not statistically significant. No significant difference is seen in the incidence of premature rupture of the membranes between the five groups. Postpartum hemorrhage occurred only in addict patients, both non-clinic and clinic (A, C).

The overall incidence of medical complications was higher and is to be expected in the addict groups, but the values are not statistically significant. Medical complications found in all groups of patients included: syphilis, gonorrhea, urinary tract infection, cellulitis, serum hepatitis, anemia, hypertension, diabetes mellitus, cardiac disease, asthma, and obesity. Table VII lists those medical complications seen most frequently. The life-style (usually prostitution) of the drug-dependent female exposes her to a higher risk of contacting hepatitis, cellulitis and other infections. Due to the lack of adequate nutrition, the drug-dependent pregnant woman more often develops anemia due to iron and/or folic acid deficiency.

Although there is no significant difference between treated and non-treated groups, the patients with prenatal care have the advantage of having their medical complications identified and treated.

TABLE VII
Medical Complications (Groups A-E)
Philadelphia General Hospital
1969-1973

GROUP	A N = 56	B N = 58	C N = 92	D N = 50	E N = 50
% Overall Medical Complications	39.3	48.3	34.8	22.0	36.0
Syphilis	10.7	12.0	12.0	0	0
Gonorrhea	3.6	3.4	3.3	0	0
Urinary Tract Infection	10.7	6.8	7.6	4.0	10.0
Cellulitis	7.1	3.4	1.1	0	0
Serum Hepatitis	9.0	6.9	1.1	0	0
Anemia	8.9	15.5	13.1	6.0	10.0

NEONATAL OUTCOME

All infants born to known addicts are initially placed in the high-risk nursery for close observation of the onset of symptoms. Drug therapy is not begun until the symptoms progress and cannot be managed by such conservative measures as swaddling the infant and administering demand feedings. To assure a more comfortable atmosphere for the infant and to prevent excessive excoriation of the knees, toes, and nose, a sheepskin is frequently used over the sheet of the isolette and later in the bassinette.

Neonatal narcotic withdrawal can readily be misdiagnosed as meningitis, gastroenteritis, hypocalcemia, symptomatic hypoglycemia and intracranial hemorrhage because of the wide variety of non-specific signs. It is most important to make an accurate differential diagnosis and then employ the appropriate treatment because all these disorders are life-threatening in the newborn. Since these conditions may exist concomitantly with the abstinence syndrome, the physician evaluates the infant further. Blood studies for calcium and sugar are drawn in these infants and, if there is evidence in the prenatal or intrapartum history of infection or asphyxia, the infant is evaluated further by complete blood count, blood culture, suprapubic tap, culture of the ear canal and lumbar puncture.

A "Neonatal Abstinence Score Sheet" (Finnegan, L.P., Kron, R.E., Connaughton, J.F., and Emich, J.P., 1973) is utilized to record the symptomatology of infants born to mothers who are known addicts or infants who begin to exhibit behavior which is suspiciously similar to symptoms of withdrawal. This specially designed scoring system for the appraisal of the infant born to the drug-dependent mother has recently been devised at the Philadelphia General Hospital and is used as a clinical and research tool. The score can monitor the passively addicted infant in a more comprehensive and precise way than has previously been described and permits a more objective clinical estimate of the withdrawal syndrome. The scoring system is then related to the dosage schedule of phenobarbital or paregoric as part of an ongoing project designed to test the comparative usefulness of recommended therapy for neonates with abstinence symptoms. Furthermore, it is useful in following the progression or diminution of symptomatology before, during and after drug therapy is instituted.

Prior to the use of this scoring system (July 1972), the decision to treat the infant with drugs was made by the nursery physician in conjunction with the nurse's evaluation of the infant's symptomatology. The choice of the specific drug to be used was left to the physician who was assigned to the infant. The available drugs were those that have been recommended as effective in neonatal abstinence. Paregoric, phenobarbital, chlorpromazine, methadone or Valium were administered in the currently recommended dosages. The amounts were then titrated to meet the clinical requirements of the individual infants.

Although many parameters delineating the outcome of the infant of the drug-dependent mother have been evaluated in the Family Center Program,

TABLE VIII
Birth Weight—Average
Philadelphia General Hospital
1969-1973

Group A	2492 grams
Group B	2545 grams
Group C	2852 grams
Group D	3032 grams
Group E	3021 grams

only a few will be presented in this paper. Most noteworthy are the statistics concerning average birth weight, infant morbidity including severity of withdrawal and other neonatal problems, and neonatal mortality.

Table VIII delineates the average birth weight of Groups A through E. The low average birth weight of Group A (2493 grams) is consistent with the results of other investigators' studies (Krause, S.O., Murray, P.M., Holmes, J.B., and Burch, R.E., 1958; Sussman, S., 1963; Perlmutter, J.F., 1967; Stern, R., 1966; Stone, M.L., Salerno, L.J., Green, M., and Zelson, C., 1971; Harper, R.G., Sia, C.G., and Blenman, S., 1973; Newman, R.G., 1973; Scott, N.R., and Ryan, J.J., 1973; Blinick, G., Wallach, R.C., and Jerez, E., 1969; Davis, R.C., and Chappel, J.N., 1973) which included "non-treated" pregnant addicts. There is a progressive increase in the average birth weights in the addict group, with Group C comparing favorably with the infants born to non-addicted mothers. The differences in birth weights in each group are statistically significant (P 0.0005).

The incidence of withdrawal symptomatology is shown in Table IX. Although there is very little difference in the overall incidence in the three groups, marked differences appear when the symptomatology is separated according to the severity. Severity of withdrawal was categorized into:

Mild—withdrawal symptomatology of mild degree not necessitating drug therapy;
Moderate—withdrawal symptomatology of moderate degree necessitating drug therapy for less than 14 days;
Severe—withdrawal symptomatology of severe degree necessitating drug therapy for longer than 14 days.

In general, Group A infants are those with heroin withdrawal, whereas Group B and C infants have methadone withdrawal. Some of the latter also were noted to have morphine in their urine toxicology studies. (Nearly 50% of methadone-treated patients in the program had "cheated" at least once.)

Severe withdrawal was most pronounced in Group A, whereas infants in Groups B and C generally had mild to moderate withdrawal. A large number of the infants born to mothers who were "treated" and were on very low dosage methadone experienced no withdrawal symptomatology.

Other neonatal problems such as infection, asphyxia neonatorum, transient tachypnea of the newborn, aspiration pneumonia, intrauterine growth retardation, and jaundice were more commonly seen in Groups A and B, whose mothers had insignificant prenatal care or none at all. The incidence of these problems was: Group A = 52%; Group B = 53%; Group C = 33%.

Fifteen of the 206 infants born to drug-dependent mothers (1969-1973) died. In Group A, 3 infants died (5%); in Group B, 8 infants died (14%), and in Group C there was one intrauterine fetal death at 32 weeks' gestation and there were 3 neonatal deaths (4%). One of these three latter infants died of severe meconium aspiration syndrome* (weight = 3650 grams), another of complications secondary to the anomaly gastroschisis (weight = 2260 grams) and the other from hydrops fetalis, primary atelectasis and subarachnoid hemorrhage (weight = 2730 grams).

In Group B, the range of birth weights in the infants who expired was 795-2268 grams. All infants died from the sequelae of their premature birth (asphyxia neonatorum, respiratory distress syndrome).

In Group A, the three infants who succumbed weighed 907, 980 and 1650 grams, respectively. The cause of death was immaturity in the first two. The third infant was born without a heartbeat and was resuscitated, but succumbed at two days of age due to severe prenatal and postnatal asphyxia.

---

* The mother was taking 120 mg of methadone daily along with an undetermined amount of heroin, and detoxification was not attempted.

TABLE IX
Withdrawal Symptomatology in 191 Infants
of Drug-Dependent Mothers

	Groups		
	A %	B %	C %
Total Withdrawal	94	92	86
Severe Withdrawal	28	13	17
Moderate Withdrawal	28	35	45
Mild Withdrawal	38	44	24
No Withdrawal	57	77	13

COMMENTS

The literature has been reviewed and the data from a large study analyzed. The review of the data demonstrates: (1) Untreated addicts have a high percentage of obstetrical complications, especially pre-eclampsia (average 10.7%) with its frequent sequelae of abruptio placenta and fetal distress. (2) Prenatal care, along with treatment of drug dependence, somewhat reduces this morbidity. (3) The incidence of low birth weight is reduced in only two reports, the first being in the infants born to patients in the intensively treated groups of the Davis and Chappel study, with an average of 25%, and the second report being that of the Philadelphia General Hospital study Group C showing 22.8%. The incidence of infant withdrawal is extremely high in all groups. However, in this study, when withdrawal symptomatology is classified according to severity, the patients in Group C demonstrated an improvement over other groups in the number of infants who underwent severe withdrawal.

Davis and Chappel reported an increased incidence of fetal mortality when the mother is detoxified or withdrawn from heroin or methadone in the last trimester. In reviewing the delivery records, we find no evidence of increased fetal distress and/or meconium stained amniotic fluid in patients so managed.

SUMMARY

The number of young women addicted to opiates has increased markedly in the past ten years. Accordingly, there has been a sharp rise in pregnancies complicated by addiction. The care of the pregnant addict and her newborn has become a major and controversial problem. There is a need for a specific approach to this particular high-risk patient and her newborn.

A comprehensive approach to the care of 206 pregnant addicts and their infants at the Philadelphia General Hospital has significantly reduced maternal and infant morbidity heretofore associated with pregnancies complicated by opiate addiction. More significantly, the incidence of obstetrical complications has been reduced to 12%, with a decrease in incidence of low birth weight to 22% and a reduction of infant morbidity to 33%.

The authors propose that application of this comprehensive type of approach to the pregnant addict is a significant factor in the successful management of these patients.

Notes

This effort was supported in part by Research Grant IROI-00325-01 from the National Institute for Mental Health and Research Grant # 1674 from the Commonwealth of Pennsylvania.

Requests for reprints should be addressed to Philadelphia General Hospital, Division of Nurseries, 700 Civic Center Boulevard, Philadelphia, Pennsylvania 19104.

We wish to acknowledge the cooperation of Dr. Harvey Weiner of the West Philadelphia Mental Health Consortium Methadone Clinic. We are also grateful to the staff of the Family Center Program, the Newborn Nurseries, and the Obstetrical Department of the Philadelphia General Hospital for their cooperation and patience in the management of these patients. Our thanks are extended to Mrs. Evelyn Delmelle for her assistance in collecting and analyzing the data on addiction.

References

Blinick, G., Wallach, R.C., and Jerez, E. Pregnancy in methadone detoxification programs. *American Journal of Obstetrics and Gynecology,* 1969, 105 (7). 997-1003.

Davis, R. C., and Chappel, J. N. Pregnancy in the context of narcotic addiction and methadone maintenance. *Proceedings of the 5th National Conference on Methadone Treatment,* 1973, March 17-19, Washington, D.C., 1146-1164.

Finnegan, L. P., Kron, R. E., Connaughton, J. F., and Emich, J. P. A scoring system for the objective evaluation of the neonatal abstinence syndrome: A new clinical and research tool. In press.

Harper, R. G., Sia, C. G., and Blenman, S.: Observations on the sudden death of infants born to addicted mothers. *Proceedings of the 5th National Conference on Methadone Treatment,* 1973, March 17-19, Washington, D.C. 1122-1127.

Krause, S. O., Murray, P. M., Holmes, J. B., and Burch, R. E. Heroin addiction among pregnant women and their newborn babies. *American Journal of Obstetrics and Gynecology,* 1958, 75 (4). 754-758.

Newman, R. G. Results of 120 deliveries of patients in the New York City methadone maintenance treatment program. *Proceedings of the 5th National Conference on Methadone Treatment,* 1973, March 17-19, Washington, D.C. 1114-1121.

Perlmutter, J. F. Drug addiction in pregnant women. *American Journal of Obstetrics and Gynecology,* 1967, 99 (4). 569-572.

Scott, N. R., and Ryan, J.J. Clinical evaluation of pregnant methadone maintenance patients and their newborn infants. *Proceedings of the 5th National Conference on Methadone Treatment,* 1973, March 17-19, Washiington D.C. 1128-1132.

Stern R. The pregnant addict. A study of 66 case histories. *American Journal of Obstetrics and Gynecology,* 1966, 94 (4). 253-257.

Stone, M. L., Salerno, L. J., Green, M., and Zelson, C. Narcotic addiction in pregnancy. *American Journal of Obstetrics and Gynecology,* 1971, 109 (5). 716-723.

Sussman, S. Narcotic and methamphetamine use during pregnancy. *American Journal of Diseases of Children,* 1963, 106 (9). 325-330.

Addictive Diseases: an International Journal 2 (1): 37-43 (1975)

Metabolic Capabilities of the Human Fetus: Drug Biotransformation

M. R. JUCHAU
Department of Pharmacology
School of Medicine
University of Washington
Seattle, Washington

INTRODUCTION

The exposure of unborn human infants to drugs and foreign chemicals which have been ingested intentionally by the mother without the sanction of qualified medical personnel represents a specialized area of concern which has received far too little emphasis until very recently. Studies dealing with the capacity of the human fetal organism to biochemically convert these and other foreign organic chemicals into other more, less or differently bioactive chemical species are even more specialized and have only just begun to receive investigative attention. However, a number of recent reviews (Pelkonen and Karki, 1973; Rane et al., 1973; Juchau, 1973; Yaffe and Juchau, 1974) have dealt with the subject, attesting to the potential importance of this area of research. The purpose of the present paper is to present a concise summary of the current status of the research in this field and to attempt to interpret the findings in terms of investigational observations made in this laboratory.

MIXED-FUNCTION OXIDATION IN HUMAN FETAL TISSUES

Although drugs and other foreign organic chemicals are commonly biotransformed via oxidation, reduction, hydrolysis and conjugation, the principal emphasis in studies of human fetal drug metabolism has been placed upon the highly interesting monooxygenase systems—in particular those linked to cytochrome P-450. Yaffe and co-workers (Yaffe et al., 1970) were the first to demonstrate that in contrast to common experimental animals, human fetal livers contain significant quantities of cytochrome P-450 as early as the first trimester of gestation. They were able to detect significant rates of mixed-function oxidation of various endogenous substrates (testosterone and sodium laurate) but attempts to demonstrate the capacity of human fetal liver microsomes to oxidatively N-demethylate aminopyrine yielded equivocal results. Other investigators also have reported negative results in attempts to detect the catalysis of oxidative demethylation reactions in preparations of human fetal hepatic tissues (Pomp et al., 1969; Juchau and Pedersen, 1973). Other investigators, however, have reported that preparations of human fetal liver microsomes could oxidatively metabolize hexobarbital, desmethylimipramine, aminopyrine, ethylmorphine, aniline, 3,4-benzpyrene, chlorpromazine and N-methylaniline at rates approaching those observed in similar preparations of adult human liver (Pelkonen et al., 1973). More recently it has been reported that diazepam was oxidatively biotransformed at comparatively rapid rates in preparations of human fetal livers at six months' gestation (Ackermann and Richter, 1974). Rane (1974) also has reported that N-oxidation of N,N-dimethylaniline would occur in the presence of human fetal liver microsomes and appropriate cofactors. Since such reactions represent potentially hazardous bioactivation mechanisms, it would appear that they should be studied in much greater detail and with more sensitive and specific assay systems to resolve some of the apparently conflicting results reported from various laboratories. Nevertheless, there does appear to be sufficient evidence to suggest that the mixed-function oxidation of certain drugs will occur in human fetal tissues, although very little is known at present concerning the substrate specificity of the enzyme systems involved.

Since mixed-function oxidation frequently leads to the formation of intermediate epoxides during the hydroxylation of aromatic compounds, we have also been concerned with the capacity of human fetal tissues to catalyze the degradation of epoxides via epoxide hydrase and glutathione S-epoxide transferase enzymes. Our studies (Juchau and Namkung, 1974) have indicated, however, that these tissues (with the exception of the placenta) contain high activities of both of these enzymes. Again, however, since only naphthalene-1,2-oxide was employed as substrate in the investigations, nothing is yet known concerning the substrate specificity of those human fetal enzymes. Studies in this area would seem to be of prime importance in view of the following considerations:

1. Unborn infants may be exposed chronically to varying levels of polycyclic aromatic hydrocarbons via inhalation of such compounds from the external environment into the lungs, particularly by mothers who smoke.
2. Several studies now have shown that human fetal tissues can actively catalyze the hydroxylation of 3-4-benzpyrene, one of the principal car-

cinogens present in cigarette smoke. Hydroxylation of the ring structure presumably involves the formation of intermediate epoxides. Epoxides may be proximate or ultimate carcinogens.

3. It is now known (Schoental, 1974) that fetal tissues are particularly susceptible to tumorigenic transformations induced by chemical agents, including polycyclic aromatic hydrocarbons. Due to the very long latent period, however, tumors may not become manifest until several decades after the initiatory event in carcinogenesis. Since chemicals (including drugs) are felt to be responsible for approximately 80% of all malignant tumors, these facts are particularly pertinent. In addition, most chemicals must be bioactivated to the active carcinogen.

4. An important new experimental observation concerns the *combined* effect of transplacental and postnatal exposures to chemicals. In experimental animals, it has been shown (Napalkov, 1973) that fetal exposure to a chemical carcinogen facilitates the effect of postnatal contact with the same or with different carcinogens. This observation may indicate that a person's lifetime risk of developing cancer might be conditioned by prenatal chemical exposures.

5. Rates of formation vs. further degradation of the epoxides in fetal tissues may be critical determinants of the transplacental carcinogenic activity of polycyclic aromatic hydrocarbons present in tobacco smoke. Rates of formation of dihydrodiols and glutathione conjugates vs. phenolic compounds may also be important, since the latter are usually cytotoxic and would also be expected to serve as substrates for highly active sulfokinase enzymes present in the fetal adrenal gland and liver. Intermediates of sulfate metabolism also can be highly electrophilic and thus may also be carcinogenic. In addition, glucuronidation mechanisms which normally would tend to inactivate phenolic compounds appear to be absent from or be very low in the human fetal liver (Rane et al., 1973).

6. Studies on human placental tissues (which are fetal in origin) indicate (Juchau and Namkung, 1974) that cigarette smoking can markedly induce the hydroxylase without markedly affecting the hydrase. Although very preliminary, this would tend to imply that the concentrations of reactive epoxides and phenolic compounds would be increased under such conditions, since induction likewise does not appear to affect the glutathione S-epoxide transferase system present in the cytosol (unpublished). Studies on K-region epoxides are clearly in order.

The above considerations serve only to illustrate a few of the many complex problems which will require investigation in order to evaluate intelligently the potential effects of prenatal drug exposure.

OTHER "PHASE I" REACTIONS IN
HUMAN FETAL TISSUES

Aside from biotransformation via the highly interesting mixed-function ox-idation reactions, appropriate drug substrates also may undergo dehydrogena-tion, reduction, hydrolysis or conjugation in human fetal tissues. (Conjugation or synthetic reactions are frequently referred to as "Phase II" reactions.) Inves-tigative efforts in this area, however, have been minimal. The reduction of aro-matic nitro groups and azo linkages proceeds at readily measurable rates in the presence of human fetal liver homogenates or homogenate subfractions and ap-propriate cofactors (Juchau, 1971; Juchau and Pedersen, 1973; Juchau et al., 1973). The fetal adrenal gland was particularly active with respect to the cataly-sis of these reduction reactions. Correspondingly high specific activities have been observed in monkey fetal adrenal glands, and primate fetal adrenals also appear to be much more active than the fetal livers with respect to drug oxida-tions in both humans and monkeys (Juchau and Pederson, 1973).

It is to be expected that suitable foreign organic substrates would be me-tabolized in human fetal tissues via hydrolysis and dehydrogenation. No system-atic investigations of these phenomenon have been undertaken to my knowl-edge, although alcohol and aldehyde dehydrogenases have been studied in human fetal liver preparations by various investigators (Pikkarainen and Raiha, 1969; Pikkarainen, 1971; Smith et al., 1971). In the case of the alcohol dehydro-genases, different isoenzymes appeared to change progressively with increasing gestational age, whereas no differences between fetal and adult aldehyde dehy-drogenases could be detected. The capacity of human fetal enzymes to catalyze hydrolytic reactions also is undoubtedly high, although essentially nothing is known concerning the substrate specificities of human fetal hydrolases. Particu-larly important may be the characteristics of B-glucuronidase and sulfatase en-zymes.

CONJUGATION OF DRUG SUBSTRATES IN THE
HUMAN FETUS

Conjugating activity in the fetus and newborn has been of particular inter-est because of the frequent occurrence of jaundice in newborn infants coupled with findings in experimental animals that enzymes involved in the formation of glucuronides appeared to be deficient in prenatal and neonatal animals. When compared with studies on drug oxidation and reduction, conjugation reactions in human fetal tissues have received little attention. Earlier reports (Dutton, 1959; Hirvonen, 1966) indicated that the human fetal kidney was more active than the fetal liver with respect to the catalysis of glucuronide formation using O-aminophenol or 4-methylumbelliferone as substrates. The activities observed, however, were very low as compared with human adult liver. Recent studies have reported negative results with respect to the capacity of the human fetal liver to catalyze glucuronidation reactions during early pregnancy (Rane et al., 1973; Chakraborty et al., 1971). 4-Methylumbelliferone, x-naphthol and p-nitrophenol were tested as aglycone acceptors.

The fetal liver and adrenal glands are extremely active with respect to the catalysis of sulfate transfer, and although no specific examples have been given, sulfurylation of foreign phenolic compounds (e.g., morphine, diethylstilbesterol) could be an important factor in human fetal pharmacology and toxicology. As previously mentioned, sulfurylation of compounds such as polycyclic aromatic hydrocarbons following their hydroxylation in fetal tissues could likewise prove to be an important regulatory mechanism. This and other conjugation reactions, such as acetylation, conjugation with amino acids and other carbohydrate moieties, and methylation should be much more intensively investigated. The possibility that human fetal tissues may contain enzyme systems which catalyze the conjugation of drug substrates with various unordinary endogenous chemicals should not be overlooked.

SUMMARY

Studies on drug metabolism in the human fetus have provided evidence that this organism possesses enzyme systems which are capable of catalyzing a wide variety of drug-biotransformation reactions. Fetal organs which appear to be particularly important in this regard are the liver, adrenal gland and placenta. However, research has indicated that other organs, including the lung, kidney, intestine, pancreas, etc., possess the capacity to catalyze certain drug-metabolic reactions. Some investigators have reported that enzymic activities observed in human fetal livers approached those measured in human adult livers. Specific activities observed in the human fetal adrenal gland were even higher for certain reactions.

Notes

Requests for reprints should be sent to Dr. M. R. Juchau, Department of Pharmacology SJ-30, School of Medicine, University of Washington, Seattle, WA 98195.

Original research reported was supported by Grant HD-04839 from the National Institute of Child Health and Human Development and CRBS-250 from the National Foundation (March of Dimes).

References

Ackermann, E., and Richter, K. Diazepam metabolism in the human fetus. *International Symposium on Perinatal Pharmacology*, 1974, p. 1 (abstract).

Chakraborty, J., Hopkins, R., and Parke, D. V. Biological oxygenation of drugs and steroids in the placenta. *Biochemical Journal*, 1971, *125*, 15-16.

Dutton, G. J. Glucuronide synthesis in fetal liver and other tissues. *Biochemical Journal*, 1959, *71*, 141-148.

Hirvonen, T. Fetal and postnatal development of glucuronide formation in mammalian tissue slices. *Sarja-Series A II, Biologia-Georaphica,* Turku, 1966.

Juchau, M. R. Drug biotransformation in the human fetus: Nitro group reduction. *Archives Internationales de Pharmacodynamie et de Therapie,* 1971, *194,* 204-216.

Juchau, M. R. Placental metabolism in relation to toxicology. *CRC Critical Reviews in Toxicology,* 1973, *2,* 125-159.

Juchau, M. R., Lee, Q. H., Louviaux, G. L., Symms, K. G., Krasner, J., and Yaffe, S. J. Oxidation and reduction of foreign compounds in tissues of the human placenta and fetus. In *Fetal Pharmacology,* 1973 (L. Boreus, ed.) Raven Press, New York, 321-335.

Juchau, M. R., and Pedersen, M. G. Drug biotransformation reactions in the human fetal adrenal gland. *Life Sciences,* 1973, *12,* 193-204.

Juchau, M. R., and Namkung, M. Studies on the biotransformation of naphthalene-1,2-oxide in fetal and placental tissue of humans and monkeys. *Drug Metabolism and Disposition,* 1974, *2,* 380-386.

Napalkov, N. P. Some general considerations on the problem of transplacental carcinogenesis. In *IARC Scientific Publication No. 4,* 1973 (L. Tomatis and U. Mohr, eds.) Lyon, 14-22.

Pelkonen, O., and Karki, N. T. Drug metabolism in human fetal tissues. *Life Sciences,* 1973, *13,* 1163-1180.

Pikkarainen, P. H. Aldehyde-oxidizing capacity during development in human and rat liver. *Annales Medicinae Experimentalis et Biologiae Fenniae,* 1971, *49,* 151-156.

Pikkarainen, P., and Raiha, N.C.R. Development of alcohol dehydrogenase in the human liver. *Pediatric Research,* 1967, *1,* 165-173.

Pomp, H., Schnoor, M., and Netter, K. J. Untersuchungen uber die Arzniemitteldemethylierung in der fetalen Leber. *Deutsche Medizinische Wochenschrift,* 1969, *94:23,* 1232-1240.

Rane, A. Drug metabolism in the human fetal liver. *International Symposium on Perinatal Pharmacology,* 1974 p. 34 (abstract).

Rane, A., Sjoqvist, F., and Orrenius, S. Drugs and fetal metabolism. *Clinical Pharmacology and Therapeutics,* 1973, *14,* 666-672.

Schoental, R. Carcinogenicity as related to age. *Annual Review of Pharmacology,* 1974, *14,* 185-205.

Smith, M., Hopkinson, D. A., and Harris, H. Development changes and polymorphism in human alcohol dehydrogenase. *Annals of Human Genetics,* 1971, *34,* 251-259.

Yaffe, S. J., and Juchau, M. R. Perinatal pharmacology. *Annual Review of Pharmacology,* 1974, *14,* 219-239.

Yaffe, S. J., Rane, A., Sjoqvist, F., Boreus, L.-O., and Orrenius, S. The presence of a monooxygenase system in human fetal liver microsomes. *Life Sciences,* 1970, *9,* 1189-1200.

DISCUSSION

Q. *Dr. Slotkin:* Concerning the possible toxicity of catechol products, are any of these compounds substrates for catechol methyltransferase and does the fetal or neonatal liver contain sufficient amounts of this enzyme to do anything to these compounds?

A. *Dr. Juchau: Catechol methyltransferase is present in relatively high concentrations, both in fetus and in the placenta. To my knowledge, however, studies of substrate specificity have not been completed. I presume that these compounds would be methylated. I do not know the relative rates of these reactions; I assume that they would proceed at relatively rapid rates, if you consider reactions involving catecholamines as a criterion.*

Q. *Dr. Neal:* Induction of benzpyrene hydroxylase, and the susceptibility to neoplasia, is a very complicated picture. I am speaking primarily of Wattenberg's work at the University of Minnesota, where he shows induction by dietary manipulation. Altered incidence of neoplasia is seen following induction of the polycyclic aromatic hydroxylases. Do you have any comments on this?

A. *Dr. Juchau: According to the current theory, the relative rates of epoxide formation versus epoxide degradation can be the determining factor for induction of neoplasias. This also remains to be demonstrated experimentally, although it does make good sense chemically. So, what has to be evaluated here are not only the rates of benzpyrene hydroxylation, (which actually give you one measure of formation of epoxides) but also to measure the glutathione conjugation rates, and the rates of epoxide hydration, which is particularly important because this is enzymically controlled and the latter is controlled by an inducible enzyme.*

Q. *Dr. Neal:* Another factor here is that benzpyrene hydroxylase may not always attack that K region, but also may hydroxylate other areas.

A. *Dr. Juchau: Absolutely—one thing that we are currently investigating in our laboratories is the biotransformation of K region epoxides, which have been more heavily implicated as carcinogenic agents and as mutagenic agents. That is a good point.*

Addictive Diseases: an International Journal 2 (1): 45-61 (1975)
© 1975 by Spectrum Publications, Inc.

Drugs of Abuse: Teratogenic and Mutagenic Considerations

MICHAEL A. EVANS
MICHEL W. STEVENS
BERNARDO MANTILLA-PLATA
RAYMOND D. HARBISON
Department of Pharmacology
Vanderbilt University
School of Medicine
Nashville, Tennessee

Teratogenic and mutagenic research in this country has been stimulated by four significant events of the past fifty years.

About the turn of the century, with the increasing awareness of the biologic effects of radiation, came the finding that pelvic x-irradiation during pregnancy could result in the birth of a malformed child. Radiation-induced malformations demonstrated the first clear association between an external agent and teratogenic response in man. Following this, Hale and co-workers (1937) reported the effects of dietary deficiencies on developing fetuses. Using a vitamin A deficient diet their studies revealed for the first time that dietary deficiency was capable of producing predictable congenital defects in newborn animals. Even more alarming, however, was the report of Gregg and co-workers (1941) that a high percentage of children born to women infected with rubella virus during the first trimester of pregnancy suffered from serious neurological defects, including blindness and deafness. Even under a mild disease state, major congenital malformations were sometimes produced when the infection occurred during the first trimester. Thus as early as the 1940's the embryo was recognized as susceptible to external influences, including inadequate diet, viral infections and radiation. However, the importance of these observations beyond the biomedical

TABLE I

Drugs of Abuse and Centrally Acting Therapeutic Agents Reported for Their Teratogenic Effects

Drug	Species	Effect	Reference
Amphetamine	mouse rabbit	Ventricular and atrial septal defects, exencephaly, cleft palate or eye defects	Nora,1968;Kasirsky, 1971
Barbituric Acid (and derivatives)	mouse rat rabbit	Malformations of the head and extremities, double vertebral centra skeletal and aortic arch defects in the offspring	Setala,1964;McColl, 1967;Persaud,1965
Cannabis	rat rabbit guinea pig	Malformed,growth retardation,syndactyly, encephlocele and reduction defects of the limbs	Persaud,1968;Geber, 1969
Chlorpromazine	mouse rat	Reduced litter size and fetal weight,reduced postnatal survival, liver and serum biochemical changes,behavioral changes	Ordy,1966;Jewett,1966
Deserpidine	rat	Malformations of limb,tail,abortion,fetal death, reduced fetal size	Tuchmann-Duplessis, 1961
Diphenylhydantoin	mouse	Cleft lip and palate,skeletal malformations	Harbison,1970
Ethinamate	mouse	Malformations,fetal death	Takano,1963
Gluthethimide	mouse rat rabbit	Malformations axial skeleton,stillbirth,reduced fertility	McColl,1963;Tuchmann Duplessis,1963
Haloperidol	mouse rat	Retarded implantation,malformations,cleft palate,etc.,fetal death	Vicki,1969
Imipramine	rat rabbit	Malformations kidney,etc.,fetal death,reduced fetal weight	Harper,1965

TABLE I (cont)

Drug	Species	Effect	Reference
Lysergic Acid Diethylamide	mouse rat hamster	Central nervous system abnormalities.congenital defects,histologic abnormalities of the lens	Auerbach,1967; Alexander,1970; Gerber,1967
Mescaline	guinea pig	Defects in central nervous system	Gerber,1967
Methadone	guinea pig	Defects in embryo (skeletal)	Gerber,1969
Methaqualone	rat	Double vertabrae centra and extra lumbar ribs in offspring	McColl,1963
Methylphenidate	mouse	Fetal death	Takano,1963
α-Methyltryptamine	rat	Malformations skeleton,etc.	Yakovleva,1966
Morphine	mouse rat	Exencephalic and axial skeletal defects, growth retardation	Friedler,1972; Iuliucci,1971
Nialamide	mouse	Implantation apparently prevented	Poulson,1963
Pemoline	mouse	Fetal death	Takano,1963
Phenelzine	mouse rabbit	Fetal death, implantations probably prevented Malformation head,limbs	Poulson,1964
Prochlorperazine	mouse rat	Malformation, eye, cleft palate, fetal death, abortion, reduced litter size	Roux,1959
Reserpine	rat rabbit	Malformation eye, etc., abortion, fetal death, reduced litter size,offspring weight, behavioral changes	Goldman,1965;Kehl, 1956
Salicylate	rat	Gastrochisis, hydrocephalus,spina bifida, ocular and facial defects	Warkany,1959

field were not fully appreciated for another twenty years when in the late 1950's a new glutethimide analog was introduced to the general public.

Thalidomide was therapeutically prescribed throughout Western Europe as a new hypnotic and tranquilizing agent. Clinical and animal studies had demonstrated that the drug was relatively safe and very effective with little or no side effects in man. Shortly after its introduction into therapy, however, there appeared an increase in infants born with phocomelia paralleling the increased usage of the drug. Finally in 1961 Lenz and co-workers reported an association between phocomelia infants and mothers receiving thalidomide at the University Pediatric Clinic in Hamburg. That report of less than fifteen years ago established the first significant association between the taking of the relatively non-toxic drug, thalidomide, and the birth of severely malformed infants. Since that forceful public recognition, a whole range of unrelated chemical agents, drugs and environmental factors have now been shown to experimentally produce congenital defects in the mammalian species. In some cases, the work in animals has been predictive of what happened in man, such as the diphenylhydantoin (DPH) induced cleft palates in children of epileptic mothers (Mirkin, 1971); in others the relationship between animal studies and man is not as well developed.

It has been estimated that close to one-half the number of children in hospital wards are there as a result of prenatally acquired malformations (Shepard, 1973). In animal studies, over 600 chemical agents and drugs have now been shown to produce congenital malformations; yet only about 20 of these are known to produce congenital defects in humans. So at present there does exist a wide variance between what is known in both animal and man and what actually exists in the clinical situation.

Table I summarizes the results from a number of animal investigations of the last fifteen years concerning the effects of drugs, some of which are abused, on the developing fetus. The pattern of usage for most of these drugs and agents is such that a high percentage of women in child-bearing age have probably had some exposure to these chemicals. Many of the agents in the table demonstrated teratogenesis at doses below visible maternal toxicity, which suggests that in man teratogenesis can be produced without maternal signs or symptoms. These teratogenic effects vary between oral malformations as shown with diphenylhydantoin to the variety of anomalies produced by some amphetamines. In addition, a number of these drugs, for example, methadone and barbituric acid, are also capable of producing changes in fetal growth which are compatible with life. What the full effect of these chemical agents are in man we still do not know, but the evidence indicates that these drugs are capable of producing teratogenesis in at least one mammalian species.

Table II is a summary from human investigations of the past fifteen years concerning the positive mutagenic effects of drugs, some of which are abused. These studies used cell cultures and lymphocytes. As illustrated, little if any-

TABLE II
Drugs of Abuse and Centrally Acting Therapeutic Agents Reported as Positive
Mutagens

Drug	Species
Caffeine	Man (HeLa Cells)
Chlordiazepoxide	Man (Leukocytes)
Diazepam	Man (Leukocytes)
LSD-25	Man (Leukocytes)
Scopolamine HBr	Man (HeLa Cells)

Barthelmess, A. Mutagenic substances in the human
environment. Chemical Mutagenesis in Mammals and Man.
Ed. F. Vogel and G. Rohtorn, New York: Springer-Verlag,
1970.

thing is yet known about this aspect of drug toxicity, particularly in the mammalian species, despite the fact that drugs of abuse represent a wide variety of chemical structures and are used by a high percentage of the population. Further knowledge in this area is critical if we are to understand the total ramifications of present-day drug usage.

Teratogenic hazards of drugs for humans are real and ominous. Although a typical therapeutic dose of thalidomide averaged about 100 mg total, patients were reported to have recovered from ingestion of as much as 14 g taken with suicidal intent. Teratogenic studies were completed in both the rat and the mouse before clinical trials, and the results demonstrated no morphological aberrations at any dose level below maternal toxicity.

In this instance, however, the human species proved to be many times more sensitive than the experimental animal to the teratogenic effects of a drug. Table III illustrates the comparative teratogenic effect of thalidomide for several different species, including man. For the rat and mouse, the minimum dose necessary to produce a teratogenic response is approximately 30 to 60 times that needed in man. In the pregnant woman, as little as one to two therapeutic doses of thalidomide given at the critical time of organogenesis has been documented as producing congenital defects in the child (Williams, 1963). Since the original correlation by Lenz in 1961, several species of monkeys have been found to be sensitive to the teratogenic effects of thalidomide; because of the specific metabolic pathways in man, however, the human species is still regarded as the most susceptible to thalidomide teratogenesis. Certainly, dosage is an important factor in any aspect of drug effect; but the variability and possible susceptibility of even a small percentage of developing fetuses to teratogenesis at low doses

TABLE III
Comparative Thalidomide Teratogenicity (mg/kg/day) Following Oral
Administration

Species	Smallest Dose Producing Defects
Man	0.5-1.0
Monkey, Cynomolgus	10
Rabbit	30
Mouse	31
Rat	50
Armadillo	100
Dog	100
Hamster	350

must be considered before full approval for clinical use is given.

Because of the many factors involved in drug-induced teratogenesis, anthropomorphizing the dose-response relationship from animal to man is difficult and arbitrary. We know that drug-induced teratogenesis is dose-related, but beyond that, little is really understood concerning the minimal dose of most drugs necessary to produce teratogenesis in man or the extent of the variability of the response in man. The only real definition we can make at present is that if a drug is teratogenic in any animal species at a dosage below maternal toxicity, then the possible hazard of teratogenicity in humans must be fully considered before the drug is released for public use.

One of the major problems in experimental teratology is defining the terms of congenital malformation. As used in animal studies, the term has meant the production of gross structural abnormalities of prenatal origin detectable by observation. In man, the term must be expanded to include not only death and morphological change, but also functional and behavioral deficits. These effects are not as easily measured, and yet they probably constitute the greatest teratogenic hazard in terms of percentage population. Certainly any drug which prevents the fullest expression of genetic character either anatomical or behavioral must be used with extreme caution in the pregnant woman. Unfortunately, our present animal models are unable to predict with any degree of certainty, the drugs which produce functional and behavioral changes in offspring.

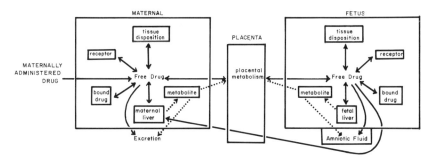

FIG. 1.   Drug disposition in a model of the maternal-placental-fetal unit.

Figure 1 illustrates some of the pharmacodynamic processes to be considered for the relationship influencing transfer of drugs and tissue disposition, and pharmacological activity between the maternal and fetal compartments. In general, any factor which can alter the level of free drug or metabolite in the maternal compartment is capable of altering the level of free drug in the fetus. The degree of placental transfer for any drug is directly proportional to the free drug concentrations in the maternal plasma. Since the fetus has deficient means for drug excretion except by way of redistribution to the maternal compartment, any metabolism of the drug to a more polar compound either in the placenta or in the fetus would act to contain that drug within the fetus.

Gillette and co-workers (1973) have demonstrated that enzymes which catalyze the reduction of nitro compounds such as nitrofurozone do exist in the fetal liver and that fetal hepatic enzymes might participate in drug-induced fetotoxicity. Further studies by Pelkonen and co-workers (1973) demonstrated that in vitro capacity of human fetal liver to metabolize 3,4 benzpyrene, aniline, aminopyrine and hexobarbital was lower than that of the liver of human adult patients with uncomplicated cholelithiosis. Because of the wide variations observed in fetal metabolism and the consideration that the fetal liver is relatively larger than the adult liver, Pelkonen suggested that there may be pregnancies in which the fetus is considerably more able to metabolize xenobiotics than the mother on the basis of body weight. Since placental transfer is preferential to lipid soluble drugs rather than the more polar drug metabolites, fetal drug metabolism can lead to an accumulation of metabolites in the fetus. However, further studies are still needed in this area to define the steady state kinetics of fetal drug levels.

A third important site of drug biotransformation, other than maternal and fetal liver, is the placenta. Drug biotransformation, including certain oxidation, reduction, hydroxylation and conjugation reactions, are quite active in placental tissues, and the capacity of the placental system to metabolize drugs increases with gestational age (Juchau, 1973). Placental oxidation of 3,4 benzpyrene and other polycyclic aromatic hydrocarbons may approach levels observed in analogous preparations of adult hepatic tissues (Juchau, 1973a).

Some general conclusions concerning fetal-placenta metabolism and concentration of drugs in the fetus can be reached on the basis of pharmacokinetic principles. Upon acute administration, when lipid soluble drugs are not rapidly cleared by the maternal liver, the activities of enzymes in the placenta and fetus may increase the final concentrations of drug metabolites in the fetus above maternal level, since excretion of drug metabolites is greatly reduced from the fetal compartment. Rane and co-workers (1973) demonstrated that at least for desipramine this is the case, and that the ultimate fetal levels of drug metabolites is increased above maternal plasma following maternal administration. Further studies with other drugs are needed to confirm this observation. A second conclusion seems to be that when slowly metabolized drugs are given repetitively to patients, the plasma level of non-metabolized drug in the fetus will be at least as high as the lowest steady state levels found in the maternal plasma.

In the maternal compartment, several important factors have now been evaluated for their effects on fetal drug concentrations and drug-induced teratogenesis. As shown in our laboratory (Harbison and Becker, 1971) hepatic drug metabolism does influence fetal drug levels and teratogenesis. Competitive inhibition of drug metabolism by concomitant drug treatment elevated maternal plasma drug levels while stimulating drug metabolism by pre-treatment with phenobarbital lowered maternal plasma drug levels. Fetal drug concentrations paralleled maternal plasma concentration. Thus, inhibition of maternal hepatic metabolism increases the concentration and prolongs the disappearance of drug from the fetus. Oral facial anomalies following inhibition of drug metabolism increased almost 100% above control, reflecting the increased fetal drug concentration. Similar but more pronounced results were seen for the incidence of skeletal anomalies. Drug-induced teratogenic effects are related to fetal drug concentration and suggest that alterations in maternal pharmacokinetics can significantly alter the production of fetal abnormalities.

Further studies in our laboratory have supported these prior results and amplify the importance of maternal drug pharmacokinetics with respect to fetal drug concentrations. For example, radiolabeled methadone was administered at a dose of 5mg/kg i.v. to day 17 pregnant mice. At two hours following administration, the animals were sacrificed, and total radioactivity was measured in maternal plasma and fetal tissue. As shown in Figure 2, pretreatment of the mother with SKF 525A, a metabolic inhibitor, and phenobarbital, a stimulator, had no effect on the maternal plasma level of methadone plus metabolites. However, in the fetus, phenobarbital pretreatment significantly lowered methadone plus metabolite levels. Treatment with SKF 525A on the other hand, significantly increased the total fetal level of drug and metabolites. Thus, alteration in the pharmacodynamics of drugs in the mother can alter the fetal concentration of the drug and its metabolites.

Other pharmacodynamic factors in the mother besides metabolism must be

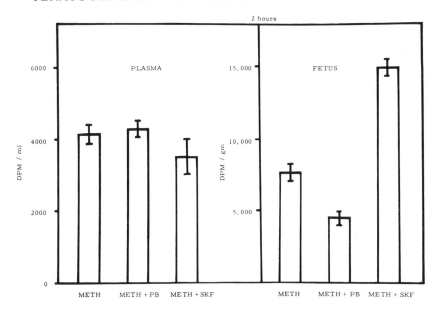

FIG. 2. Carbon-14 concentration, methadone plus metabolites (ordinate), of maternal plasma and whole fetus 2 hr following administration of 14C-methadone (5 mg/kg, i.v.) to day 17 pregnant mice. The type of pretreatment is shown on the abscissa: none (METH); phenobarbital 50 mg/kg, i.p. bid for 4 days prior to methadone treatment (METH + PB); SKF 525A (40 mg/kg) 1 hr prior to treatment (METH + SKF). Each bar represents the mean + S.E.

considered. These include the ratio of bound to free drug in the plasma and tissue deposition. Alteration of plasma protein binding by other drugs or environmental factors would certainly be expected to influence the fetal level of drug. Also any change in the excretion rate of a drug which would tend to increase or decrease the free plasma level could also alter the fetal drug level.

Until a few years ago, the placental membranes were regarded as impermeable, particularly for drugs and chemical agents. However, experimental research has demonstrated that the placental membrane is readily permeable by most chemicals and drugs. The ability of free drugs or metabolites to cross the placenta is modulated by numerous factors, including lipid solubility, molecular weights and age of the placenta. Studies of placental blood flow and the exchange of various molecules and ions across the amniotic membranes have been conducted both in utero and in isolated tissue. Small molecules with a molecular weight of less than 1,000 appear to pass readily between fetal and maternal blood. Most therapeutic agents, particularly those associated with central nervous system effects, have a molecular weight ranging from 250 to 400 and a high lipid to water solution, and thus appear to meet the criteria for rapid diffusion.

Table IV lists some of the drugs that have been shown to cross the human placenta barrier and their subsequent adverse effects in the fetus. Most of these agents were studied in late pregnancy, and the effects noted in the fetus are mainly toxicological rather than teratological. Some of the effects have been

TABLE IV

Drugs That Cross the Human Placental Barrier and That May Endanger the Fetus

Drug	Adverse Effects	Reference
Acetophenetidin	Methemoglobinemia	Adamson, 1966
Anesthetics (volatile)	Depressed fetal respiration	Sapeika, 1960
Barbiturates	Depressed respiration	Sapeika, 1960
Chloral Hydrate (large doses)	Fetal death	Sapeika, 1960
Chlorpromazine	Neonatal jaundice, mortality? and prolonged extrapyramidal signs	Martin, 1971
Dextroamphetamine Sulfate (Dexedrine)	Transposition of vessels?	Nora, 1965
Heroin	Initial neonatal addiction, neonatal death; respiratory depression	Apgar, 1964
Lysergic Acid Diethylamide (LSD)	Chromosomal damage; stunted offspring	Smart, 1968
Mepivacaine (carbocaine)	Fetal bradycardia; neonatal depression	Gordon, 1968
Methadone	Fetal respiratory depression	Smith, 1949
Morphine	Initial neonatal addiction; respiratory depression, neonatal death	Apgar, 1969
Nicotine (smoking)	Small neonates	Warbany, 1968
Phenobarbital (in excess)	Neonatal hemorrhage and death	Apgar, 1969
Quinine	Deafness, thrombocytopenia	Lenz, 1966
Reserpine	Nasal block, respiratory obstruction	Shirkey, 1966
Salicylates (aspirin)	Neonatal bleeding	Apgar, 1969
Thiazides (Chlorothiazide, Methylclothiazide, etc.)	Neonatal death, thrombocytopenia	Rodriguez, 1964

well documented, such as the fetal withdrawal syndrome resulting from maternal heroin ingestion; others like dextroamphetamine-induced inversion of greater vessels need further study.

In animals, an extensive list is available concerning the different types of drugs capable of crossing the placenta and causing fetal damage. Table V illustrates some of the prototype drugs which cross the placental barrier. The extensiveness of this list suggests that the problem of placental transfer in humans is more acute than probably realized. One of the major factors also influencing placental transfer of drugs is the gestational age of the fetus. Stevens and Harbison (1974) demonstrated that during early development of the mouse fetus, placental transfer of DPH was high, reflecting the early development of the placenta. By day 14, however, fetal levels of DPH decreased more than 50% but significantly increased at parturition time. The biphasic nature of this placental transfer of drugs is consistent with the concept of placental development, maturation and death. Preliminary studies conducted for methadone placental transfer have indicated similar findings for influence of gestational age. Radiolabeled methadone was administered at a dosage of 5 mg/kg i.v. to pregnant mice at three gestational ages: day 13, corresponding to late organ development; day 17, reflecting the fetal growth and maturation period; and day 19, corresponding to the period of parturition. The animals were sacrificed at 4 hours following drug administration, and total methadone plus metabolites were measured in the fetal tissues. Figure 3 illustrates that increasing transfer of methadone to the fetus is observed with increasing gestational age, indicating that placental development can affect transfer of methadone.

Until recently, the effects of drugs and chemical agents on the newborn had not been well studied with respect to potency. Initial studies with methadone in this laboratory have suggested that the susceptibility of the newborn to drugs

TABLE V
Drugs That Cross the Placental Barrier of Animals and May Require
Evaluation of Effects on the Human Fetus

Alcohol	Barbiturates	LSD (Lysergic Acid Diethylamide)
Alkaloids	Caffeine	Meprobamate
Amphetamine	Chlorpromazine (Thorazine)	Phenothiazines
Anesthetic Gases	Diphenylhydantoin (Dilantin)	Salicylates (Aspirin)
Antihistamines	Imipramine	

Ginsberg, J. Placental drug transfer. Annual Review of Pharmacology, 1971, 11: 387-407.

Sarteschi, P., Cassano, G.B., and Placidi, G.F. Placental penetration and foetal uptake of neuropharmacological agents. Advances in Theoretical and Clinical Research, 1973, 6: 50-58.

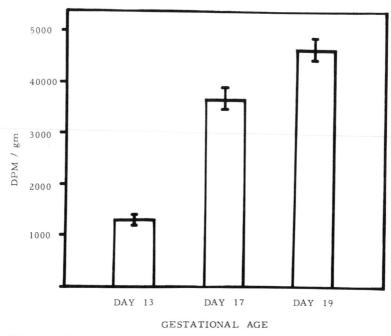

FIG. 3.   Carbon-14 concentration, methadone plus metabolites (ordinate), or whole fetus, 4 hr following administration of 14C-methadone to pregnant mice at various gestational ages (abscissa). Each bar represents the mean + S.E.

and chemical agents is greatly increased when compared to that in the adult animal. Methadone was administered intraperiotoneally to both adult and newborn rats of 3 to 7 days of age. The adult median lethal dosage was calculated as 15.2 mg/kg, which is good agreement with other published results (Henderson, 1948). Newborn median lethal dosage for rats, however, was reduced to 4.1 mg/kg of body weight, indicating a four-fold increase in sensitivity of the newborn to toxic effects of methadone. A review of newborn and adult median lethal dosage by Goldenthal (1971) indicate that for a number of CNS drugs, the adult was approximately 3 to 5 times less sensitive to the toxic drug effects than the newborns. Thus, drug levels in the adult which are not considered to be harmful may have a serious toxicological effect in the newborn due to the increase in susceptibility. The reason for this increase in sensitivity is probably due to four major factors:

1. Reduced hepatic enzyme function for efficient metabolism of the drug.
2. Reduced plasma protein level in the fetus or newborn which would increase the level of free drug.
3. A relative non-functional blood brain barrier at this early stage of development.
4. Susceptibility of growing tissue and cells to drugs and chemical agents is probably greater than that of the mature tissue and cells.

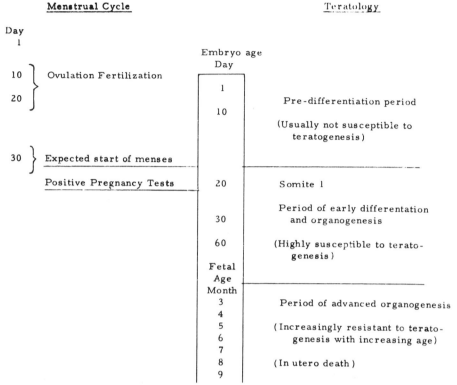

FIG. 4.   Relationship of ovulation cycle in the adult human female to teratogenic susceptibility. The diagram applies to a regular 28-day ovulation cycle.

Probably the most critical factor involved in drug-induced teratogenesis is
the in utero age of the developing fetus. Figure 4 shows the relationship of the
ovulation cycle in the adult female to teratogenic susceptibility. Organogenesis
in humans begins about the twentieth day of gestation (the first somite stage)
and continues for the most part through the third month. A continuing process
of finer morphologic and biochemical differentiation goes on throughout the
second trimester, and the last three months are devoted primarily to growth
with further biochemical development. The risk of morphologic anomalies is
therefore greater during the first trimester (day 20 - day 90), i.e., during the
period of greatest organ development.

In animals, studies (Harbison and Becker, 1972) demonstrated that the
teratogenic effects of DPH in the rat were determined by fetal age at the time of
drug administration. If administered during early gestation (day 7 - 10), hydronephrosis was the prominent morphological observation. However, administration on days 10 through 14 resulted in cleft palate formation. In humans, it is
also suggested that malformations produced by thalidomide are dependent on

58   EVANS, STEVENS, MANTILLA-PLATA, HARBISON

the fetal age at administration (Goldstein et al., 1974). On days 21 to 22 of gestation, anotia was the principal teratogenic response produced by thalidomide; from days 24 to 27, phocomelia of the arms was observed; and on days 28 to 30 of fetal age, phocomelia of the legs was noted. This differentiation of drug-induced effect with fetal age reflects the "cinematographic sequences" of development. The implication of these findings suggest that ingestion of drugs during later development may induce subtle biochemical defects. Certainly, further research is needed in this area if we are to understand the full effect of drugs on the fetus. Since pregnancy is not recognized until at least twenty days after fertilization, an unacceptable large proportion of human embryos will have been exposed to the risk of malformation before pregnancy is recognized. Therefore, contraindication of a drug during pregnancy is not enough for prevention of teratogenic effects in the fetus.

In summary, studies have indicated that during the early period of development, the placental membrane is very permeable by most drugs and chemicals, and it is not until later development that the placenta matures and is a barrier to high fetal levels of drug. Interaction of drugs in the pregnant animal following multiple drug administration has been shown to influence the fetal level of drug, so that multiple drug use during early organogenesis could act to greatly increase the teratogenic response. Also, environmental factors, such as pollutants, stress, and noises, could interact to increase the teratogenic response to a particular drug.

The human fetus in utero is not an ideal sequestered environment nourished by a placenta which maintains optimal fetal homeostasis. Fetal development is sensitive to a number of external agents, including drugs and chemicals, and changes in the maternal disposition of drugs can greatly influence drug teratogenesis. We now need to further explore the mechanism by which teratogenesis is brought about by agents which are generally abused and the relationship of the various factors that are involved in fetal development. It is indeed surprising that while more than 600 agents have been shown to produce teratogenesis in animals, only 20 of them are documented in man. Either human fetal development differs considerably from animal models or we have failed to detect their incidence in man.

Note

This study was supported in part by DA 00141.

References

Adamson, K. The effects of pharmacological agents upon the fetus and newborn. *American Journal of Obstetrics and Gynecology,* 1966, *96,* 437-460.
Alexander, G.J., Gold, G., Miles, B., and Alexander, R.B. Lysergic acid diethylamide intake in pregnancy: Fetal damage in rats. *Journal of Pharmacology and Experimental Therapeutics,* 1970, *173,* 48-59.

Apgar, V. Drugs in pregnancy. *Journal of the American Medical Association*, 1964, *190*, 840-841.

Auerbach, R., and Rugowski, J.A. Lysergic acid diethylamide: Effects on embryos. *Science*, 1967, *157*, 1325-1326.

Barthelmess, A. Mutagenic substances in the human environment. *Chemical Mutagenesis in Mammals and Man*. New York: Springer-Verlag, 1970.

Friedler, G., and Cocrin, J. Growth retardation in offspring of female rats treated with morphine prior to conception. *Science*, 1972, *175*, 654-655.

Geber, W.F. Congenital malformation induced by mescaline, lysergic acid and bromolysergic acid in the hamster. *Science*, 1967, *158*, 265-266.

Geber, W.F., and Schramm, L.C. Comparative teratogenicity of morphine, heroin and methadone in the hamster. *Pharmacologist*, 1969, *11*, 248.

Geber, W.F., and Schramm, L.C. Effects of marihuana extract on fetal hamsters and rabbits. *Toxicology and Applied Pharmacology*, 1969a, *14*, 276-282.

Gillette, J.R., Menard, R.H., and Stripp, B. Active products of fetal drug metabolism. *Clinical Pharmacology and Experimental Therapeutics*, 1973, *14*, 680-692.

Ginsberg, J. Placental drug transfer. *Annual Review of Pharmacology*, 1971, *11*, 387-407.

Goldenthal, E.I. A compilation of LD 50 values in newborn and adult animals. *Toxicology and Applied Pharmacology*, 1971, *18*, 185-207.

Goldman, A.S., and Yokovic, W.C. Teratogenic action in rats of reserpine. *Proceedings of the Society of Experimental Biology and Medicine*, 1965, *118*, 857-862.

Goldstein, A., Aronow, L., and Kalman, S.M. *Principles of Drug Action*, New York: John Wiley and Sons, 1974.

Gordon, H.R. Fetal bradycardia after paracervical block. *New England Journal of Medicine*, 1968, *279*, 910-914.

Gregg, N.M. Congenital cataract following German measles in the mother. *Transaction of the Ophthalmology Society of Australia*, 1941, *3*, 35-46.

Hale, F. Relation of maternal vitamin A deficiency to microphthalmia in pigs. *Texas State Journal of Medicine*, 1937, *33*, 228-232.

Harbison, R.D., and Becker, B.A. Relation of dosage and time of administration of diphenylhydantoin to its teratogenic effect in mice. *Teratology*, 1969, *2*, 305-312.

Harbison, R.D., and Becker, B.A. Effects of phenobarbital and SKF 525A pretreatment on diphenylhydantoin disposition in pregnant mice. *Toxicology and Applied Pharmocology*, 1971, *20*, 573-581.

Harbison, R.D., and Becker, B.A. Diphenylhydantoin teratogenicity in rats. *Toxicology and Applied Pharmacology*, 1972, *22*, 193-200.

Harper, K.H., Palmer, A.K., and Davies, R.E. Effect of imipramine upon the pregnancy of laboratory animals. *Arzneim. Forsch.*, 1965, *15*, 1218-1221.

Henderson, F.G., and Chen, K.K. Effect of age upon toxicity of methadone. *Proceedings of the Society of Experimental Biological Medicine*, 1948, *68*, 350-351.

Iuliucci, J.D., and Gautieri, R.F. Morphine-induced fetal malformations. *Journal of Pharmaceutical Sciences*, 1971, *60*, 420-424.

Jewett, R.E., and Norton. S. Fetal effects of chlorpromazine. *Experimental Neurology*, 1966, *14*, 33-37.

Juchau, M.R. Placental metabolism in relation to toxicology *CRC Critical Review in Toxicology*, 1973a, September, 125-158.

Juchau, M.R., Lee, Q.H., and Louviaux, G.L., Symms, K.G., Krasner, J., and Yaffe, S.J. Oxidation and reduction of foreign compounds in tissue of the human placenta and fetus. *Fetal Pharmacology*, New York: Raven Press, 1973.

Kasirsky, G., and Tansy, M.F. Teratogenic effects of methamphetamine in mice and rabbits. *Teratology*, 1971, *4*, 131-134.

Kehl, R., Audibert, A., Gage, C., and Amager, J. Action de la reserpine. *C.R. Soc. Biol.*, 1956, *150*, 2196-2199.

60   EVANS, STEVENS, MANTILLA-PLATA, HARBISON

Lenz, W. Malformations caused by drugs in pregnancy. *American Journal of Disabled Children,* 1966, 112.

Lenz, W., and Knapp, K. Thalidomide embryopathy. *Archives of Environmental Health,* 1962, *5,* 100-105.

Martin, E.W. *Patient response, Hazards of Medication,* Philadelphia: Lippincott, 1971, 271-284.

McColl, J.D., Globus, M., and Robinson, S. Drug induced skeletal malformations in the rat. *Experientia,* 1963, *19,* 183-184.

McColl, J.D., Robinson, S., and Globus, M. Effects of some therapeutic agents on the rabbit fetus. *Toxicology and Applied Pharmacology,* 1967, *10,* 244-252.

Mirkin, B.L. Diphenylhydantoin: Placental transport, fetal localization, neonatal metabolism and possible teratogenic effects. *Journal of Pediatrics,* 1971, *78,* 329-337.

Nora, J.A. Dextroamphetamine teratogenicity. *Lancet,* 1965, *2,* 1021.

Nora, J.A., Sommerville, R.J., and Fraser, F.C. Homologies for congenital heart diseases. *Teratology,* 1968, *1,* 413-416.

Orly, J.M., Somorajski, T., Collins, R.L., and Rolsten, C. Teratogenic effects of promazine. *Journal of Pharmacology and Experimental Therapeutics,* 1966, *151,* 110-117.

Pelkonen, O., Kaltiala, F.H., Larmi, T.K.I., and Karki, N.T. Comparison of activities of drug metabolizing enzymes in human fetal and adult livers. *Clinical Pharmacology and Experimental Therapeutics,* 1973, *14,* 840-846.

Persaud, T.V.N. Tierexperimentelle Untersuchungen zur Frage der Teratogenen Wirkung von Barbituraten. *Acta Biological Med. Ger.,* 1965, *14,* 89-90.

Persaud, T.V.N., and Ellington, A.C. Teratogenic activity of cannabis resin. *Lancet,* 1968, *2,* 406-407.

Poulson, E., and Robson, J.M. Teratogenic effects of nialamide. *Journal of Endocrinology,* 1963, *27,* 147-149.

Poulson, E. and Robson, J.M. Effect of phenelzine and some related compounds on pregnancy and on sexual development. *Journal of Endocrinology,* 1964, *30,* 205-215.

Rane, A., von Bahr, C., Orrenius, S., and Sjoqvist, F. Drug metabolism in the human fetus. *Fetal Pharmacology,* New York: Raven Press, 1973.

Rodriguez, S.U. Neonatal thrombocytopenia associated with ante-partum administration of thiazide drugs. *New England Journal of Medicine,* 1964, *270,* 881-884.

Roux, C. Action teratogene de la prochlorpamazine. *Archives French Pediatrics,* 1959, *16,* 968-971.

Sapeika, B.A. The passage of drugs across the placenta. *South African Medical Journal,* 1960, *34,* 34-55.

Sarteschi, P., Cassano, G.B., and Placidi, G.F. Placental penetration and foetal uptake of neuropharmacological agents. *Advances in Theoretical and Clinical Research,* 1973, *6,* 50-58.

Setala, K., and Nyyssonen, O. Hypnotic sodium pentobarbital as a teratogen in mice. *Naturwissenschaften,* 1964, *51,* 412.

Shepard, T.H. *Catalog of Teratogenic Agents,* Baltimore: The Johns Hopkins University Press, 1973.

Shirkey, H.C. Drugs and children. *Journal of the American Medical Association,* 1966, *196,* 418-421.

Smart, R.C. The chromosomal and teratogenic effects of lysergic acid diethylamide. *Canadian Medical Association Journal,* 1968, *99,* 805-810.

Smith, E.J. A report on the comparative study of newer drugs used for obstetrical anesthesia. *Americal Journal of Obstetrics and Gynecology,* 1949, *58,* 695-702.

Stevens, M.W., and Harbison, R.D. Placental transfer of diphenylhydantoin: Effects of species, gestational age and route of administration. *Teratology,* 1974, *9,* 317-326.

Takano, K., Tanimura, T., and Nishimura, H. Teratological studies with ethinamate. *Proceedings Congress of the Anatomical Research Association of Japan,* 1963, *3,* 2.

Tuchmann-Duplessis, H., and Mercier-Parot, L. Malformations foetales chez le rat traite par de fortes doses de deserpidine. *C.R. Soc. Biol.,* 1961, *155,* 2291-2293.

Tuchmann-Duplessis, H., and Mercier-Parot, L. Repercussion d'un somnifere, le glutethimide, sur la gestation et le developpement foetal du rat, de la souris et du lapin. *C.R. Acad. Sci.* (Paris), 1963, *256,* 1841-1843.

Vichi, F. Neuroleptic drugs in experimental teratogenesis. *Teratology, Proceedings of a Symposium.* Amsterdam: Excerpta Medica Foundation, 1969.

Warkany, J. *Drugs and Teratology in Pediatric Therapy,* St. Louis: Mosby, 1968.

Warkany, J., and Tokacs, E. Experimental production of congenital malformations in rats by salicylate poisoning. *American Journal of Pathology,* 1959, *35,* 315-331.

Williams, R.T. Teratogenic effects of thalidomide and related substances. *Lancet,* 1963, *1,* 723.

Yakovleva, A.I., and Sorokina, M.N. Teratogenic effects of some adrenergic drugs. *Farmakol. Toksik,* 1966, *29,* 224-229.

Addictive Diseases: an International Journal 2 (1): 63-77 (1975)

Cytogenetic Risks to the Offspring of Pregnant Addicts

CYRIL A. L. ABRAMS
Department of Pediatrics
the Roosevelt Hospital and the
College of Physicians and Surgeons
Columbia University, New York, N.Y.

In recent years it has been clearly shown that a variety of physical, chemical and pharmacological agents have the ability to induce structural changes in the chromosomes of somatic cells and gametes, in vivo as well as in vitro (Shaw, 1970). Many forms of radiant energy, including gamma rays, X-rays and ultraviolet light, isotopes derived from radiactive fallout, isotopes used in diagnostic medicine, air and water pollutants, food ingredients, substances added as food preservatives, chemicals in our immediate environment, and a variety of pharmaceutical products have been proven to be, or are suspected of being, able to damage chromosomes in plants, animals and man. Furthermore, a large number of these environmental agents have been screened in specific test systems for mutagenic and teratogenic effects, and some have shown a close correlation between their mutagenic potential and their ability to cause chromosomal damage (Kihlman, 1966; Epstein and Shafner, 1968). Viruses are well known for their ability to cause fragmentation of chromosomes and probably constitute the most important and ubiquitous class of clastogen, or chromosome-breaking agent. A number of pharmacological compounds are now being implicated as chromosome-breaking agents, among which the hallucinogens and narcotic addictive drugs are preeminent.

The ability of psychoactive drugs to cause chromosome damage in laboratory animals and humans has been well documented. These findings have brought an added dimension to the field of drug administration in general and the problem of narcotic addiction in particular. In the narcotic culture of today, widespread use of addictive drugs by women during their reproductive years raises the questions whether chromosome damage can occur directly in the fetus from exposure to the drug in utero, and whether drug-induced chromosomal aberrations in the gametes of addicted parents can be transmitted to their progeny. It is also pertinent to ask to what extent drug-induced chromosomal damage in the germ cells of the fetus constitutes a genetic hazard for future generations. Chromosomal aberrations in the germ cells of mice treated with LSD have been described by several investigators (Skakkeback, Philip and Rafaelsen, 1968; Cohen and Mukherjee, 1968; Jagiello and Polani, 1969).

Structural abnormalities in chromosomes arise from breakage of the whole chromosome or of one of the chromatids, depending on what stage of the cell cycle the damage occurs. Aberrations are thus generally regarded as either chromosome or chromatid in type. More specifically they are classified as chromatid breaks, isochromatid breaks, fragments, gaps, deletions, rings, dicentrics, exchange figures and markers. They may be defined as follows:

Chromatid break: A clear visual discontinuity of chromatin material in a single chromatid with displacement of the distal segment from the axis of the proximal portion.

Isochromatid break: This has the same characteristics as a chromatid break, but both chromatids are involved at the same level.

Fragment: A chromatid break with the distal portion appearing as a non-aligned piece of chromatin material close to the proximal segment or lying free at a distance from the proximal portion.

Gap: A pale, attenuated, chromatic region appearing as a discontinuity of chromatin material without displacement of the distal portion.

Deletion: A chromatid break with loss of the broken-off portion resulting in unequal lengths of the sister chromatids.

Ring: This is a structural rearrangement and represents the joining together of the chromatid ends of a single chromosome following the occurrence of a double break. It is scored as two breaks.

Dicentric: This structural rearrangement is a functionally single chromosome with two centromeres formed by the fusion of portions of two chromosomes. It is scored as two breaks.

Exchange figure: This is a complex rearrangement produced by translocations and combinations of two or more chromosomes which results in the formation of a triradial or quadriradial figure. It is scored as two or three breaks.

Marker: This is an atypical, unidentifiable chromosome shorter or longer than a normal chromosome.

Thus, chromosomes which have been damaged may become shortened, lengthened or structurally altered in a variety of ways with corresponding genetic effects, namely, loss or addition of genes, or changes in gene order and linkage groups.

The first report of chromosome damage due to LSD appeared in 1967, when Cohen and his co-workers demonstrated that the addition of LSD to cultures of normal human lymphocytes resulted in an increased frequency of chromosomal aberrations (Cohen, Marinello and Back, 1967). While these in vitro observations have been confirmed by other workers (Bick, 1970), contradictory findings have been reported from different laboratories regarding the effects of LSD in vivo, and the question whether significant chromosome damage occurs in individuals using illicit or pure LSD remains controversial.

Few reports have been published of chromosome studies in newborn infants who were exposed to psychoactive drugs in utero. In one study (Cohen, Hirschhorn et al., 1968), a statistically significant increase in mean chromosomal breakage rate was found in infants exposed to LSD in utero compared with controls. Included in this study was a group of children whose mothers had used LSD prior to conception but not during pregnancy. These children also showed an increased frequency of chromosomal aberrations over controls. However, the use of multiple drugs, including opiates, by the mothers before and during pregnancy, gives rise to difficulties in interpreting the data. In five additional studies on infants who had been exposed to LSD in utero, increased chromosomal breakage rates are reported in three (Egozcue, Irwin and Maruffo, 1968; Hulten, Lindsten et al., 1968; Jacobson and Berlin, 1972), and no unusual chromosome damage in two (Sato and Pergament, 1968; Dumars, 1971). Some of the children in these various reports were found to have chromosomal aberrations as long as 6 months, 18 months, 28 months, 34 months and 5 years after birth. Furthermore, several showed evidence of Philadelphia-like chromosomes (Cohen, Hirschhorn et al., 1968; Egozcue, Irwin and Maruffo, 1968). One case of 13 trisomy with D/D translocation in the offspring of an LSD user has been recorded (Hsu, Strauss, Hirschhorn, 1972).

Opiates have received little attention regarding their effects on chromosomes, and reports in the literature are as scanty as those on LSD are profuse (Table I). In one study of 22 ex-addicts who had used multiple drugs, including opiates, Amarose and Schuster found the incidence of chromosomal abnormalities in peripheral blood lymphocytes to be higher than in bone marrow cells, and higher than in the peripheral blood lymphocytes of normal controls (Amarose and Schuster, 1971). In a combined in vivo and in vitro study, Falek and co-workers found a statistically significant increase in chromosome abnormalities in a group of 16 drug users on a methadone maintenance program. In addition to chromosome breaks, dicentrics were observed in 6 patients and an exchange figure in one patient. These patients also abused other drugs, but not LSD. The in vitro study, however, in which morphine, quinine and methadone were added to cultures of human leucocytes, revealed no difference in frequency of chromo-

TABLE I
Opiates and Chromosomes

Literature reference	Drug exposure	Type of exposure	Chromosome Abnormalities
Amarose and Schuster (1971)	Opiates, amphet, barbit, psychedelics	In vivo	Increased frequency in peripheral blood of drug user
Falek et al (1972)	Methadone	a) In vivo	a) Increased frequency in peripheral blood of drug user
		b) In vitro	b) None
Kushnick (1972)	Heroin and Cocaine	In vivo	45/X0 in offspring
Abrams and Liao (1972)	Heroin and Methadone	In vivo	Increased frequency in peripheral blood of offspring

some damage between treated and untreated cultures (Falek, et al., 1972). There is one report in the literature of an XO chromosomal abnormality in an infant born to an addict who used heroin and cocaine. (Kushnick, Robinson and Tsao, 1972), and a study in our own laboratory revealed an increased incidence of chromosomal aberrations in the offspring of women who were addicted to heroin during pregnancy (Abrams and Liao, 1972).

Over the past three and a half years we have studied the peripheral blood chromosomes of 34 newborn infants who had been exposed to heroin and methadone in utero, and of 22 control infants whose mothers did not use drugs in pregnancy. The first part of the study was undertaken in 1970-71, when methadone treatment was less prevalent than now and infants born to pregnant addicts were exposed predominantly to heroin in utero. The second part of the study covers the period 1972-74, when many pregnant addicts were enrolled in methadone maintenance programs and their infants were exposed predominantly to methadone in utero.

MATERIAL AND METHODS

In the first study, 16 drug-exposed infants were compared with 14 controls. The drug-exposed group ranged in age from 12 hours to 31 days at the time of chromosome analysis. A history of heroin use by the mothers during pregnancy was obtained in all instances, but the total dose taken could not be estimated with any degree of accuracy. Multiple drugs were apparently not used, but ten mothers did receive methadone during pregnancy, in most instances for brief periods only before they resorted to heroin again. Eight of the 16 infants showed withdrawal symptoms at birth indicating transplacental passage of the drug, and 5 had received treatment with Valium, Thorazine and paregoric before blood samples were obtained for chromosomal analysis. One baby had a viral illness. This was identified as a herpes simplex infection which had been acquired in utero. No evidence of concomitant infection was observed in the other infants at the time of blood sampling.

The control infants ranged in age from one to 13 days. All were healthy and none had received any medication   other than a routine Vitamin K injection, as did the heroin-exposed babies, prior to chromosome analysis.

Uniform procedures for blood sampling, culturing and harvesting were followed. Triplicate cultures from the test and control babies were set up in parallel on the same day, and after 72 hours of culture, chromosomes were prepared on slides in accordance with standard techniques. One hundred suitable metaphase spreads per subject were analyzed and chromosome aberrations were classified according to the criteria previously described. In this pilot study the slides were not evaluated on a blind basis and the identity of the index and control babies was known to the observer.

TABLE II
Chromosomal Aberrations in Newborn Infants Exposed to Heroin in Utero

Patient	Age (days)	Sex	Total cells analyzed	Type & frequency of Chromosomal aberrations								No. of chromosomal aberrations	No. of cells with chromosomal aberrations	Remarks	
				CB	ICB	Gap	Dic	Ring	Frag	Del	Biz			Mother (during pregnancy)	Infant (before blood sampling)
1	4	M	100	9	2	6	1	...	1	...	...	19	17	Methadone	Chlorpromazine
2	8	F	100	1	...	1	...	...	1	...	...	3	3	Methadone	
3	1	M	100	6	...	2	1	...	5	3	...	17	10	Methadone	Opiates
4	31	F	100	9	...	4	3	...	3	...	...	19	14	Methadone	
5	12	M	100	3	...	2	4	...	3	...	...	12	10	Methadone & Virus	Virus
6	9	M	100	3	...	...	...	...	...	...	...	3	3	Methadone	Diazepam
7	7	F	100	7	2	...	5	1	2	1	...	18	18	Methadone	
8	3	F	100	3	...	2	7	...	3	...	1	16	12	Methadone	
9	14	F	100	...	1	...	...	...	1	...	2	4	3	Methadone	
10	10	F	100	4	...	2	3	...	1	1	...	11	10		
11	5	F	100	7	1	...	2	...	2	...	...	10	10	Methadone	Diazepam
12	3	M	100	3	...	2	1	...	2	...	...	8	6	Methadone	
13	1	M	100	3	...	4	...	...	...	...	...	7	7	Methadone	
14	4	M	100	3	1	1	2	...	...	...	...	7	6	Methadone	Diazepam
15	1/2	M	100	5	1	...	1	...	3	...	...	10	9	Methadone (in labor)	
16	3	M	100	15	1	2	1	...	2	...	...	20	17		Diazepam
											Mean:	11.5	9.7		

Results of First Study

Thirteen of the 16 (81%) heroin-exposed infants showed a high incidence of chromosomal aberrations in multiple cells. The distribution and frequency of chromosomal aberrations, and of cells with chromosomal aberrations, in the heroin-exposed babies is seen in *Table II*. One hundred cells in each subject were scored for 9 different types of chromosomal aberration. The number of aberrations per patient ranged from 3 to 20 per 100 cells analyzed, with a mean value of 11.5. The total number of cells showing chromosomal aberrations per patient ranged from 3 to 18, with a mean value of 9.7 per 100 cells analyzed. These mean values were 6.7 and 6.0 times higher, respectively, than the mean values in the control infants, whose findings are shown in *Table III*. Total chromosomal aberrations and total number of cells with chromosomal aberrations ranged from 1 to 6 per 100 cells analyzed in both categories, with mean values of 1.7 and 1.6, respectively, which are much lower than in the heroin group.

Table IV compares the type and frequency of individual chromosomal aberrations in the 2 groups of babies in greater detail. Among the 1600 cells analyzed in the 16 heroin-exposed babies, 81 chromatid breaks were found in 15 patients, 29 dicentrics in 11 patients, 28 fragments in 13 patients, 28 gaps in 11 patients, 9 isochromatid breaks in 7 patients, 5 deletions in 3 patients, 3 markers in 2 patients and 1 ring in 1 patient. Among the 1400 cells analyzed in the 14 control babies, 20 chromatid breaks were found in 9 patients and 4 gaps in 2 patients. No structural rearrangements were observed. The presence of dicentrics, markers and a ring in the heroin group is especially noteworthy, for the reasons previously mentioned.

The difference in mean values between the 2 groups was found to be statistically significant (P 0.0001), as shown in Table V.

The second study comprised 18 infants who had been exposed predominantly to methadone in utero and 8 control infants who had no drug exposure in utero. In the drug-exposed group almost all the babies were between 1 and 7 days of age at the time of blood sampling. In 2 infants, cultures were unsuccessful at birth and could only be re-done in follow-up at age 7 weeks and 6 months, respectively. All mothers, except one, were taking methadone in doses ranging from 5 mg to 110 mg per day. The majority were taking over 50 mg a day. Seven mothers admitted to intermittent heroin use during pregnancy. Barbiturates were found in the urine of 3 babies, and cocaine in the urine of 1 baby, at birth. One mother who took heroin in the last month of pregnancy gave no history of methadone use previously. One mother had received isoniazide and ethambutol for tuberculosis while pregnant. Thirteen babies had withdrawal symptoms. All the babies, except one, had chromosome analysis before treatment was initiated. This infant had already been treated with Thorazine when chromosome analysis was done at age 7 weeks. The control infants ranged in age from 1 to 10 days and all were healthy.

TABLE III

Chromosomal Aberrations in Control Infants

Patient	Age (days)	Sex	Total cells analyzed	Type & frequency of Chromosomal aberrations								No. of chromosomal aberrations	No. of cells with chromosomal aberrations
				CB	ICB	Gap	Dic	Ring	Frag	Del	Biz		
1	2	M	100	1	...	...	...	...	...	...	...	1	1
2	1	F	100	...	...	...	...	...	...	...	...	...	...
3	2	M	100	...	...	...	...	...	...	...	...	...	...
4	5	F	100	1	...	...	...	...	...	...	...	1	1
5	3	F	100	...	...	...	...	...	...	...	...	...	...
6	2	F	100	2	...	...	...	...	...	...	...	2	2
7	3	F	100	5	...	...	...	...	...	...	...	5	5
8	3	F	100	3	...	...	...	...	3	...	...	6	6
9	3	F	100	1	...	...	...	1	...	...	...	2	1
10	5	F	100	3	...	...	...	...	...	...	...	3	3
11	13	M	100	2	...	...	...	...	...	...	...	2	2
12	3	F	100	2	...	...	...	...	...	...	...	2	2
13	13	M	100	...	...	...	...	...	...	...	...	...	...
14	10	F	100	...	...	...	...	...	...	...	...	...	...
											Mean:	1.7	1.6

Procedures for blood sampling, culturing, harvesting and scoring of chromosomal aberrations were the same as in the first study. In this study the culture tubes and slides were evaluated on a blind basis, and the identity of the index and control subjects was not known to the person analyzing the slides.

Results of Second Study

Among the 1800 cells analyzed in the 18 methadone-exposed babies, 30 chromatid breaks were found in 12 infants, 29 fragments in 7 infants, 9 dicentrics in 2 infants, 5 isochromatid breaks in 4 infants, 2 gaps in 1 infant, 2 markers in 1 infant, 1 ring in 1 infant and 1 quadricentric in 1 infant. The total number of aberrations was 79, and the mean number of aberrations was 4.4 per 100 cells, or 0.044 per cell. The mean number of *cells* with aberrations was 2.4 per 100 cells. Among the 800 cells analyzed in the 8 control babies, 13 chromatid breaks were found in 5 infants, 5 fragments in 5 infants, 4 isochromatid breaks in 4 infants, and 4 gaps in 4 infants. No structural rearrangements were observed. The total number of aberrations was 26, and the mean number of aberrations was 3.2 per 100 cells, or 0.032 per cell. The mean number of cells with aberrations was 3.1 per 100 cells.

The difference in mean values between the methadone-exposed and control infants is statistically not significant.

The increased incidence of structural rearrangements in the methadone group is of particular interest, however, since these aberrations rarely occur spontaneously in man.

DISCUSSION

The results of our studies must be interpreted with caution, since the pregnant addict is exposed to a variety of factors which can damage chromosomes in the fetus. These factors include nutritional deficiencies and infections, to which the heroin addict is especially prone, chemical impurities in the "bag" of heroin, and abuse of multiple drugs. Any or all of these noxious influences may have contributed to the high incidence of chromosomal abnormalities found in the group of heroin-exposed infants in our study. By the same token, the low incidence of chromosomal abnormalities in the methadone-exposed group may reflect the improved life-style of the methadone-treated mother, which closely approaches normal, and the elimination of those adverse environmental factors peculiar to the heroin addict. However, the presence of chromosomal rearrangements, such as dicentric and ring chromosomes in the offspring of methadone-treated women, whose drug exposure is predominantly methadone, even when other drugs are abused, leads one to suspect that methadone may be capable of causing significant chromosome damage in the fetus during pregnancy. It should be pointed out that chromosomal rearrangements, which can be trans-

TABLE IV
Type and Frequency of Chromosomal Aberrations in Offspring of Pregnant Addicts
(1970-71)

	HEROIN		CONTROL	
	Aberrations (n=1600 cells)	Patients (n=16)	Aberrations (n=1400 cells)	Patients (n=14)
CB	81	15/16	20	9/14
Dic	29	11/16	0	-
Frag	28	13/16	0	-
Gaps	28	11/16	4	2/14
ICB	9	7/16	0	-
Del	5	3/16	0	-
Biz	3	2/16	0	-
Ring	1	1/16	0	-
Total chromosomal aberrations	184		24	
Mean chromosomal aberrations	11.5/100 cells 0.115/cell		1.7/100 cells 0.017/cell	
Total cells with chromosomal aberrations	155		23	
Mean cells with chromosomal aberrations	9.7/100 cells		1.6/100 cells	

mitted to future generations, are considered more significant cytogenetic effects than breaks and fragments which usually produce non-viable cells.

The growing evidence that chromosomal aberrations can be induced experimentally by addictive drugs in vivo and in vitro, and that chromosomal aberrations occur in the circulating leucocytes of drug users and their offspring, focuses attention on an issue of a more fundamental nature, namely, the genetic and other hazards implicit in damage to the genome. If chromosome damage is found in the peripheral blood, the important question arises whether it might also be present in the germ cells.

Damage to the genetic apparatus of the germ cells has far-reaching implications from a mutagenic and teratogenic point of view, and its relevance to the present-day epidemic of drug addiction is a cause for much concern. Widespread use of drugs that damage chromosomes may well constitute a serious genetic hazard to future generations by increasing the damage to the human gene pool and thereby increasing the mutagenic load in the population. Such effects could result in an increased frequency of spontaneous abortions, an increased frequency of birth defects, an increased incidence of postnatal morbidity and mortality, and an increased incidence of chromosomal aberrations in the population at large.

TABLE V
Comparison of Chromosomal Aberrations in Heroin-exposed and Control
Infants

	Heroin (n=16)	Control (n=14)	Difference
Mean no chromosome aberrations per 100 cells analyzed	11.5	1.7	9.8*
Mean no. cells with chromosome aberrations per 100 cells analyzed	9.7	1.6	8.1*

*Statistically significant: P<0.0001 (Wilcoxon Rank Sum Test)

A further problem to be considered in drug-induced chromosome damage is the potential danger of malignant change in a cell with a chromosomal aberration. It is well known that chromosomal aberrations are found in individuals with established neoplastic disease, and in some instances their presence in normal health predisposes to the later development of malignant disease. Children affected by Bloom's syndrome, Fanconi's anemia and ataxia telangiectasia characteristically display an abnormal degree of chromosome breakage in their peripheral leucocytes and show a marked propensity to develop leukemia and other lymphoproliferative disease. The question thus arises whether chromosome aberrations induced by exogenous agents increase the risk of malignant disorders in affected individuals. The increased incidence of leukemia in individuals harboring damaged chromosomes many years after exposure to excessive radiation lends support to this hypothesis and is indeed a portent of the risks involved (Court Brown and Doll, 1965).

It is thus a matter of some urgency for large-scale cytogenetic studies to be undertaken on population groups at risk, so that the vulnerability of chromosomes to drugs can be more fully explored, the possible effects of chromosomal damage better determined, and the potential dangers of drug abuse from a genetic standpoint more clearly defined.

Summary and Conclusions

Our studies may be summarized as follows:
1. Infants exposed predominantly to heroin in utero showed a significant increase in the frequency of chromosomal aberrations in their peripheral blood

compared with controls, whereas infants exposed predominantly to methadone in utero did not.

2. Adverse environmental factors which may have contributed to the abnormal cytogenetic findings in the heroin-exposed infants were less prominent in the methadone-exposed infants.

3. The presence of chromosomal rearrangements in both groups of drug-exposed infants leads us to suspect that heroin and methadone can induce chromosome damage in vivo, and permits us to infer that these drugs are potentially harmful to the fetus from the cytogenetic point of view

SUMMARY

Peripheral blood chromosomes were studied in 34 newborn infants who had been exposed to heroin and methadone *in utero*, and in 22 newborn controls. Those infants (16) exposed predominantly to heroin showed a significant increase in the frequency of chromosomal aberrations compared with 14 controls (p 0.0001), whereas those (18) exposed predominantly to methadone showed no significant difference in the incidence of chromosomal aberrations compared with 8 controls. Chromosomal rearrangements (dicentrics, rings, markers) were observed, however, in both drug-exposed groups, which leads us to suspect that heroin and methadone can induce chromosome damage in vivo, and permits us to infer that these drugs are potentially harmful to the fetus from the cytogenetic point of view.

Acknowledgements

Thanks are due to Maria Freda, Lana Fleischmann, Eleanor Newman and Ruth Lynch for their valuable technical and secretarial assistance. The author also expresses his thanks to Dr. Lucy Swift, St. Luke's Hospital, New York City, for her collaboration in this study.

Notes

This study was supported by grants AM05531 and MH-21920 from the NIH.

Requests for reprints should be addressed to Cyril A.L. Adams, The Roosevelt Hospital, 428 West 59th Street, New York, N.Y. 10019.

References

Abrams, C.A.L., and Liao, Pei-yu. Chromosomal aberrations in newborns exposed to heroin in utero. *J. Clin. Invest.* 1972, *51*, 1a (abstract # 2).

Amarose, A.P., and Schuster, C.R. Chromosomal analyses of bone marrow and peripheral blood in subjects with a history of illicit drug use. *Archives of General Psychiatry*, 1971,*25*, 181-186.

Bick, Y.A.E. Comparison of the effects of LSD, Heliotrine and X-irradiation on chromosome breakage, and the effects of LSD on the rate of cell division. *Nature*, 1970, *226*, 1165-1167.

Cohen, M.M., Marinello, M.J., and Back, N. Chromosomal damage in human leukocytes induced by lysergic acid diethylamide. *Science*, 1967, *155*, 1417-1419.

Cohen, M.M., Hirschhorn, K., Verbo, S., Frosch, W.A., and Groeschel, M.M. The effect of LSD-25 on the chromosomes of children exposed in utero. *Pediatric Research*, 1968, *2*, 486-492.

Cohen, M.M., and Mukherjee, A.B. Meiotic chromosome damage induced by LSD-25. *Nature*, 1968, *219*, 1072-1074.

Court Brown, W.M., and Doll, R. Mortality from cancer and other causes after radiotherapy for ankylosing spondylitis. *British Medical Journal*, 1965, *2*, 1327-1332.

Dumars, K.W. Parental drug usage: Effect upon chromosomes of progeny. *Pediatrics*, 1971, *47*, 1037-1041.

Egozcue, J., Irwin, S., and Maruffo, C.A. Chromosomal damage in LSD users. *Journal of the American Medical Association*, 1968, *204*, 214-218.

Epstein, S.S., and Shafner, H. Chemical mutagens in the human environment. *Nature*, 1968, *219*, 385-387.

Falek, A., Jordan, R.B., King, B.J., Arnold, P.J., and Skelton, W.D. Human chromosomes and opiates. *Archives of General Psychiatry*, 1972, *27*, 511-515.

Hsu, L.Y., Strauss, L., and Hirschhorn, K. Chromosome abnormality in offspring of LSD user: D-trisomy with translocation. *Journal of the American Medical Association*, 1970, *211*, 987-990.

Hulten, M., Lindsten, J., Lidberg, L., and Ekelund, H. Studies on mitotic and meiotic chromosomes in subjects exposed to LSD. *Ann. Genet. (Paris)*, 1968, *11*, 201-210.

Jacobson, C.B., and Berlin, C.M. Possible reproductive detriment in LSD users. *Journal of the American Medical Association*, 1972, *222*, 1367-1373.

Jagiello, G., and Polani, P.E. Mouse germ cells and LSD-25. *Cytogenetics*, 1969, *8*, 136-147.

Kihlman, B.A. *Actions of Chemicals on Dividing Cells*. Englewood Cliffs, N.J., Prentice-Hall, 1966.

Kushnik, T., Robinson, M., and Tsao, C. 45,X chromosome abnormality in the offspring of a narcotic addict. *American Journal of Diseases of Children*, 1972. *124*, 772-773.

Sato, H., and Pergament, E. Is lysergide a teratogen? *Lancet*, 1968, *1*, 639-640.

Shaw, M.W. Human chromosome damage by chemical agents. *Annual Review of Medicine*, 1970, *21*, 409-432.

Skakkeback, N.E., Philip, J., and Rafaelson, O.J. LSD in mice: Abnormalities in meiotic chromosomes. *Science*, 1968, *160*, 1246-1248.

DISCUSSION

Q. *Dr. Zelson*: We, too, have been interested in the studies of the chromosomes, but, unfortunately, our results are a little different from those of Dr. Abrams. We have 40 controlled mothers, 22 heroin mothers, and 27 methadone mothers; and we have 47 controlled babies, 39 heroin babies, and 47 methadone babies. We were studying the mitotic index in which we were interested at that time, but the question of chromosomal breakage also was studied carefully. Two hundred cells were counted each time. The karyotypes were done within the first 24 hours of birth and, among these, we found that there was one abnormality in the mother. She had a translocation type of abnormality. We had one baby with a translocation and one Klinefelters. All the others were perfectly normal. We have a chromosome breakage rate of between 1 and 2 percent. Now, I do not understand or know why the difference is so great, because we followed this very carefully, and we have discussed this many times, and our geneticist could not find the breaks as described by you. Incidentally, among the methadone babies, there were 19 males and 27 females. So if you want a female baby, take methadone. The controls were 24 males and 22 females, which is more or less normal. In the heroin group, there were 17 males and 21 females. This is not statistically significant but interesting.

A. *Dr. Abrams: The only comment I can make on that is that it is interesting. The discrepancies in data seem to apply to many drug studies, and I understand those negative findings very well. The only thing is that one has to use one's own controls. We do know that in the normal population you can even get an occasional dicentric, and an occasional acentric fragment. That may contradict our own findings in a way. However, when you use your own controls under parallel circumstances, and find these abnormalities in one group and not in the other, we feel that this is significant. We cannot draw any definitive conclusions from it. The numbers are still small, and we still have a rather small study. We have about 15 more patient's slides waiting to be studied, so I think it is still a little controversial. We just feel suspicious that those drugs are doing something to the chromosomes. Of course, we do not see in normals, and even in our routine karyotyping of patients just off-the-wards, we do not run into these peculiar looking chromosomes.*

Q. *Dr. Braude:* Do you think that perhaps the differences would be due to length of exposures of the mother, or maybe different doses? We recently had a small group meeting of geneticists, because we are all interested, obviously, in genetic problems. It seems that, for certain drugs of abuse, you find some differences up to a certain dose. When the dose is exceeded, there is a kind of cytotoxicity which comes into the picture. Have you seen any of this?

A. *Dr. Abrams: Would that be an in vitro study possibly, because, as you increase the dose, it will prevent the cells from multiplying and you would not see any damage. That is true as you increase the dose. But, I suspect in vivo, this is not the case. A certain population of cells will be killed, but another population will be damaged. A spectrum from damage to death will exist at all doses.*

Q. *Dr. Solish:* Did you look at the chromosomes of the mothers of those babies that had the high frequency of aberrations; and if so, did the incidence of breaks or abnormalities of the mother have any relationship to those of the baby? The other question that I would like to ask is, did you with any of these babies have a chance to follow up—in other words, to repeat the karyotype at some later date to see what happens? There may be a great deal of healing in that period of time and, therefore, the changes we see in some instances may have something to do with the time in which the karyotypes are done.

A. *Dr. Abrams: This is true. The first question is no, we have not studied the mothers at all. We have limited ourselves purely to the newborn infant. We do have a follow-up clinic and we have been obtaining chromosomes. They are not included in this group and I do not even think any of them have been analyzed* *yet. They have been prepared as slides, but it is a slow, tedious process. I do not know, but we are looking into that. This is part of an ongoing study and we hope to have the answer to that within the coming year in the follow-ups.*

Q. *Dr. Rementeria:* I was wondering what you would think of the findings of previous heroin studies, where they found neither any increased congenital anomalies in the heroin group compared to the controlled groups, nor your findings of increased chromosomal breakages with the use of heroin. How would you make the two studies compatible?

A. *Dr. Abrams: Are you talking about clinical congenital abnormalities and how to reconcile the two?*

A. *Dr. Rementeria:* Right.

A. *Dr. Abrams:* What you see in the peripheral blood does not necessarily reflect what is happening in the gametes. Go back even further; for the child to develop a congenital anomaly, the damage must either be in the zygote or in the pre-zygote at the time of conception, or soon after. But once the whole fetus is formed, any damage occurring later is unlikely to cause clinical abnormalities. Beyond that critical period of formation, say, in the first trimester, one could say that there may be circulating abnormal chromosomes.

Addictive Diseases: an International Journal 2 (1): 79-88 (1975)
© 1975 by Spectrum Publications, Inc.

The Fetal Alcohol Syndrome

KENNETH LYONS JONES
Department of Pediatrics
University of California, San Diego

INTRODUCTION

A pattern of altered growth and morphogenesis, referred to as the fetal alcohol syndrome, has now been reported in 16 unrelated children, all of whom were born to severe chronic alcoholic women who continued to drink heavily throughout their pregnancy. (Jones, et al., 1973; Jones, and Smith, 1973; Ferrier et al., 1973; Hall and Orenstein, 1974; Palmer et al., 1974)

HISTORICAL REVIEW

Since the initial discrimination of this disorder, historical evidence has been brought to light indicating that an association between maternal alcoholism and serious problems in the offspring is not a new observation. Evidence is even available from classical Greek and Roman mythology suggesting that maternal alcoholism at the time of conception can lead to serious problems in fetal development. This led to an ancient Carthaginian ritual forbidding the drinking of wine by the bridal couple on their wedding night in order that defective children might not be conceived. (Haggard and Jellinek, 1942.)

In 1834, a select committee of the British House of Commons was established to investigate drunkenness, prior to the establishment in that same year of an Alcoholic Licensure Act. Evidence presented to that committee indicated that infants born to alcoholic mothers sometimes had a "starved, shriveled, and imperfect look." (Report on Evidence of Drunkenness presented to the House of Commons by the Select Committee, 1834.)

In 1900, Sullivan investigated female alcoholics at the Liverpool Prison. He was able to document an increased frequency of early fetal death and early infant mortality in their offspring. (Sullivan, 1900.) Other investigators have

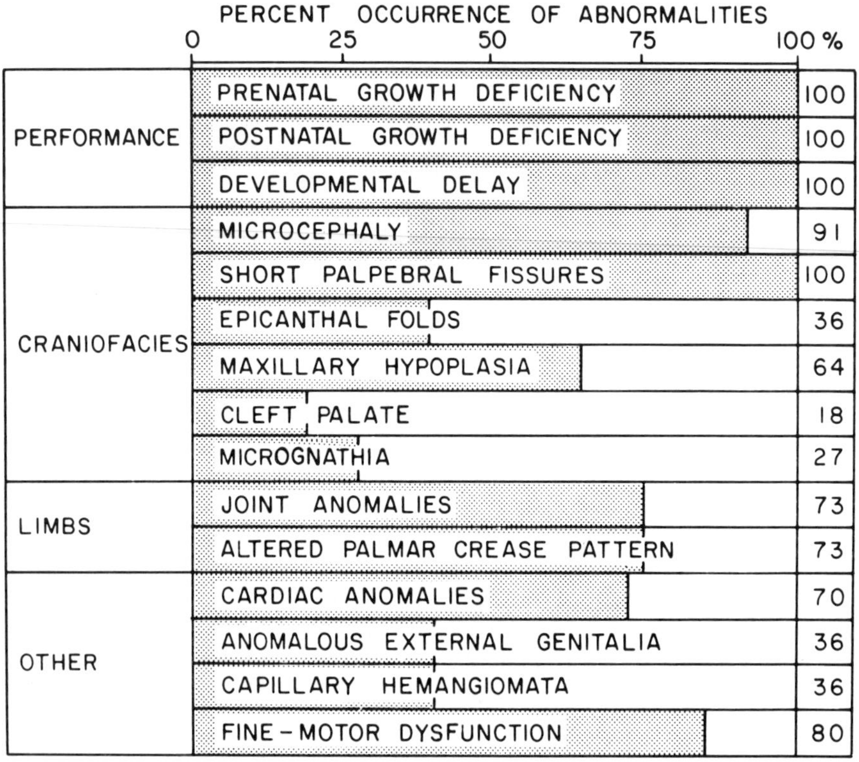

PERCENT OCCURRENCE OF ABNORMALITIES

		100
PERFORMANCE	PRENATAL GROWTH DEFICIENCY	100
	POSTNATAL GROWTH DEFICIENCY	100
	DEVELOPMENTAL DELAY	100
CRANIOFACIES	MICROCEPHALY	91
	SHORT PALPEBRAL FISSURES	100
	EPICANTHAL FOLDS	36
	MAXILLARY HYPOPLASIA	64
	CLEFT PALATE	18
	MICROGNATHIA	27
LIMBS	JOINT ANOMALIES	73
	ALTERED PALMAR CREASE PATTERN	73
OTHER	CARDIAC ANOMALIES	70
	ANOMALOUS EXTERNAL GENITALIA	36
	CAPILLARY HEMANGIOMATA	36
	FINE-MOTOR DYSFUNCTION	80

FIG. 1.   The pattern of abnormalities in the initial 11 patients evaluated with the fetal alcohol syndrome.

found increased frequency of prematurity, and decreased weight of surviving children born to chronic alcoholic mothers.

Animal experiments relative to the effects of ethanol on early morphogenesis have led to variable results (Sandor, 1968). However, recent experiments by St. Saudor have demonstrated ethanol-induced dysmorphogenesis in chick as well as albino rat embryos (Sandor, 1968; Sandor, 0000, Sandor and Amels, 1971). This consisted, in the developing chick, of deformed brain vesicles and spinal cord, abnormal development of somites and retardation of general growth and stage of morphogenesis (Sandor, 1968). Interpreting from these animal studies, he warned in 1968, and again, as recently as 1972, that there exists "a serious danger signal of prenatal risk of ethanol intoxication during early pregnancy in humans" (Sandor and Amels, 1971).

CLINICAL PICTURE

Features shared by the initial eleven children evaluated with this disorder are summarized in Figure 1. Three of the affected children, one from each of the

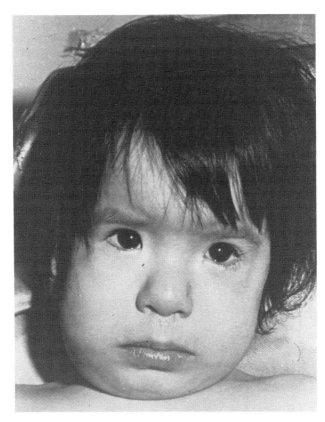

FIG. 2. A 1-year-old American Indian girl. Note the short palpebral fissures and maxillary hypoplasia.

ethnic groups in which this syndrome has been described, are illustrated in Figures 2-4.

The prenatal growth deficiency has been more severe with regard to birth length than birth weight. This is in direct contrast to most studies of generalized maternal undernutrition, in which the newborn infants are underweight for their length.

The immutable nature of the prenatal effect on growth rate is demonstrated by the consistency and severity of the postnatal growth deficiency. In the patients who could be followed after one year of age, linear growth rate was 65% of normal, while the average rate of weight gain was only 38% of normal, despite the fact that six of the children were hospitalized on numerous occasions for failure to thrive, during which time adequate caloric intake was well documented, and despite the fact that three of them were in excellent foster-care placement.

Intelligence quotients ranged from below 50 to 83 , with an average I.Q. of 63.

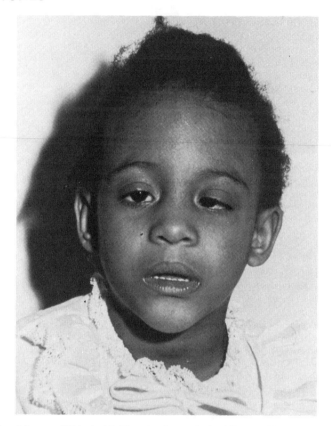

FIG. 3.   A 3-year-old black girl. Note the short palpebral fissures, bilateral ptosis, and strabismus on the left.

With regard to the microcephaly, head circumference was less than the third percentile for chronologic age at birth in 10 of the 11 patients, and in all but one, evaluated at one year of age, it was below the third percentile not only for chronologic age, but for height age as well.

The joint anomalies were variable, and consisted of congenital hip dislocation in three patients; inability to completely extend the elbows in three patients; camptodactyly of the fingers in three; clinodactyly of toes in two; and inability to completely flex the metacarpal-phalangeal joints in two patients.

Altered palmar crease patterns were variable, and consisted of the following: rudimentary palmar creases, aberrant alignment of palmar creases, or a single upper palmar crease.

Cardiac anomalies consisted of an atrial septal defect in one patient, a patent ductus arteriosus in one patient, and six of the children had grade 3-4 out of 6 systolic murmurs interpreted as representing ventricular septal defects.

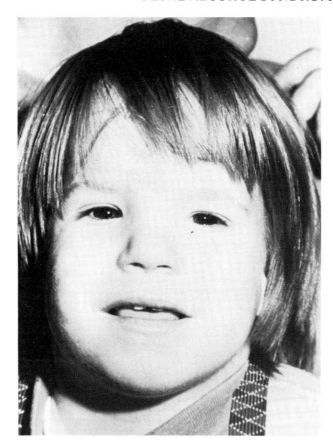

FIG. 4.   A 2-year-old white boy. Note the short palpebral fissures and maxillary hypoplasia.

Anomalies of the external genitalia consisted of hypoplastic labia majora in three patients, and a septated vagina in one.

Fine motor dysfunction was manifest by a weak grasp in some patients, poor eye-hand coordination in others, and by tremulousness in the newborn period.

Two children with the Fetal Alcohol Syndrome have been identified in the newborn period. Both had serious problems with neonatal respiratory adaptation. One had difficulty with the initiation of respirations, and was noted in the delivery room to have "alcohol on his breath." The other, depicted in Figure 5, had multiple apneic episodes, culminating in death at five days of age. The findings in the brain noted at the autopsy of that child are of special pertinence. There were extensive developmental anomalies which resulted primarily from aberrations of neuronal migration, and thereby in multiple heterotopias

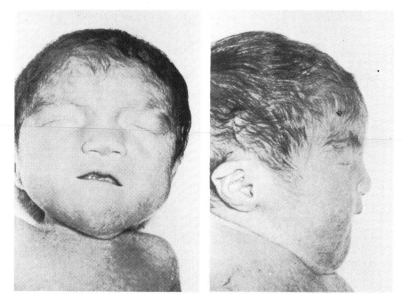

FIG. 5. A necropsy picture of a 5-day-old American Indian girl. Note the short palpebral fissures, the flat facies, and hirsutism.

throughout the leptomeninges and cerebral mantle, as well as the subependymal regions.

Some of the functional and structural abnormalities in this syndrome, such as microcephaly, development delay and fine motor dysfunction may all be secondarily related to the type of malorientation of the brain observed in this patient. Even the joint anomalies could well be related to neurologic impairment of the fetus, including diminished movement in utero, resulting from this type of malorientation of brain structure.

ETIOLOGY

The similarity of the overall pattern of malformation in these children suggests a singular etiology most likely environmentally determined by some as yet unknown effect of the maternal alcoholism. Regarding direct toxicity, the most obvious possibility is ethanol itself. There is good evidence in humans and other animals that ethanol freely crosses the placental barrier. Animal studies have shown it to be distributed in the amniotic fluid and throughout multiple fetal tissues, at least during late gestation. Other direct toxic possibilities include one of the breakdown products of ethanol, such as acetaldehyde, or an unknown toxic agent in the alcoholic beverages which were consumed. Indirect deficiency states include the effect of generalized maternal undernutrition or deficiency of a specific nutrient or vitamin.

OUTCOME OF PREGNANCY IN OFFSPRING OF
CHRONIC ALCOHOLIC WOMEN

All the children evaluated up to the present time with the fetal alcohol syndrome have been ascertained on the basis of their problems in growth and morphogenesis. A study has recently been completed, the purpose of which has been to set forth the incidence and nature of problems of morphogenesis and function in the offspring of a group of women who were ascertained purely by the history of chronic alcohoism (Jones et al., 1974). The total sample of 23 was drawn from the Collaborative Perinatal Project of the National Institute of Neurologic Disease and Stroke. This has been a prospective study of 55,000 pregnant women and their offspring, followed up to seven years postnatally in 12 medical centers. Two non-alcoholic control women were matched for socioeconomic group, maternal education, race, maternal age, parity, marital status, and instution where the mother and child were followed. The results of this study suggest the overwhelming magnitude of the handicapping problems that maternal alcoholism can impose on the developing fetus. Four of the 23 offspring of women who drank heavily prior to and during pregnancy died prior to one week of age, a perinatal mortality of 17%, as opposed to 2% for the control group.

The most frequent problem noted in the surviving children of women who drank prior to and during pregnancy was deficient intellectual performance at 7 years of age, manifested by an I.Q. of 79 or below, occurring in 44% of the children, as opposed to 9% of their matched controls. With respect to prenatal growth deficiency, a greater percent of infants born to alcoholic mothers were below the third percentile for head circumference, length, and weight than their matched controls. In addition, there were structural anomalies such as short palpebral fissures, ptosis and strabismus, as well as joint anomalies and cardiac murmurs. All occurred more frequently in infants born to alcoholic mothers than controls.

Relative to the incidence of the Fetal Alcohol Syndrome, 6 of the 19 surviving children born to chronically alcoholic women (32%) had enough abnormal features to suggest the possibility of the Fetal Alcohol Syndrome from the physical findings alone, whereas not one of the matched controls was so affected.

The frequency of the adverse outcome of pregnancy for chronically alcoholic women from this study was 43%: 4 who died in the newborn period and 6 with the Fetal Alcohol Syndrome, as opposed to 2 percent of their matched controls. Because of the magnitude of this risk, it is recommended that serious consideration be given toward early termination of pregnancy in severe, chronically alcoholic women.

Conclusion

Further studies are now clearly indicated, relative to the amount and duration of maternal alcoholism necessary to result in offspring with the Fetal Alcohol Syndrome. In addition, the total spectrum of the disorder needs to be more completely delineated. Finally, more basic studies must be performed relative to the specific cause and possible prevention of this tragic disorder.

SUMMARY

An association between chronic maternal alcoholism and a unique pattern of malformation in the offspring, referred to as the fetal alcohol syndrome, has recently been documented. The principal features of the disorder are prenatal onset growth deficiency, microcephaly, developmental delay, short palpebral fissures, cardiac defects, and joint anomalies.

The frequency of adverse outcome in the offspring of chronic alcoholic women is sufficiently high (43%) to merit serious consideration of pregnancy termination in such women.

Notes

Requests for reprints should be addressed to Kenneth Lyons Jones, Department of Pediatrics, University Hospital, 225 West Dickinson, San Diego, Calif. 92103.

References

Ferrier, P.E., Nicod, I., and Ferrier, S. Fetal alcohol syndrome. *Lancet* 2:1496, December, 1973

Haggard, H.W., and Jellinek, E.M. *Alcohol Explored.* Garden City, New York: Doubleday, Doran and Company, Inc., 1942

Hall, B.D., and Orenstein, W.A. Noonan's phenotype in an offspring of an alcoholic mother. *Lancet* 1:680, April, 1974

Jones, K.L., Smith, D.W., Streissguth, A.P., and Myrianthopoulos, N.C. Outcome in offspring of chronic alcoholic women. *Lancet* I:1,076-1,078, June, 1974

Jones, K.L., and Smith, D.W. Recognition of the fetal alcohol syndrome in early infancy. *Lancet* 1:999-1001, November, 1973

Jones, K.L., Smith, D.W., Ulleland, C.N., and Streissguth, A.P. Pattern of malformation in offspring of chronic alcoholic mothers. *Lancet* 1:1267-1271, June 1973

Palmer, R.H., Ouellette, E.M., Warner, L., and Leichtman, S.R. Congenital malformations in offspring of a chronic alcoholic mother. *Pediatrics* V:53:490-494, April, 1974

Report on Evidence of Drunkenness presented to the House of Commons by the Select Committee, 1834

Sandor, S. The influence of aethyl-alcohol on the development of the chick embryo. *Rev. roum. Embryol. Cytol. Ser Embryol.* 1, 5, 51-76, 1968

Sandor, S. The influence of aethyl-alcohol on the developing chick embryo. II ibid, 167-171

Sandor, S., and Amels, D. The action of aethanol on the praenatal development of albino rats. *Rev. roum. Embryol. Cytol. Ser Embryol.* 8:105-118, 1971

Sullivan, W.C. The children of the female drunkard. *Med. Temp. Rev.*, 3:72-79, 1900

DISCUSSION

Q. *Dr. Connaughton*: As an obstetrician, we give alcohol, as you know, to a lot of women who are pregnant. We give alcohol intravenously to women who are in premature labor; and sometimes we start it as early as 32 weeks and they will have three or four courses of IV alcohol and then they will be told to drink up to a pint or more of alcohol a day. Have you had any experience with these women and their babies?

A. *Dr. Jones*: No. I would just like to stress right now that the Fetal Alcohol Syndrome, to the extent that the children we have seen with this disorder, has occurred only in women who are very severe, chronically alcoholic women. Of the initial eight that we evaluated, five had delirium tremens; two of them had cirrhosis of the liver, and so on. These are severe chronic alcoholics, and severe chronic alcoholics who drink throughout the pregnancy. The malformations that we have seen in this disorder indicate that a problem in development was occurring early in pregnancy. As far as what happens after 32 weeks, the only study that I am aware of, looking in any way at the offspring of women who have been on alcohol drips to suppress labor, was a study in which bone marrow studies were done, up to two or three months of age in the offspring of women who have been on heavy alcohol drips. This was done because in chronic alcoholic adults there are large cytoplasmic inclusions that are present in the bone marrow after an alcoholic binge, which usually disappears after two to three weeks. They looked for the cytoplasmic inclusions in the offspring of women who were on alcohol drips and, after two or three months of doing bone marrow studies in these children, they still had cytoplasmic inclusions in their bone marrow. The implication is that alcohol certainly is getting distributed throughout multiple fetal tissues at this stage of gestation, but I am relatively sure that it is not leading to the Fetal Alcohol Syndrome. What it is doing as far as future development is concerned, I really cannot say.

Q. *Dr. Roloff*: You have described an important sign to recognize in the so-called short palpebral fissures. From your slides, I wondered whether you have standardized this, because I was of the impression that maybe it was an increased intercanthral distance rather than short palprebral fissures.

A. *Dr. Jones*: In fact, the intercanthral distance in these babies is completely normal, and it looks like there is an increased intercanthral distance because the palprebral fissures are short. The palprebral fissures in normal newborns vary between 1.8 cm and about 2.1 cm. Among the babies whose pictures I showed you, the palprebral fissure size was approximately 1.3 cm. This is a great difference in terms of palpebral fissure size.

Q. *Dr. Grover*: I think you have evidence that alcohol is having some effects on fetal brain development as demonstrated by your pictures of the brain with "holes" through it and convolutions filled with cells. Physicochemical studies with ethanol and a lot of other alcohols have demonstrated changes in membrane conformation. If you have some kind of probe in the membrane, you can measure membrane structure changes when you add ethanol to these membranes. What happens is that you get changes in the membrane conformation and fluidization of the membrane; and what this does many times is to change the permeability to a lot of different ions and that could be a generalized effect on many organ systems.

A. *Dr. Jones*: That is fascinating, thank you.

Addictive Diseases: an International Journal 2 (1): 89-99 (1975)

Heat-Stable Alkaline Phosphatase in Methadone-Maintained Pregnancies

RITA G. HARPER
Departments of Pediatrics and
Obstetrics and Gynecology
Cornell University Medical College
North Shore University Hospital
Manhasset, New York

ELLEN FEINGOLD
Department of Obstetrics and Gynecology
State University of New York
Downstate Medical Center
Brooklyn, N.Y.

GEORGE SOLISH
Department of Obstetrics and Gynecology
State University of New York,
Downstate Medical Center
Brooklyn, N.Y.

MYRON SOKAL
Department of Pediatrics
Cornell University Medical College
North Shore University Hospital
Manhasset, N.Y.

INTRODUCTION

Review of the addiction literature reveals that the effects of methadone and heroin during pregnancy have been studied primarily in relation to clinical parameters, i.e., withdrawal, jaundice, birth weight, respiratory distress, etc. (Harper et al., 1974; Reddy et al., 1971; Rajegowda et al., 1972; Zelson et al., 1971; Nathenson et al., 1972; and Glass et al., 1971). More subtle studies of placental integrity under the influence of heroin or methadone and independent of fetal outcome have not yet been reported.

One enzyme, placental heat-stable alkaline phosphatase (HSAP), has been reported to be of value as an indicator of placental function (Quigley et al., 1970; Hunter et al., 1970; and Curzon et al., 1968). This enzyme, HSAP, is

89

produced primarily by the syncytiotrophoblastic layer of the placenta (Wislocki et al., 1946; Boyer, 1961; and Beck et al., 1950). It is elevated in maternal serum in normal pregnancy in progressively increasing amounts and falls after delivery (Quigley et al., 1970; Hunter et al., 1970; Curzon et al., 1968; and McMaster et al., 1964). The enzyme is heat stable (Neale et al., 1965 and Kaplan, 1972). The physiological function has not yet been determined for placental, or indeed, any other alkaline phosphatase. Attempts have been made to correlate HSAP with toxemic pregnancies (Bagga et al., 1969 and Benster, 1970), fetal demise (Hunter, 1969), and placental damage (Hunter, 1969).

Since rising values might reflect subtle placental damage, we elected to study this enzyme in methadone-maintained addicts throughout pregnancy.

STUDY GROUP

At State University of New York, Downstate Medical Center, a Family and Maternity Care Program for pregnant addicts and their spouses has been in operation since 1971 (Harper et al., 1974 and Kissen et al., 1973). From this large addicted population, we selected thirty pregnant methadone-maintained addicts and sequentially monitored their HSAP levels throughout pregnancy along with the HSAP levels of matched non-addicted pregnant controls.

The pregnant addicts were selected on the basis of their being:

1. historically known addicts, currently methadone-maintained or drug-free in the Family and Maternity Care Program;
2. pregnant; and
3. willing to have their blood drawn every two weeks and their urines monitored for drugs of abuse frequently during the pregnancy. Women were not included in the study group if they had known concurrent medical problems, i.e., diabetes.

The data from women who developed obstetric complications, i.e., preeclampsia, or who had less than three successive HSAP determinations prior to delivery, were deleted at the end of the study.

Controls were selected from the General Obstetric Clinic of State University of New York, Downstate Medical Center. The controls were selected on the basis of their being:

1. historically known non-addicts;
2. pregnant; and
3. willing to have their blood drawn every two weeks and their urines monitored for drugs of abuse frequently during pregnancy. Exclusions were made on the same basis as for addicted participants.

METHADONE-MAINTAINED PATIENTS

During the first seven months of the study, seventeen methadone-maintained patients were delivered. Two methadone-maintained patients, however, developed preeclampsia, and three had less than three sequential determinations for HSAP. The data from these five patients were deleted, leaving data from twelve methadone-maintained patients. One of the included methadone-maintained patients became drug-free by the thirtieth week of pregnancy. This drug-free patient was added to the drug-free group. There then were eleven methadone-maintained patients who had delivered within the time period who had three or more sequential determinations.

The methadone-maintained women ranged from twenty to thirty years of age. Seven were white; four were black. All had a previous history of opiate addiction ranging from two to seven years. Parity ranged from nullipara to para five. All except two had been started on methadone maintenance in our Family and Maternity Care Program prior to the twentieth week of pregnancy; the two who were not in our program by the twentieth week of pregnancy had been on street methadone and were on methadone administered by the program by the thirtieth week. The starting methadone dose ranged from 20 mg/day to 90 mg/day (Table I). A clinical attempt was made to detoxify all patients during their pregnancy without regard to the research protocol.

The urinary drug screen for morphine-quinine, barbiturates, cocaine, amphetamine, and methaqualone revealed that the urines of two methadone-maintained addicted patients exhibited drugs of abuse once, two patients twice, and one patient three times in two hundred eighty-two urines examined (Table II).

DRUG-FREE

Three historically addicted and currently drug-free patients delivered during the study period. One, however, was not included because of insufficient HSAP determinations. The two remaining women were both white. One was twenty-one years of age, the other thirty-one years of age. Both were para one (Table III).

The urine of the two drug-free patients was screened seventy-nine times for drugs of abuse (Table II). One woman's urine showed methadone until she completed detoxification at the thirtieth week of pregnancy; her urine was completely negative for drugs thereafter. The other woman had detoxified prior to conception and her urine was drug-free through all of pregnancy.

CONTROL PATIENTS

Five controls delivered within the study period. The control group ranged from twenty-one to thirty-five years of age. Three were black and two were

TABLE I
Age, Race and Drug History of 11 Methadone-Maintained Patients

	AGE	RACE	DRUG Hx	START METH MAINT (WKS GEST)	STARTING DOSE (mg/24 hr.)	DOSE AT DELIVERY (mg/24 hr.)
METHADONE-MAINTAINED PATIENTS						
LB	25	W	heroin - 4 yrs	<20	90	30
			amphet, meth			
			x 1 yr			
LH	28	W	heroin - 3 yrs	<20	60	15
SB	28	W	heroin - 6 yrs	<20	20	5
SC	30	W	heroin - 7 yrs	<20	50	10
			meth x 4 yrs			
MP	30	B	heroin - 5 yrs	<20	70	30
			meth x 2 yrs			
TA	23	B	heroin - 3 yrs	<20	40	40
			meth x 2 yrs			
TH	23	B	heroin - 5 yrs	<20	90	60
			Quaalude, meth,			
			cocaine x 6 mos			
AM	20	W	heroin - 3 yrs	<20	25	15
			meth x 1 yr			
CP	25	B	heroin - 3 yrs	<20	80	45
			meth x 2 yrs			
CN	21	W	heroin - 2 yrs	str meth*	30	30
			meth x 1 yr	28		
EC	24	W	heroin - 5 yrs	str meth*	30	40
				30		

*str meth = street methadone

white. Parity ranged from nullipara to para four. None had a history of drug addiction (Table III).

Sixty-two urines analyzed were completely negative for drugs of abuse throughout the pregnancy (Table II).

METHOD

Blood was obtained from the subjects by venipuncture, and samples were centrifuged immediately after drawing and the serum was incubated at 56°C for one hour in a water bath. After cooling, the HSAP level was determined by Hansen's modification of the method of Kind and King (Hansen, 1966).

TABLE II
Urine Drug Screen

	# OF URINES SCREENED	POSITIVE URINES
METHADONE-MAINTAINED PATIENTS		
LB	37	Amphet x 1
LH	10	None
SB	27	Morphine-Quinine x 2 Doriden x 1
SC	47	None
MP	31	Amphet x 1 Morphine-Quinine x 1
TA	25	Barbit x 1
TH	30	Barbit x 2
AM	36	None
CP	9	None
CN	18	None
EC	12	None
TOTAL	282	
DRUG-FREE PATIENTS		
AG	66	None
EF	13	None
TOTAL	79	
CONTROL PATIENTS		
SM	13	None
YT	12	None
NZ	13	None
MF	10	None
PK	14	None
TOTAL	62	

RESULTS

The mean level of HSAP rose gradually through pregnancy in normal control patients and showed a wide range of levels (Figure 1). Our mean level agreed closely with the previous published reports of Quigley et al. (1970) and Hunter et al. (1970). The mean level of HSAP of the drug-free patients was similar to that of the controls (Figure 2).

The mean level of HSAP rose gradually throughout pregnancy in methadone-maintained women. Although the mean HSAP level of the methadone-

TABLE III

Age, Race and Drug History of 2 Drug-Free Patients and 5 Controls

	AGE	RACE	DRUG Hx	START METH MAINT (WKS GEST)	STARTING DOSE (mg/24 hr)	DOSE AT DELIVERY (mg/24 hr)
DRUG-FREE PATIENTS						
AG	21	W	heroin - 3 yrs	20	30	0
			meth x 2 yrs			
EF	31	W	heroin - 11 yrs	0	0	0
			meth x 3 yrs			
CONTROL PATIENTS						
SM	35	W	None	0	0	0
YT	25	B	None	0	0	0
NZ	21	W	None	0	0	0
MF	35	B	None	0	0	0
PK	30	B	None	0	0	0

maintained patients was above the level of the controls at all weeks of gestation, this level was not statistically significant (Figure 3).

However, if the methadone patients were divided into two groups: (1) those who received greater than 60 mg/day of methadone at twenty weeks of gestation, and (2) those who received 60 mg/day or less at twenty weeks of gestation, 81% of the determinations exceeded the normal control standard deviation for those receiving the higher dose, while only 20% of those receiving the lower dose exceeded the normal control standard deviation (Figure 4).

No correlation of HSAP was found with birth weight, placental weight, Apgar scores, and length of time on heroin.

The mean cord blood level in the controls was 2.2 King Armstrong units. That of the infants born to methadone-maintained mothers was 2.6 King Armstrong units.

The decay curves post partum of normal controls, drug-free, and methadone-maintained mothers showed no difference (Figure 5).

Comments

Heat-stable alkaline phosphatase rises progressively throughout pregnancy in the serum of methadone-maintained pregnant patients in a manner similar to normal controls and to drug-free patients who once were addicted.

Those patients who started with greater than 60 mg of methadone/day appear to have an increased incidence of elevated HSAP levels. These higher levels

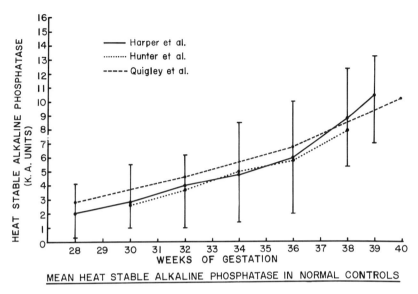

MEAN HEAT STABLE ALKALINE PHOSPHATASE IN NORMAL CONTROLS

FIG. 1

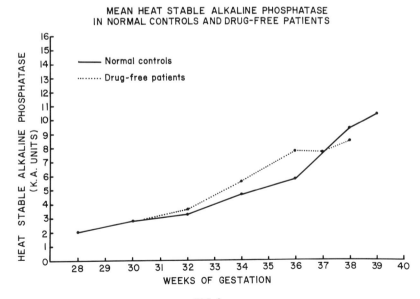

FIG. 2

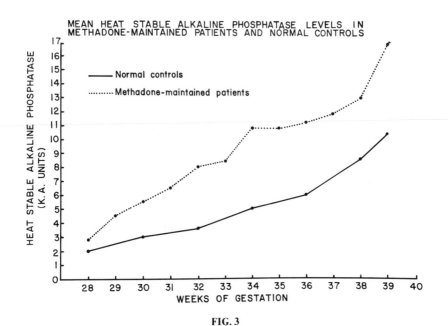

FIG. 3

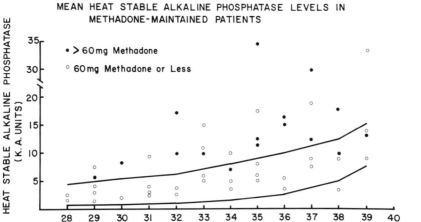

FIG. 4

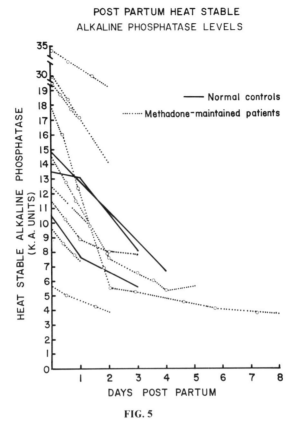

POST PARTUM HEAT STABLE
ALKALINE PHOSPHATASE LEVELS

—— Normal controls

········· Methadone-maintained patients

FIG. 5

suggest that methadone may affect the maternal-placental-fetal unit in more subtle ways than have previously been considered.

Heat-stable alkaline phosphatase cannot be used as a marker to differentiate those pregnancies which are methadone-maintained from those which are drug-free.

There was no correlation between the HSAP level and fetal outcome. This is not surprising, since even massive placental damage does not always result in fetal damage or demise.

The similar decay curves of HSAP post partum indicate that both methadone-maintained women and normal controls metabolize HSAP at the same rate.

At present, studies of placental function are continuing in our laboratory which may further elucidate subtle changes in methadone-maintained pregnancies.

SUMMARY

Heat-stable alkaline phosphatase (HSAP) levels were serially determined in eleven methadone-maintained patients, two drug-free patients, and five normal controls. The mean level of HSAP rose progressively in all three groups. The HSAP levels from patients who were maintained on greater than 60 mg of methadone/day at the beginning of the study exceeded the standard deviation of normal controls in 81% of the determinations. Only 20% of the determinations for HSAP of those maintained on 60 mg of methadone/day or less exceeded the standard deviation of normal controls. These higher levels of HSAP in women receiving higher doses of methadone during pregnancy suggest that methadone during pregnancy may affect the maternal-placental-fetal unit in more subtle ways than has previously been considered.

Notes

Requests for reprints should be addressed to Rita G. Harper, North Shore University Hospital, 300 Community Drive, Manhasset, New York 11030.

References

Bagga, O.P., Mullick, V.D., Madan, P., and Dewan, S. Total serum alkaline phosphatase and its isoenzymes in normal and toxemic pregnancies. *American Journal of Obstetrics and Gynecology*, 1969, *104*. 850-855.

Beck, E., and Clark, L.C. Plasma alkaline phosphatase. *American Journal of Obstetrics and Gynecology*, 1950, *60*. 731-740.

Benster, B. Serum heat-stable alkaline phosphatase in pregnancy complicated by hypertension. *The Journal of Obstetrics and Gynaecology of the British Commonwealth*, 1970, *77*. 990-993.

Boyer, S.H. Alkaline phosphatase in human sera and placentae. *Science*, 1961, *134*. 1002-1004.

Curzen, P., and Morris, I. Heat stable alkaline phosphatase in maternal serum. *The Journal of Obstetrics and Gynaecology of the British Commonwealth*, 1968, *75*. 151-157.

Glass, L., Rajegowda, B.K., and Evans, H.E. Absence of respiratory distress syndrome in premature infants of heroin-addicted mothers. *Lancet*, 1971, *2*. 685-686.

Hansen, P.W. A simplification of Kind and King's method for determination of serum phosphatase. *Scandinavian Journal of Clinical and Laboratory Investigation*, 1966, *18*. 353-356.

Harper, R.G., Solish, G.I., Purow, H.M., Sang, E., and Panepinto, W.C. The effect of a methadone treatment program upon pregnant heroin addicts and their newborn infants. *Pediatrics*, 1974, *54*. 300-305.

Hunter, P.J., Pinkerton, J.H.M., and Johnston, H. Serum placental alkaline phosphatase in normal pregnancy and preeclampsia. *Obstetrics and Gynecology*, 1970. *36*. 536-546.

Hunter, R.J. Serum heat stable alkaline phosphatase: An index of placental function. *The Journal of Obstetrics and Gynaecology of the British Commonwealth*, 1969, *76*. 1057-1069.

Kaplan, M.M. Alkaline phosphatase. *The New England Journal of Medicine*, 1972, *286*. 200-202.

Kissin, B., and Sang, E. Treatment of heroin addiction. *New York State Journal of Medicine*, 1973, *73*. 1059-1065.

McMaster, Y., Tennant, R., Clubb, J.S., Neale, F.C., and Posen, S. The mechanism of the elevation of serum alkaline phosphatase in pregnancy. *The Journal of Obstetrics and Gynaecology of the British Commonwealth*, 1964, *71*. 735-739.

Nathenson, G., Cohen, M.I., Litt, I.F., and McNamara, H. The effect of maternal heroin addiction on neonatal jaundice. *The Journal of Pediatrics*, 1972, *81*. 899-903.

Neale, F.C., Clubb, J.S., Hotchkis, D., and Posen, S. Heat stability of human placental alkaline phosphatase. *The Journal of Clinical Pathology*, 1965, *18*. 359-363.

Quigley, G.J., Richards, R.T., and Shier, K.J. Heat-stable alkaline phosphatase. *American Journal of Obstetrics and Gynecology*, 1970, *106*. 340-351.

Rajegowda, B.K., Glass, L., Evans, H.E., Maso, G., Swartz, D.P., and Leblanc, W. *The Journal of Pediatrics*, 1972, *81*. 532-534.

Reddy, A.M., Harper, R.G., and Stern, G. Observations on heroin and methadone withdrawal in the newborn. *Pediatrics*, 1971, *48*. 353-358.

Wislocki, G.B., and Dempsey, E.W. Histochemical age-changes in normal and pathological placental villi. *Endocrinology*, 1946, *38*. 90-109.

Zelson, C., Rubio, E., and Wasserman, E. Neonatal narcotic addiction: 10 year observation. *Pediatrics*, 1971, *48*. 178-188.

DISCUSSION

Q. *Dr. Glass*: Regarding the amniocentesis on the methadone women, did you have the opportunity to do L/S ratios on the amniotic fluid, systematically?

A.*Dr. Harper:* Yes, but we do not have the results of this.

Q. *Dr. Glass*: Do you find any statistical difference between them?

A. *Dr. Harper: No, I did not say that: we do not have the results at this time. We did notice that the quantity of heat-stable alkaline phosphatase in the amniotic fluid was directly dependent upon whether or not the baby was in any sort of difficulty, and if the baby passed meconium. The level of heat-stable alkaline phosphatase was considerably higher than in those babies where the amniotic fluid was clear.*

Q. *Dr. Glass*: What I am considering is the possible maturational effect of methadone on amniotic fluid phospholipids.

A. *Dr. Harper: We are in the process of putting together a series of reports of infants who have been maintained on methadone throughout their pregnancy, and who, in fact, did develop respiratory distress syndrome, but we do not have the results at this time.*

Addictive Diseases: an International Journal 2 (1): 101-112 (1975)
© 1975 by Spectrum Publications, Inc.

Clinical Observations on Metha-done-Maintained Pregnancies

ROY C. DAVIS
Medical-Psychiatric Department
Illinois Drug Abuse Programs
Chicago, Illinois

JOHN N. CHAPPEL
Department of Psychiatry

ALFONSO MEJIA-ZELAYA
Department of Obstetrics and Gynecology

JOHN MADDEN
Department of Pediatrics
University of Chicago
Pritzker School of Medicine
Chicago, Illinois

INTRODUCTION

Prior to the widespread use of methadone maintenance as a treatment adjunct, few alternatives were available for the treatment of pregnant narcotic addicts. Attempts to provide standard prenatal care without specific treatment for the addiction have met with a high incidence of loss from treatment, both obstetrical and medical complications as well as poor maternal and neonatal follow-up (Stone et al., 1971; Krause et al., 1958; Stern, 1966). High rates of prematurity, low-birthweight infants and neonatal deaths were often reported (Cobrink and Hood, 1959; Goodfriend et al., 1956). Several recent studies (Nichtern, 1973; Wilson et al., 1973) have shown that infants of mothers whose addiction has gone untreated are at high risk for developmental and behavioral disorders. Experience with hospitalization and rapid medical detoxification has resulted in loss from treatment and a return to the use of illicit drugs before delivery for over 66% of the pregnant addicts treated in this manner (Blinick et al., 1969; Davis and Chappel, 1973).

Reports on methadone-maintained pregnancies reveal a decreased incidence of prematurity and low-birthweight infants, fewer medical and obstetrical complications as well as significantly improved treatment retention rates (Davis and Chappel, 1973; Statzer and Wardell, 1972; Davis, R., et al., 1974; Blinick et al., 1973). Drug abuse treatment facilities providing intensive psychosocial support have reported reduced incidence of illicit drug use, increased ability to achieve abstinence by delivery and a higher rate of stable, intact families who are providing good care for their newborns (Davis, R., et al., 1974; Sang et al., 1973; Rothstein and Gould, 1974). Infants with intrauterine exposure to methadone have shown significantly depressed visual orientation and following responses, although mental and psychomotor development has been within normal limits (Ramer and Lodge, 1974).

Complications in methadone-maintained pregnancies include an increase in the frequency, severity and length of treatable neonatal withdrawal syndrome (Davis, R., et al., 1974; Zelson, 1973; Davis, M., et al., 1973), continued use of illicit narcotics in programs where adequate psychosocial supports are not available (Statzer and Wardell, 1972), and frequent abuse of hypnotics and sedatives, especially alcohol (Davis, R. et al., 1974; Ramer and Lodge, 1974; Davis, M., et al., 1973). Prejudicial and irrational staff attitudes toward the methadone-maintained mother have also been noted to interfere with effective treatment (Distasio and Nesbitt, 1974).

In contrast to earlier reports (Wallach et al., 1969), there is a growing body of literature indicating a positive correlation between maternal methadone dose and the incidence and severity of the neonatal narcotic withdrawal syndrome (Davis, R., et al., 1974; Davis, M., et al., 1973). Although a wide range of dosage regimes and withdrawal techniques are being practiced, most programs now make concerted efforts to reduce dosages by delivery. One exception to this is the Methadone Maintenance Treatment Program in New York which maintains its pregnant patients on doses of 80-120 mg on the rationale that high doses deter continued illicit narcotics use (Newman, 1973). Also in New York, the Kings County Addictive Diseases Hospital, using a low-dose to abstinence regime in a comprehensive maternity and family care unit, reports increased treatment retention and rehabilitation rates complicated by a 20% incidence of perinatal mortality (Sang et al., 1973). Mondanaro and her colleagues (1974) in San Francisco, increase the patients' dose from 20 to 50 or 60 mg to eliminate drug hunger. Psychosocial support is initiated and then dosages are gradually reduced to 30-40 mg by delivery. Programs in both Chicago (Davis, R., et al., 1974) and Boston (Rothstein and Gould, 1974) recommend that patients be maintained on the lowest possible dose that will suppress withdrawal symptoms and not have the mother substituting other dangerous drugs. Dose reduction in the third trimester has been associated with intrauterine fetal withdrawal (Zuspan et al., 1974) and fatal meconium aspiration (Rementeria and Nunag, 1973; Madden and Chappel, 1974). Several investigators have also stressed the importance of individual and community variables such as the availability and quality of street drugs, the patient's age, living circumstances, history of addiction and quality of interpersonal and medical resources as indicators in determining dosage levels and treatment goals (Davis, R., et al., 1974; Sang et al., 1973; Rothstein and Gould, 1974).

This paper reports on 218 pregnancies followed by the Illinois Drug Abuse Programs (I.D.A.P.) from January 1969 to March 1974. The I.D.A.P. is multimodality and community-based, offering residential and outpatient units which use both methadone and abstinence approaches.

CLINICAL PROCEDURES

All patients were accepted without screening, if evidence of narcotic addiction was present. Each had available the full range of treatment modalities offered by the I.D.A.P. All patients were subject to urine monitoring and screening for illicit drug use three times weekly. Methadone was utilized in the lowest doses necessary to suppress withdrawal symptoms in either the pregnant women or the developing fetus. The women were encouraged to tolerate slight discomfort if necessary while doses were adequately stabilized. Gradual withdrawal was available upon request and in consultation with the patient's obstetrician. The women were treated in one of four groups based on the treatment available at the time and on the woman's preference.

Group I   *General Methadone Maintenance* (N = 41)
These women received regular treatment, including methadone, in clinics of the I.D.A.P. No other intervention was made, either because it was not available during the early years of the program or because additional help was refused. Having had little or no prenatal care, patients in this group tended to enter treatment for addiction in the late second or third trimester.

Group II   *I.D.A.P. Psychosocial Support* (N = 48)
This group was formed in response to poor results obtained during our early experience with Group I. In addition to normal addiction treatment services these women received: 1) regular weekly individual or marital counseling focused on the conflicts and problems of pregnancy; 2) prenatal classes and groups at the I.D.A.P.; 3) liaison with medical, legal and welfare agencies on behalf of the woman.

Group III   *Interagency Psychosocial Support* (N = 96)*
These women received interagency care provided by staff of the I.D.A.P.

---

* Data on this group were reported at the National Conference on Drug Abuse, March, 1974, Chicago, Illinois.

Table I
Demographic Characteristics

	Group I (N=41)	Group II (N=48)	Group III (N=96)	Group IV (N=33)
Average Age	27.2	27.0	25.0	24.7
Average Gravidity	4.0	4.4	4.1	3.3
Average Parity	1.9	2.5	2.2	2.3
Average Years of Heroin Use	5.9	6.7	4.2	3.9
MARITAL STATUS				
Single	2 (4.9%)	6 (12.5%)	11 (11.5%)	9 (27.3%)
Married	17 (41.5%)	13 (27.1%)	27 (28.1%)	4 (12.1%)
Common-law	13 (31.7%)	19 (39.5%)	39 (40.6%)	12 (36.4%)
Separated	5 (12.2%)	6 (12.5%)	19 (19.8%)	6 (18.2%)
Divorced	1 (2.4%)	2 (4.2%)	0	1 (3.0%)
Widowed	0	1 (2.1%)	0	0
Unknown	3*(7.3%)	1*(2.1%)	0	1*(3.0%)
RACE				
Caucasian	9 (22.0%)	4 (8.3%)	12 (12.5%)	4 (12.2%)
Negro	18 (44.0%)	42 (87.5%)	78 (81.3%)	29 (87.8%)
Hispanic	7 (17.0%)	2 (4.2%)	5 (5.2%)	0
Other	0	0	1 (1.0%)	0
Unknown	7*(17.0%)	0	0	0

* Interviewers failed to record data.

and the University of Chicago Hospitals. A team of physicians, nurses, social workers, addiction counselors, a nutritionist and a psychologist ran a weekly prenatal clinic for women from all I.D.A.P. clinics. A 24-hour paging service and transportation to the hospitals and clinics were available. Treatment teamwork was characterized by frequent, ongoing coordinated contact between specialized I.D.A.P. staff and the obstetric, pediatric and social service staff of the University of Chicago.

Group IV   *Heroin Deliveries* (N = 33)
This group of patients received no treatment for their heroin addiction prior to delivery. They do not, however, compose a typical street group

since 12 of the 33 were hospitalized prior to delivery while participating in a research project in another Chicago area hospital.

None of these groups was controlled for such critical factors as secondary drug use or addictions during pregnancy or prior to entry into treatment.

FINDINGS

The I.D.A.P. has treated approximately 12,200 addicts in the past six years. Of these, 2,856 (23.4%) were females, the majority of whom were of child-bearing age. Through March of 1974, 223 (7.8%) either entered methadone treatment while pregnant or conceived while receiving methadone. Table I de-lineates some of the demographic characteristics of the population reported on in this paper.

In the last two years the average age of the pregnant patients treated in the I.D.A.P. (i.e., Group III) has dropped from 26.9 to 25.0 years, while the frequency with which women have conceived on methadone has increased by 24.9% over the previous four years.

Table II shows the pregnancy results according to treatment group. Group I had a noticeably higher rate of fetal wastage and perinatal mortality than did Groups II, III and IV. Group IV had a considerably higher incidence of low-birthweight infants than did the methadone-treated groups and shows an average birthweight of less than 2,500 grams. The incidence of congenital ano-malies among all the groups was no greater than in the general population.

Of the 185 methadone-treated pregnancies in Groups I, II, and III, the two groups receiving psychosocial support had substantially higher treatment reten-tion rates at the time of delivery. Group I retained only 27 (68.5%) women in treatment at delivery, while Group II retained 48 (100.0%) and Group III re-tained 90 (93.9%).

The pregnancy results for the patients in Group III were analyzed accord-ing to length of fetal exposure to methadone. Forty-nine women conceived while in methadone treatment while 9 entered treatment in the first trimester, and 21 and 16 entered in the second and third trimester of pregnancy respectively. The relative effects of length of exposure to methadone are shown in Table III.

There was no pronounced relationship found in regard to trimester of entry into treatment and average birthweight or incidence of low-birthweight infants. There was, however, a higher incidence of fetal loss and perinatal mortality among women who did not conceive on methadone. The difference is particu-larly noticeable between the group that conceived on methadone and those that entered treatment in the third trimester. The proportion of infants who required treatment for withdrawal was approximately 9 to 10% higher among women who were not in treatment at conception. The average length of treatment was reduced for infants whose mothers entered treatment in their third trimester.

Of the 90 women who were in treatment at delivery in Group III, 5 were

TABLE II
Pregnancy Outcome

	Group I (N=41)	Group II (N=48)	Group III (N=96)	Group IV (N=33)
Viable				
Infants	16	41	81	30
Twins	0	0	1 set	1 set
Spontaneous				
Abortions	7	1	3	0
Perinatal				
Mortalities	6	5	7	2
Fetal Deaths	0 (31.7%)	1 (12.5%)	2 (one due to trauma) (13.0%)	0 (6.7%)
Results Unknown	12*	0	4	1
Average				
Birthweight	2594 gms.	2783 gms.	2707 gms.	2473 gms.
Low-birthweight				
Infants	6 (22.7%)	13 (29.5%)	21 (23.5%)	15 (45.5%)
	(Birthweight unknown in 15 cases)	(Birthweight unknown in 2 cases)	(Birthweight unknown in 5 cases)	(Birthweight unknown in 1 case)

*The high incidence of unknown results is related to the high rate
of loss from treatment in Group I.

abstinent, 18 were on less than 20 mg of methadone, while 335 were on 21-40 mg
and 32 were on more than 40 mg. The average dose at delivery was 35.7 mg.
Table IV presents the pregnancy results and infant morbidity rates analyzed according to the maternal dose of methadone at delivery.

Eighty-two of the infants born to the 90 women in Group III were exposed
to the possibility of chemotherapeutic treatment for withdrawal. Forty-four
(53.7%) required treatment. The incidence of infants requiring treatment increased as the maternal methadone dose increased. There are emphatic differences between the low and moderate dose groups and between the low and
high dose groups.

Twenty-four (13.0%) of the women in all three of the treatment groups were
clinically observed to have been abusing central nervous system depressants,

TABLE III
Pregnancy Results and Infant Morbidity Relative to Length of Exposure to
Methadone

	Conceived on Methadone (N=49)[*]	Entered Treatment at <26 Weeks Gestation (N=30)	Entered Treatment at >25 Weeks Gestation (N=16)
Viable Infants	45	24	11
Twins	1 set	0	0
Spontaneous Abortions	1 ⎫	2 ⎫	0 ⎫
Stillborns	1 ⎬(6.2%)	0 ⎬(14.2%)	1 ⎬(26.7%)
Neonatal Deaths	1 ⎭	2 ⎭	3 ⎭
Results Unknown	1	2	1
Infants Treated for Withdrawal	22 (45.8%)	15 (57.7%)	8 (57.1%)
Average Length of Infant Treatment	13.9 days	13.9 days	8.1 days

[*]One woman achieved abstinence just prior to conception and thus is not included in these statistics.

most commonly alcohol and barbiturates, while receiving methadone treatment. The incidence of fetal wastage and perinatal loss observed in this group was 41.7% as compared to a 12.3% loss rate in methadone-treated pregnancies not obviously complicated by C.N.S. depressant abuse.

DISCUSSION AND SUGGESTED HYPOTHESES

Several hypotheses have been generated by our clinical experience with these patients. This review has supported recent reports (Stone et al., 1971; Blinick et al., 1973) that the prevalence of pregnancy in narcotics addiction, particularly among younger women on methadone, is increasing. These findings may represent an increased probability of conception due to the stabilization of life-styles accompanied by heightened desire for family life and/or the action of methadone-influenced metabolic processes. Like much of the other data report-

TABLE IV
Outcome According to Maternal Methadone Dose

	Delivery on 20 mg or Less (N=23)	Delivery on 21-40 mg. (N=35)	Delivery on More than 40 mg. (N=32)
Viable			
Infants	19	32	26
Twins	0	0	0
Spontaneous			
Abortions	1 ⎫	1 ⎫	1 ⎫
Stillborns	0 ⎬ (13.6%)	2 ⎬ (8.5%)	0 ⎬ (13.3%)
Neonatal	⎪	⎪	⎪
Deaths	2 ⎭	0 ⎭	3 ⎭
Results			
Unknown	1	0	2
Low-birthweight			
Infants	6 (28.5%)	6 (17.6%)	7 (24.2%)
Infants Treated			
for Withdrawal	4 (19.0%)	20 (62.5%)	20 (69.0%)
Average Length of			
Infant Treatment	11.7 days	13.6 days	13.7 days

ed in these studies, however, these figures may simply reflect the greater accessibility investigators have to data related to methadone-treated pregnancies as compared to heroin-addicted pregnancies.

Stresses that cause the expectant addict to continue to abuse drugs, avoid prenatal care and drop out of treatment seem to be effectively managed through a program of psychosocial support which includes:

1. Individual and marital counseling by both professionals and paraprofessionals related to the conflicts and problems involved in the methadone-maintained pregnancy;
2. Prenatal classes and groups designed specifically to educate patients and help them work through the issues related to drug use during pregnancy;
3. Frequent collaboration with the staff of the prenatal clinics and hospitals concerning management problems and prejudicial attitudes;
4. Material assistance in the form of financial aid or transportation to and from prenatal clinics and hospitals, etc.

Table II indicates that the incidence of fetal wastage and perinatal loss in methadone-maintained pregnancies is higher among women who do not receive this support as part of their treatment. This suggests the hypothesis that methadone alone does not adequately alter life-styles which adversely affect pregnancy outcome.

The various frequencies of infant morbidity shown in Table IV are consistent with the hypotheses of other investigators (Davis, M., et al., 1973 ; Zelson et al., 1973) that the incidence and severity of treatable neonatal narcotic withdrawal syndrome is positively correlated with the maternal methadone dose.

The higher rate of infant mortality among women who entered treatment in their third trimester (see Table III) and/or complicated their pregnancy through secondary use or addiction to barbiturates or alcohol casts doubts on the conclusions of other investigators (Zelson et al., 1973) who attribute greater toxicity to methadone than to illicit heroin. Studies which control for addiction history, maternal dose of heroin and methadone during pregnancy, date of entry into treatment, and secondary drug use are lacking and therefore preclude such conclusions. An alternative hypothesis might be that active addicts are less able to support large habits in the street in the last trimester and thus that the high rates of infant mortality are related to high doses of heroin and its adulterants, supplemented by methadone and other drugs.

The use of methadone in the treatment of the heroin-addicted pregnancy is an important adjunct in avoiding the high rate of loss from treatment incurred during rapid detoxification and the legal and medical hazards of continued heroin abuse. It warrants the continued attention of both the medical practitioner and researcher.

Notes

Supported in part by the Maternal Child Health Service, Health Services and Mental Health Administration, Grant No. MC-R-170168-02.

Requests for reprints should be addressed to Roy C. Davis, D.Mn., Medical-Psychiatric Department, Illinois Drug Abuse Programs, 1440 South Indiana Avenue, Chicago, Illinois 60605.

The authors gratefully acknowledge the assistance of Dr. Edward C. Senay of the I.D.A.P. and the University of Chicago and Dr. Frederick Zuspan also of the University of Chicago.

References

Blinick, G., Jerez, E., and Wallach, R.C. Methadone maintenance: pregnancy and progeny. *Journal of the American Medical Association*, 1973 *July*, 477-479.

Blinick, G., Wallach, R.C., and Jerez, E. Pregnancy in narcotic addicts treated by medical withdrawal. *American Journal of Obstetrics and Gynecology*, 1969, *December*, 997-1003.

Cobrink, R.W., Hood, T. Jr., and Chusid, E. The effect of maternal narcotic addiction on the newborn infant. *Pediatrics, August*, 288-304.

Davis, R.C., and Chappel, J.N. Pregnancy in the context of addiction and methadone maintenance. *Proceedings of the Fifth National Conference on Methadone Treatment*, 1973, *2*, 1146-1152.

Davis, R.C., Chappel, J.N., Cohn, S., and Mejia-Zelaya, A. An interagency approach in managing pregnant narcotics addicts. *Proceedings of the National Conference on Drug Abuse*, 1974, *1*, (In Press).

Davis, M.M., Brown, B.S., and Glendinning, S.T. Neonatal effects of heroin addiction and methadone treated pregnancies: preliminary report on 70 live births. *Proceedings of the Fifth National Conference on Methadone Treatment*, 1973, *2*, 1153-1164.

Distasio, C.A., and Nesbitt, S.J. Problems of the pregnant/post-partal opioid-dependent patient: perspectives for change. *Proceedings of the National Conference on Drug Abuse*, 1974, *1*, (In Press).

Goodfriend, M.J., Shey, I.A., and Klein, M.D. The effects of maternal narcotic addiction on the newborn. *American Journal of Obstetrics and Gynecology*, 1956, *71*(1), 29-36.

Krause, S.O., Murray, P.M., Holmes, J.B., and Burch, R.E. Heroin addiction among pregnant women and their newborn babies. *American Journal of Obstetrics and Gynecology*, 1958, *75*, 754-758.

Madden, J., and Chappel, J.N. Neonatal mortality associated with maternal methadone withdrawal. *Proceedings of the National Conference on Drug Abuse*, 1974, *1*, (In Press).

Mondanaro, J. Methadone maintenance and slow detoxification in pregnant women. *Proceedings of the National Conference on Drug Abuse*, 1974, *1*, (In Press).

Newman, R. Results of 120 deliveries of patients in the New York City methadone maintenance treatment program. *Proceedings of the Fifth National Conference on Methadone Treatment*, 1973, *2*, 1114-1121.

Nichtern, S. The children of drug users. *Journal of American Academic Child Psychiatry*, 1973, *January*, 24-31.

Ramer, C., and Lodge, A. Neonatal addiction. *Proceedings of the National Conference on Drug Abuse*, 1974, *1*, (In Press).

Rementeria, J.L., and Nunag, N.N. Narcotic withdrawal in pregnancy: stillbirth incidence with a case report. *American Journal of Obstetrics and Gynecology*, 1973, *August*, 1152-1156.

Rothstein, R., and Gould, J. Born with a habit: infants of drug-addicted mothers. *Pediatric Clinics of North America*, 1974, *May*, 307-321.

Sang, E., Panepinto, W.C., and Kissin, B. Low-dose methadone to abstinence in a maternity-family care program. *Proceedings of the Fifth National Conference on Methadone Treatment*, 1973, *2*, 1165-1171.

Statzer, D.E., and Wardell, J.N. Heroin addiction during pregnancy. *American Journal of Obstetrics and Gynecology*, 1972, *May*, 273-278.

Stern, R. The pregnant addict. *American Journal of Obstetrics and Gynecology*, 1966, *January*, 253-257.

Stone, M., Salerno, L., Green, M., and Zelson, C. Narcotic addiction in pregnancy. *American Journal of Obstetrics and Gynecology*, 1971, *March*, 716-723.

Wallach. R.C., Jerez, E., and Blinick, G. Pregnancy and menstrual function in narcotics addicts treated with methadone: the methadone maintenance program. *American Journal of Obstetrics and Gynecology*, 1969, *105*, 1226-1229.

Wilson, G.S., Desmond, M.M., and Verniaud, W.M. Early development of infants of heroin-addicted mothers. *American Journal of Diseases of Children*, 1973, *October*, 457-462.

Zelson, C., Lee, S.J., and Casalino, M. Neonatal narcotic addiction: comparative effects of maternal intake of heroin and methadone. *New England Journal of Medicine*, 1973, *December*, 1216-1220.

Zuspan, F.P., Gumpel, J.A., Mejia-Zelaya, A., Madden, J., and Davis, R. Fetal methadone withdrawal: serial amniotic fluid amine alterations. *Proceedings of the National Conference on Drug Abuse*, 1974, *1*, (In Press).

DISCUSSION

Q. *Dr. Harper:* I may have misunderstood you, but in the beginning I thought you were talking about the addictive disease service of Downstate Medical Center. I think, though, that you have some figures that are not quite true, since this is our group. We, to the best of my knowledge, have never reported a 20 percent mortality in infants whose mothers were maintained on methadone. Quite the opposite, we have a paper coming out this month which shows that in the first 51 of our infants delivered, we had three infants who died, one from cytomegalic-inclusion disease, one from a diaphragmatic hernia, and the other from neonatal meningitis. None of these were really associated with the addiction per se.

A. *Dr. Davis:* The 20% figure reflects the *total* perinatal loss *not just neonatal deaths reported in your study.*

Q. *Dr. Harper:* We do, however, agree with you that the concept of low-dose methadone abstinence in methadone-maintained patients, coupled with massive psychosocial support, can substantially reduce the incidence of obstetrical complications in women during pregnancy. The problems associated with women signing out, the problems associated with no shows in pre-clinic visits, the problems associated with preeclampsia, and things of this nature can be substantially reduced. However, at least in our program, we were unable to show any reduction at all in the incidence of withdrawal in the newborn.

A. *Dr. Davis: Yes, I might say that we have been making efforts to emulate the way that your project works. You have substantially different results than they did, for example, in Detroit, where there was a high rate of postpartum loss from treatment.*

Q. *Dr. Harper:* I think you have to realize that in this program that if four addicts have one counselor, so that it is virtually almost a one-to-one relationship, that the addict is able to call the pediatrician or the obstetrician virtually any time. It is a totally interpersonal relationship.

A. *Dr. Davis: This is facilitated by the geographic proximity of the facilities.*

Q. *Dr. Harper:* It is not that the geographic location is so close, but the telephone is very close. So I would say that the psychosocial support in this group was absolutely massive, and I think that is some of the reason why 80 percent of the people who arrived on the doorstep were still in the program one year later. Of the 20 percent who dropped out, the whereabouts of half were known. They had moved to a different city and they were in a program there; but they were not within our confines of follow-up. So I do think that you can build interpersonal relationships once you have some way of beginning to communicate with the addict.

Q. *Dr. Roloff:* I would like to hear from you on problems that we have. You referred to "encouraging the patients to tolerate the discomfort associated with low-level maintenance." We have some problem with them showing up at other medical facilities for tranquilizers and a number of other drugs. Our other problem is prejudicial attitudes. This is a two-way street, there also are prejudicial attitudes on the part of free clinics and against the smaller traditional medical facilities.

A. *Dr. Davis: In answer to the first question, in terms of tolerating the slight discomfort that I mentioned, we do intensive counseling with the patient, and what we try to do is first give them a basic knowledge about what drug use during pregnancy means. We try to establish strong positive relationships. We also try to make the patient an ally in terms of her own treatment by asking, "Are you ready for a reduction?" If she comes in complaining of discomfort and perhaps asking for other drugs, we explain what the complications of that might be, and we ask: "Do you want this? What other supports do you have?" A major kind of paradigm that we use is transferring those needs which are met by chemical drug support to interpersonal support. We also try to bring in the family of the patient. Those kinds of things are very important. In terms of the prejudicial attitudes, they go both ways. A pregnant narcotic addict quite often perceives the medical establishment as an enemy, as one who should be manipulated in order to get more drugs. We try to use a paraprofessional team approach with that; that is, a professional and a paraprofessional go into the more traditional medical health facility with the pregnant addict or to visit her while she is there in the hospital. We have the professional staff member talk with the professional staff of the hospital, use the paraprofessional or addiction counselor to break down the cultural, racial, and background barriers of the pregnant addict, to work with the hospital staff, and pretty soon we get better communication going.*

Q. *Dr. Solish:* Among the women who became drug-free during pregnancy, and who were on methadone or on heroin and became drug-free before delivery, did any of those babies have withdrawal symptoms?

A. *Dr. Davis: Clinically, I can only say that none of the five infants who were delivered by abstinent mothers received chemotherapeutic support for withdrawal.*

Addictive Diseases: an International Journal 2 (1): 113-121 (1975)

Neonatal Abstinence Syndrome: Recognition and Diagnosis

MURDINA M. DESMOND
GERALDINE S. WILSON
Department of Pediatrics
Baylor College of Medicine
Newborn Nursery and High Risk Clinic
Jefferson Davis Hospital
Maternity and Infant Care Project
City of Houston Health Department
Houston, Texas

Our assignment in this symposium is to discuss the detection and diagnosis of the abstinence syndrome in the neonate, and to outline the constellation of physical findings and clinical behaviors which make consideration of this entity practical.

The *abstinence syndrome* may be defined as a generalized disorder characterized by signs and symptoms of central nervous system excitation together with respiratory and gastrointestinal dysfunction, which arises in the transitional period following delivery and is associated with a history of continuing utilization of drugs of addictive potential by the mother during pregnancy. Its origins lie in an abnormal intrauterine environment. A series of steps appear to be necessary for its genesis and for the infant's recovery.

1. Growth and survival of the fetus in an intrauterine environment rendered abnormal by the continuing or episodic transfer of drugs of addictive potential from maternal to fetal circulations.
2. Biochemical adaptation (development of tolerance?) of the fetus to the presence of the abnormal agent in its tissues.
3. Abrupt removal of the source of drug with delivery.

113

4. Continuing metabolism and excretion of the drug by the infant. Withdrawal or abstinence signs occur when critically low tissue levels have been reached.
5. Recovery from the abstinence syndrome is gradual and occurs when the infant has reprogrammed his metabolism to the absence of the dependence-producing agent.

How may a diagnosis be made?
1. A history of abnormal drug usage in the mother during pregnancy.
2. Signs of the abstinence syndrome in the infant after birth.
3. Detection of the drug or its metabolites in the tissue fluids of the mother, or in the amniotic fluid, or the fluids or tissues of the infant. Detection of the drug or its metabolites in the infant should not be necessary for the diagnosis, since at the time signs of abstinence appear, evidence of the drug may be absent. It is the *absence* of a significant amount of the drug which is causal in this transitional disorder.
4. In a theoretical sense, the signs and symptoms of abstinence or withdrawal should be completely and temporarily relieved by administration of the drug involved in the initial dependence.

Withdrawal effects have been described following the maternal use of an increasing variety of drugs. The material presented here is based on the literature and the authors' experience with infants of mothers addicted to heroine, methadone, and barbiturates.

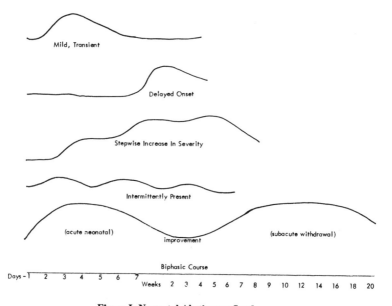

Figure I: Neonatal Abstinence Syndrome

Infants of heroin addicts often show evidence of fetal distress prior to delivery with meconium passage prior to birth (Naeye 1973).

In general, one-minute apgar scores may be low, but the majority fall within ranges expected for the nursery population involved.

Growth retardation is present in a high percentage (30 - 40%) of infants born to mothers addicted to heroin (Zelson, 1971). The percentage incidence of small-for-dates infants born to mothers on methadone during part or all of pregnancy has not been uniform in all sections of the country (Zelson, 1973; Lipsitz, 1974).

The time of onset of withdrawal varies from birth to two weeks of age, but the great majority appear within 72 hours of birth (Zelson, 1971). The type of drugs, or drugs, utilized by the mother, her dosage, the timing of the last dose before delivery, the character of labor, the type and amount of anesthesia and analgesia given during labor, the maturity, nutrition and presence or absence of intrinsic disease in the infant, may all play a role in determining the time of onset in the individual infant.

Signs of abstinence occur in a spectrum of severity, at one end so mild as to be difficult to distinguish from standard neonatal clinical behavior, and at the other, so severe as to be life-threatening if permitted to continue.

Because of variation in time of onset and variation in degrees of severity, a range of types of clinical course may be delineated (Figure 1).

The signs and symptoms are outlined in Table I.

Complications are outlined in Table II.

In the typical patient, the neurologic signs appear early and are predominant. Usually the first signs are an anxious expression, restlessness, overactivity, tremors, and constant crying. The infant appears miserable and as if in pain. The gastrointestinal signs tend to become more prominent after the first day. In a single patient we have noted severe gastrointestinal symptoms in the absence of neurologic signs, a finding similar to that reported earlier by Kunstadter in 1958.

Signs which tend to persist into infancy include hyperphagia and increased oral drive, sweating, hyperacusis, irregular sleep patterns and poor tolerance to "holding" or to abrupt changes of position in space.

Our data (Table III) suggest that the percentage of overt symptomatology is higher among infants of heroin and methadone addicts who appear undergrown at birth. A higher percentage of such infants in our institution have required drug therapy. In the immature infants, on the other hand, a larger percentage were classified as having mild signs, requiring no therapy. In this immature group, no infants were classified as having severe signs. We have been impressed by the marked episodic nature of the neural hyperexcitability in the immature infant. The infants appear restless and overactive for short periods, lapsing quickly into periods of lethargy and inactivity. Sustained tremors are not seen in immature infants until they reach gestational ages when tone is

TABLE I

CLINICAL MANIFESTATIONS OF ABSTINENCE SYNDROME	COMMENTS
CNS – related	
Frantic anxiety Restlessness, overactivity in prone or supine	early – episodic; at peak may be constant later – increasing prior to feeding
Crying – continuous, shrill, outcries	
Tremors, myoclonic jerks, flinging movements	tremor sustained only in infants of 37 weeks or more. May appear late in immature
Hypertonus	present generally in accordance with gestational age but tonicity may be briefly present in the immature
Spontaneous reflex activity mouthing, rooting, attempting to suck fingers or nearest object spontaneous Moros, startles, crossed extension	
Fever	generally associated with ↑ activity and excitation
Sneezing, hiccups, yawning	yawning may be late sign
Response disproportionate to stimulus (sound, abrupt changes of body in space)	
"Hard to hold" – failure to mold to body	respond to swaddling and upright position

TABLE I (continued)

CLINICAL MANIFESTATIONS OF ABSTINENCE SYNDROME	COMMENTS
Respiratory	
Irregular respiration, often rapid	may hyperventilate to alkalosis (Klain 1972)
Excessive secretions	
Gastrointestinal	
Suck	
Suck disorganized, poor closure around nipple depressed, short duration appear very hungry	may improve or be depressed by therapy
sensitive gag	
vomiting, regurgitation	
hyperphagia – with infatigable suck reflex	rarely may occur in absence of neurologic findings
loose stools	gradual onset, late to disappear
diarrhea	may appear 2-5th day and last up to 2-3 months
Dermatologic	
flushing with crying	
sudden circumoral pallor with cessation of cry and brief periods of immobility	early
scratches on face	2-3rd day
abrasions over pressure points	may last variable period up to months
excessive sweating	
mottling – peripheral	may persist into infancy

TABLE II

COMPLICATIONS OF ABSTINENCE SYNDROME

	Commentary
Jaundice — ↑ Infants of methadone mothers ↓ Infants of heroin or barbiturate mothers	
Infection	related to maternal infections and long hospital stay
Biochemical disturbances hypoglycemia, hypocalcemia electrolyte imbalances dehydration	– more frequent in S.G.A. and immature subjects – hyperventilation, poor feeding and diarrhea
Respiratory problems aspiration pneumonia	high incidence meconium staining A.F. vomiting and regurgitation
respiratory distress – rare in heroin addicted mothers (Glass 1971)	induction of surfactant (Taeusch 1973) abstinence signs may follow recovery from IRDS
nasal congestion	
Convulsions	occur with hypoglycemia, hypocalcemia, anoxia, etc. and in absence of above. Incidence controversial
Thermal instability	
Shock (neuronal exhaustion?)	

TABLE III:
Abstinence Syndrome in 117 Consecutive Infants Born to Mothers Addicted to
Heroin, Methadone or Combinations of These Drugs

	Wt.over 2500 gms. Gestation 37 wks. or more (N = 85)	Wt. 2500 gms. or less Gestation 37 wks. or more (N = 15)	Gestation under 37 wks. (N = 17, LGA = 1)
	%	%	%
Abstinence Syndrome present	74.1	93.3	70.6
Mild – no medication given	18.9	20.0	41.2
All – medication given	55.3	73.3	29.4
Severe – increasing dosages required to control syndrome	31.8	33.3	0.0

present in upper and lower extremities. Neural excitation is expressed by slow truncal movements, large flinging movements and wide flapping tremors at the appropriate gestational ages.

DIFFERENTIAL DIAGNOSIS

The *differential diagnosis* of the neonatal abstinence syndrome includes any entity which manifests itself by restlessness and central nervous system hyperexcitability. These entities include: the first reactivity period after birth, states associated with severe pain, septicemia, encephalitis (particularly congenital viral), meningitis, post-anoxic CNS irritation, hypoglycemia, hypocalcemia, hypomagnesia, pyridoxine dependency, hyperthyroidism, cerebral hemorrhage, polycythemia, the early stages of congestive heart failure and inborn errors of metabolism.

UNRESOLVED QUESTIONS

Unresolved questions abound for the clinician and investigator in considerations of the neonatal abstinence syndrome. Some of these controversial areas are:

The *absence of abstinence syndrome* in 10 - 25% of infants in which it might be expected to occur.

The *incidence of convulsions* complicating the abstinence syndrome is reported variously by different authors (Zelson, 1973). Convulsions are unquestionably known to occur when metabolic disturbances complicate the abstinence syndrome. They also occur in the absence of any known additional factor. Perhaps some of the controversy results from confusion surrounding the definition of neonatal seizure. Convulsions may perhaps be a function of maternal dosage, or may be characteristic of a particular drug or drugs, as described by Zelson (1973) for methadone.

The *increase of severity of symptoms* after improvement has taken place and the sudden reappearance of difficulties after the infant has been discharged from the hospital (subacute withdrawal, Desmond, 1972). Is this related to maternal use of multiple drugs of varying excretion rates, a spurious recovery after treatment with long-acting slowly excreted drugs, or to environmental triggering factors?

The *duration of the effects* of drug exposure and abstinence syndrome on the developing brain.

CONCLUSIONS

1. The neonatal abstinence syndrome is a generalized disorder characterized by CNS excitation, autonomic imbalance, respiratory and gastrointestinal dysfunction which arises in the transitional period in infants born to mothers utilizing drugs of addictive potential during pregnancy.

2. The signs are non-specific and occur in a spectrum of severity.

3. Although CNS excitation is usually predominant, gastrointestinal manifestations may occur alone.

4. Physical signs may be modified by immaturity or co-existing disease.

5. Signs which persist into infancy include hyperphagis, hyperacusis, sweating, diarrhea and irregular sleep patterns.

Notes

This paper was supported by Maternity and Infant Care Project Grant No. 06H-000-016-09, American Legion Erna and Albert Siegmund Child Welfare and Rehabilitation Foundation, and United States Public Health Service Grant No. RR-00188.
Request for reprints should be addressed to Dr. M.M. Desmond, M.D., Dept. of Pediatrics, Baylor College of Medicine, Houston, Texas 77025.

References

Behrendt, H., and Green, M. Nature of the sweating deficit of prematurely born neonates: observations on babies with the heroin withdrawal syndrome. *N. Eng. J. Med.*, 1972, *June, Vol. 286*, No. 26, 1376-1379.

Desmond, M. M., Schwanecke, R. P., Wilson, G. S., Yasunaga, S., and Burgdorff, I. Maternal barbiturate utilization and neonatal withdrawal symptomatology. *Pediatrics*, 1972, *February, Vol. 80*, No. 2, 190-197.

Glass, L., Rajegswda, B., and Evans, H. Absence of respiratory distress syndrome in premature infants of heroin-addicted mothers. *Lancet*, 1971, *Sept.*, 685-686.

Klain, D., Krauss, A., and Auld, P. Tachypnea and alkalosis in infants of narcotic-addicted mothers. *N.Y.S. J. Med.*, 1972, *Feb.*, 367-368.

Kunstadter, R. H., Klein, R. I., Lundeen, E. C., Witz, W., and Morrison, M. Narcotic withdrawal symptoms in newborn infants. *JAMA*, 1958, *October, Vol. 168*, 1008-1010.
Lipsitz, P. J., and Blatman, S. Newborn infants of mothers on methadone maintenance. *N.Y.S. J. Med.*, 1974, *June, Vol. 74*, No. 6, 994-999.
Naeye, R. L., Blanc, W., Leblanc, W., and Khatamee, M. A. Fetal complications of maternal heroin addiction: Abnormal growth, infections, and episodes of stress. *Pediatrics*, 1973, *December, Vol. 83*, No. 6, 1055-1061.
Pierson, P., Howard, P., and Kleber, H. Sudden deaths in infants born to methadone-maintained addicts. *JAMA*, 1972, *June, Vol. 220*, No. 220, 1733-1734.
Taeusch, H., Carson, S., Wang, N., and Avery, M. Heroin induction of lung maturation and growth retardation in fetal rabbits. *Pediatrics*, 1973, *May, Vol. 82*, No. 5, 869-875.
Zelson, C., Rubio, E., and Wasserman, E. Neonatal narcotic addiction: 10 year observation. *Pediatrics*, 1971, *August, Vol. 48*, No. 2, 178-188.
Zelson, C., Sook, J., and Casalino, M. Neonatal narcotic addiction: Comparative effects of maternal intake of heroin and methadone. *N. Eng. J. Med.*, 1973, *December, Vol. 289*, No. 23, 1216-1220.

DISCUSSION

Q. Dr. Kandall: In the management of the upper tract symptomatology, we have been building a large experience with babies who are symptomatic, as was the last baby you showed, for up to four to six months of age. Do you maintain those babies on therapy? We have found that symptoms persist no matter what we do. We stopped therapy of the babies and they improved in four to six months.

A. Dr. Desmond: *We have had some interesting experiences with trying it. We found that it was very difficult to give a mother, who is an addict, sedation for the baby. We tried every way we knew to avoid it. We used the swaddling techniques and support of the mother. We admit them to the hospital for a study if it seems to be too protracted. We have tried to avoid this if at all possible.*

Q. Dr. Zelson: I would like to commend Dr. Desmond for her presentation. I think it brings out all the facts that we usually see. I just want to relate something to show you how bad these babies can be after they leave the hospital. We have a contract with a social service agency and a foster home care agency to take care of our babies for us. We pay them a good deal of money and at the end of one year they decided not to take these babies any more because they found that there were problems almost through the entire year. They just could not handle them. The crying, the irritability, the restlessness, the activity, and difficulty with feeding made it too difficult; and regardless of what you did with these babies, they did not respond.

Addictive Diseases: an International Journal 2 (1): 123-139 (1975)

Biomedical Applications of Vapor Phase Analysis

EUGENE HEATH
J. THROCK WATSON
Department of Pharmacology
School of Medicine
Vanderbilt University
Nashville, Tennessee

GAS CHROMATOGRAPHY

Vapor phase analysis is attractive because some techniques such as gas chromatography are themselves separation techniques which bolster the specificity of the analytical method. Complex mixtures can be resolved into individual components because the different constituents interact differently with partitioning phases in a gas chromatographic column and thus elute or emerge from the column at discrete time intervals following application or injection of the mixture onto the column (see Figure 1). The sample is injected into the gas chromatograph with a microliter syringe; the sample aliquot is usually 2-3 microliters of dilute solution. The solvent and solute are immediately vaporized (the temperature of the gas chromatograph can be adjusted to any temperature between 50° and 300° C) and forced into the column with a constant flow of inert carrier gas (helium, nitrogen, etc.). Since the various components of the sample are retained by the GC partitioning phase to different extents, these components emerge from the column at different time intervals relative to the time of injection. It is this characteristic "retention time" under controlled conditions of flow, temperature, partitioning phase, etc., that is used in a qualitative sense to identify a substance.

Quantitative uses of gas chromatography depend to some extent on the type of detector employed, but in general, the chromatographic process operates

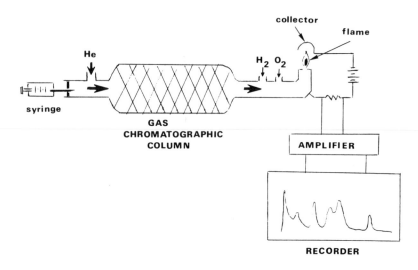

FIG. 1.   Schematic of gas chromatograph equipped with a flame ionization detector.

efficiently on femtomole (10^{-15}) to nanomole (10^{-9}) quantities of material. The flame ionization detector (FID) has practical sensitivity for as little as 50-100 ngm of material injected on column. This type of detector is shown schematically in Figure 1. The organic compound in vapor form flows into a hydrogen flame and during combustion produces positive and negative ions which are collected by electrodes in the region of the flame. An electrical signal is generated which is proportional in magnitude to the quantity of organic compound entering the FID. This signal is recorded to give an elution profile of various compounds from the GC column. The FID is useful because it is rugged and gives a linear response over a dynamic range of 3-5 orders of magnitude. It is not selective in that it will produce a signal from any compound that is combustible.

Electron capture detectors are both selective and sensitive. They operate by supplying a constant source of electrons or beta particles from a radioactive source to an electrode of the detector. Compounds emerging from the GC column can then "capture" or "trap" these free beta particles and prevent them from reaching the detector electrode. The dimunition of this "standing" or constant electron current indicates the emergence of the compound(s) capable of electron capture. It is this feature of electron capture that is the basis of selectivity for this detector. The compound must be electrophilic; halogenated compounds are very readily detected by the electron capture detector (ECD). As little as 5-20 picograms of DDT (Wilson et al., 1973) in an aliquot of biological extract can be detected by ECD. Some drugs which contain halogens can be quantified selectively by ECD. The sensitivity of ECD for drugs is not always outstanding; for example, assays for chlorpromazine (Sekerke et al., 1973) based on ECD have sensitivity only slightly better than that using FID. Although 20-30 ngm of chlorpromazine injected on column may be required to produce a readily discernible ECD peak, the ECD method for chlorpromazine still maintains good selectivity for chlorpromazine against biological background.

Probably the most versatile, selective detector which also has high sensitivity for monitoring a gas chromatograph is the mass spectrometer. Qualitative and quantitative applications of combined GC-MS are presented in another section.

SAMPLE PREPARATION

A principal requirement for vapor phase analysis is that the compound of interest be volatile or have adequate vapor pressure (30 torr) at the operating temperature of the GC or GC-MS without undergoing thermal decomposition. Since most drugs and hormones of interest do not meet this criterion some means of derivatization must be employed to replace hydrogen atoms which are capable of hydrogen bonding. There are a variety of acylating and silanizing reagents available which react with hydroxy, amino, and carboxyl functional groups to produce derivatives with suitable vapor phase properties. More detailed accounts of derivatization can be found elsewhere (McNair and Bonelli, 1969; Pierce, 1968).

COMBINED GAS CHROMATOGRAPHY — MASS SPECTROMETRY

Gas chromatographic data can be ambiguous, especially when dealing with unknown samples or complex mixtures, such as those of biological origin, because of the probability of two or more of the components having the same retention time under given gas chromatographic conditions. In these cases it is desirable to obtain accompanying characteristic data to identify the components in question; these data are often available from the combined application of gas chromatography-mass spectrometry (GC-MS). GC-MS is possible because any compound that is amenable to analysis by GC is also suitable for analysis by mass spectrometry. Combined, tandem operation of the two instruments is now possible because problems associated with differences in operating pressure (1 atm for GC, 10^{-10} atm for MS) have been overcome with the use of molecular separators (McFadden, 1973; Watson, 1969) or with improved vacuum systems.

OPERATING PRINCIPLES

Mass spectroscopy is a destructive analytical technique. The fragmentation pattern or mode of unimolecular decomposition of a molecular ion as portrayed by the mass spectrum often reveals characteristic information about a molecule which can be related to the molecular structure of the original, intact molecule.

The mode of operation in mass spectroscopy is indicated schematically in Figure 2. A sample inlet system channels the sample vapor into the ion source which is maintained under vacuum (10^{-6} to 10^{-8} atm). A small fraction (less than 0.1%) of the neutral molecules randomly diffuse into the ionization region where they are bombarded with or interact with an electron beam. These molecules receive sufficient internal energy to exceed their ionization potential so that not only is an electron expelled, resulting in a positively charged ion, but many of these molecular ions decompose into more stable fragment ions in an effort to dissipate the excess internal energy. The assemblage of ions (molecular and fragment ions) thus formed in the ionization region can then be analyzed according to m/e. This is accomplished by accelerating the entire group of ions from the ion source through a negative electric field (-4000 volts) into a magnetic field. All of the ions in the total ion beam receive the same kinetic energy (4000 volts) during acceleration, but since the ions have different masses, they will have different velocities (K.E. = $1/2 \, mv^2$). The trajectories of these various ions having different masses, and thus different velocities, will be affected differently within the region of the magnetic field. For example, the trajectory of an ion of low mass/charge (m/e) will suffer a greater curvature because it has a higher velocity than an ion of high m/e. Thus the total ion beam is resolved into several discrete ion beams within the magnetic field. For any given value of the magnetic and electric fields, only ions of a certain m/e value (M_2 in Figure 2) follow a trajectory leading to the detector. The complete mass spectrum is obtained from the mass spectrometer by sweeping the magnitude of the magnetic field, thereby drawing the ion current of one m/e value after another across the slits of the detector. Since the value of m/e $= k \, H^2/V$ where H is the magnetic field and V is the accelerating voltage, the mass spectrum could also be obtained by sweeping the magnitude of the accelerating voltage. This technique of electric scanning is not very practical for complete scans from magnetic instruments but alteration of the accelerating voltage (Sweeley et al., 1966) is useful in ion monitoring (Falkner, Sweetman, and Watson, 1975) over a limited mass range.

The quadrupole mass spectrometer is rapidly becoming more prominent in analytical laboratories. The quadrupole has no magnetic field, but rather uses a combination of DC and RF (radio-frequency) fields applied between four parallel rods to serve as a "mass filter" to resolve the total ion beam into discrete ion currents of individual m/e values. The ionization source is comparable to that described above. More detailed descriptions of the quadrupole can be found in other reviews (McFadden, 1973; Watson, 1969).

Regardless of the type of mass analyzer employed for the separation of ions the means of forming these ions can be common to all instruments. Electron ionization (EI) is the most common because it usually yields the most information about the compound being analyzed. Ions are formed by bombarding the molecule with high energy electrons (70 eV). With this method, 80 to 90% of the total ions formed are fragment ions; only a small percentage are ions of the in-

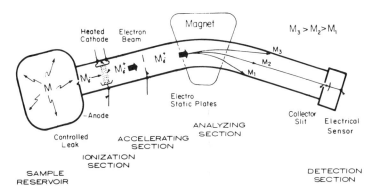

FIG. 2.   Schematic of magnetic single-focusing mass spectrometer. Reproduced, with permission, from "Gas Chromatography and Mass Spectroscopy" by J. T. Watson, *Ancillary Techniques of Gas Chromatography.* Copyright 1969 by John Wiley and Sons.

tact molecule (molecular ion). Chemical ionization, on the other hand, is a more gentle process in which the ions are formed by charge transfer from an ionized reagent gas, e.g., CH_5^+, etc., from methane. Chemical ionization characteristically produces more ions which contain the intact molecule and fewer fragment ions than does EI. The ions most commonly found are those of $m/e = M + 1$ or $M - 1$ where M is the molecular weight of the compound; in these cases the molecular ion either gains or loses a proton (Munson, 1971). CI mass spectra are thus often less complex than EI spectra and are especially useful in analyzing mixtures.

QUALITATIVE AND QUANTITATIVE APPLICATIONS

There are three general methods used in GC-MS. The most common is to scan the complete spectrum whenever a GC peak elutes from the column into the mass spectrometer. The emergence of compound(s) from the GC is usually detected by the use of a total ion monitor which is located between the ion source and the magnetic field and can be adjusted to monitor a portion of the total ion beam. In combined GC-MS it is important that the mass spectrum be obtained and recorded rapidly (i.e., a scan from m/e 40 to m/e 600 in 2 to 4 seconds) so that the sample pressure will not change significantly during the scan and thus not distort the authentic relative abundance of the ions in the mass spectrum. In addition, rapid scanning permits several, consecutive scans to be obtained during the emergence of a given compound from the gas chromatograph. The consecutively obtained mass spectra permit the investigator to ascertain whether a given GC peak is due to a single component or they can be used to identify components of a mixture which are not completely resolved by the gas chromatograph (Figure 3). Although 16 β-hydroxy-dehydroepiandrosterone-TMS and 16-oxo-androstenediol-TMS are not completely separated by

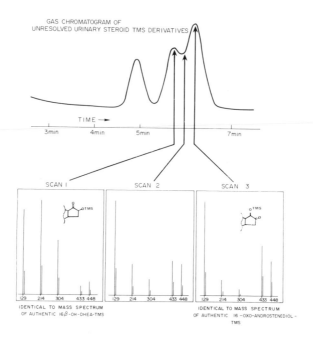

FIG. 3. Gas chromatogram of unresolved urinary steriod TMS derivatives illustrating mass spectra obtained at indicated time intervals.

gas chromatography, mass spectra which were identical with those of the pure, authentic compounds could be obtained at the extremes of the unresolved doublet (scan 1 and 3, Figure 3); scan 2 is a mixture of the mass spectra of these two compounds.

Other investigators, however, utilize another technique, repetitive scanning, in which the complete spectrum is scanned every few seconds throughout the GC separation, and all of this data is stored by a computer for future reference. This procedure eliminates operator decisions concerning whether certain peaks should be scanned and ensures that all data are recorded for off-line evaluation and interpretation. The chronological sequence of these several hundred consecutively recorded mass spectra is presented in a readily intelligible format by a plot of the total ion current of each spectrum versus spectrum index number (Figure 4). This histogram is especially helpful to the investigator in his initial evaluation of the data, in that he can readily determine which of the mass spectra in the computer contains data of major components of the sample mixture. Further, the investigator can use the computer to determine whether a given compound or class of compounds is present in the sample mixture as evidenced by its characteristic ion(s). Since all of the ions in each consecutively recorded mass spectrum are stored in the computer, the investigator can request that the computer search each recorded mass spectrum for a particular ion and, if found,

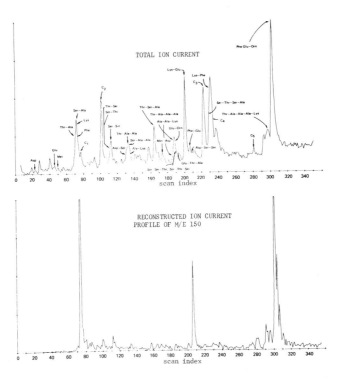

FIG. 4.   Total ionization plot generated by computer from consecutively scanned mass spectra of silylated amino alcohols (upper panel). Mass chromatogram showing the ion current profile of m/e 150 (lower panel) reconstructed from the same mass spectra indicated in the total ionization plot Reproduced, with permission, from "Sequence Determination of Proteins and Peptides by GC-MS-Computer Analysis of Complex Hydrolysis Mixtures" by Forster et al., 1973, *Techniques of Combined Gas Chromatography/Mass Spectrometry: Applications in Organic Analysis.* Copyright 1973 by John Wiley and Sons.

plot its relative abundance in each spectrum versus spectrum index number. An example of this procedure is presented in Figure 4 which shows the reconstructed profile or histogram of the ion current of m/e 150. The investigator may then devote his full attention to spectra 74, 207, and 303, since these correspond to the three major peaks indicated in Figure 4. This example illustrates the utility of mass chromatography (Hites and Biemann, 1970; Forster et al., 1973) in reducing a large quantity of data. Repetitive scanning is not designed for ultimate sensitivity but to facilitate identification of compounds or metabolites. This method requires a relatively large quantity of each compound (100-200 ng) to be injected into the mass spectrometer since the abundance of any particular ion is measured for only a brief period of time. The sensitivity can be increased by limiting the range of the scan to only a few ions (e.g., start at m/e 100 and scan to 110).

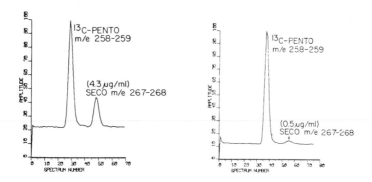

FIG. 5. Analysis of Secobarbital in maternal plasma (left panel) and infant's plasma (right panel), using pentobarbital 2,4(6),5-13C as the internal standard. Reproduced, with permission, from "Use of Stable Isotopes in Measuring Low Concentrations of Drugs and Drug Metabolites by GC-MS-COM Procedures" by Horning et al., 1973b, *Clinical Chemistry,* Volume 19. Copyright © 1973 by American Association of Clinical Chemists.

Quantitative analyses of secobarbital in both maternal and neonatal plasma in a mother-infant pair have been measured using the technique of repetitive scanning. The internal standard 2,4,5-13C-pentobarbital, was added to 0.1 ml of plasma and analyzed for the concentration of secobarbital in both the mother and infant. The mother had received 195 mg one hour before delivery. Venous blood was obtained from the mother at the time of delivery, and blood from the femoral vein was obtained from the infant 69 hours after delivery. An extract of the plasma was then derivatized and injected into a gas chromatograph-mass spectrometer (using chemical ionization). The effluent from the gas chromatograph was then repetitively scanned and stored by a computer. With the proper computer programs it was then possible to select the ions m/e 267 for secobarbital and 258 for the internal standard, 13C-pentobarbital, and to plot the relative abundance of these selected ion current profiles for quantification (Figure 5). The concentration of secobarbital was 4.3 µg/ml in the mother's plasma and 0.5µg/ml in the infant's plasma (Horning et al., 1973b).

Repetitive scanning has been used to identify drugs which were taken by acutely poisoned patients. Using a special type of separator, the organic extracts of gastric aspirate, urine and blood from 21 overdose and 15 heroin/morphine addicts were analyzed. The sensitivity of the method was 5µg/ml of fluid and it was possible to identify 35 different drugs within 10 minutes after sample acquisition (Boerner et al., 1973). This procedure has enabled the identification of four components in illicit opium samples (Smith, 1973) and allowed the urine extracts from carcinoid patients to be monitored for indole acids (Weinkam, 1974).

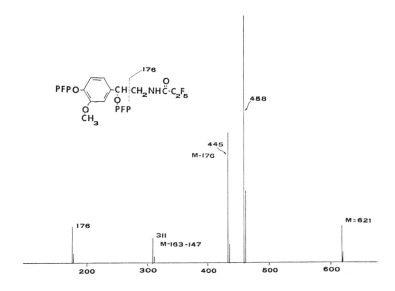

FIG. 6.   Mass spectrum of normetanephrine as the pentafluropropionyl derivative.

SELECTED ION MONITORING

One of the principal goals of gas chromatography-mass spectrometry is its potential for high sensitivity, and, in this respect, selected ion monitoring (SIM) is capable of greater sensitivity than repetitive scanning. This is due primarily to the fact that in SIM the output from the electron multiplier can be integrated over a longer time interval, thus enhancing the signal to noise ratio. To a limited extent, the more ions of a given mass spectrum that one monitors, the greater confidence one has that the corresponding compound is present in the sample. On the other hand, monitoring a large number of ions leads to a poorer statistical representation of any given single ion. Since SIM is ordinarily employed in cases where high sensitivity is important, only 2 or 3 ions for each compound of interest are usually selected.

An example for SIM is that which has been used for normetanephrine (Heath et al., 1974). The mass spectrum of normetanephrine as the pentafluropropionyl derivative (Figure 6) is characterized by two relatively intense ions (m/e 445 and 458). If the mass spectrometer monitors only these two ions, it is possible to detect and quantify normetanephrine (Figure 7). The total ion current chromatogram from a urine extract shows no peak for normetanephrine; however, by monitoring ions 445 and 458, normetanephrine in this urine extract is readily discernible and easily quantified.

Investigation of the plasma levels of amobarbital and its metabolite, 3-hydroxyamobarbital, in newborn infants was accomplished by SIM (Draffan et al., 1973; Krauer et al., 1973). The sensitivity of the method was such that 2-100

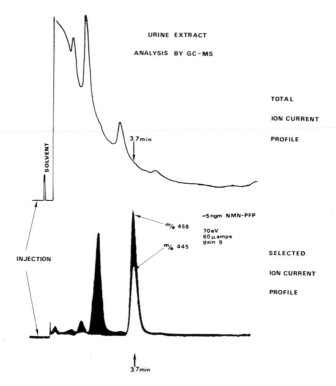

FIG. 7. Comparison of the total ion current profile (upper panel) and the selected ion current profiles (lower panel) of m/e 445 and 458 from the same biological sample containing a trace of nor-metanephrine (NMN). Reproduced, with permission, from "Application of New Analytical Techniques to Pharmacology" by J. T. Watson, *Annual Review of Pharmacology*, Volume 13. Copyright © 1973 by Annual Reviews Inc.

ng of amobarbital and 5-100 ng of 3-hydroxyamobarbital could be quantified in 0.1 ml of plasma. With butabarbital as the internal standard for amobarbital, both substances were quantified as their N,N-dimethyl derivatives by monitoring the ion current at m/e 169. Similarly, the ion of m/e 169 was monitored for the metabolite, but in order to monitor the internal standard, phenobarbital; the ion current at m/e 175 was also monitored. Plasma half-lives were determined in both mother and infant following administration of 200 mg of amobarbital intramuscularly to the mother 0.7 to 3.5 hours before delivery (Figure 8). The mean plasma half-life of amobarbital in the infants was found to be more than twice that in the mothers. The accuracy of the method was 10 ng ± 5.2% for amobarbital and 15 ng ± 7% for 3-hydroxyamobarbital per ml of plasma.

SIM has been used to measure carbamazepine (Tegretol) in humans (Palmer et al., 1973). Quantitative gas chromatographic analysis has been used for the measurement of steady state levels of this drug, but detailed pharmacokinetic evaluation has not been studied in adults or children. The standard

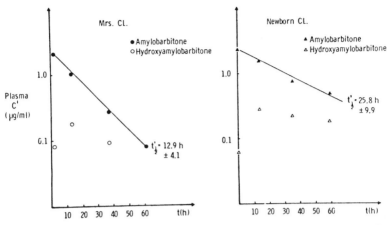

FIG. 8.   Plasma concentrations of amobarbital and hydroxyamobarbital in a mother (left panel) and her newborn child (right panel) after a single injection of 200 mg sodium amobarbital intramuscularly to the mother before delivery. Reproduced, with permission, from "Elimination Kinetics of Amobarbital in Mothers and their Newborn Infants" by Krauer, et al., 1973, *Clinical Pharmacology and Therapeutics*, Volume 14. Copyright © 1973 by the C.B. Mosby Co.

curve for the measurement of carbamazepine ranged from 50 to 500 ng/ml of plasma when the reduced form of carbamezepine (10,11-dihydroxycarbamazepine) was used as an internal standard. It was found that peak plasma concentrations occurred at 6 to 8 hours after a single oral dose of 200 mg. This concentration remained constant for about 24 hours before declining monoexponentially over the succeeding 6 days. The plasma half-life was 34.8 to 37.2 hours in this limited study.

Another CNS depressant (methaqualone) has also been measured using SIM methodology (Alvan et al., 1973). It has been previously thought that the half-life of this drug was 4 to 5 hours in man. These investigators monitored methaqualone levels for over 80 hours and demonstrated that the earlier estimates of the half-life was actually calculated on the alpha and not the beta phase of the elimination of the drug (Figure 9). With the sensitivity of their method (100 ng/ml to 5 μg/ml) their estimate of the half-life was on the order of 19.6-41.5 hours for the beta phase.

Two relatively recent advances have been made in the measurement of morphine using deuterium labeled internal standards. A quantitative SIM assay using chemical ionization has been developed in which two fragment ions were monitored for the TMS derivatives of both morphine and the internal standard, morphine-d_3. Although only one pair of ions (m/e 340, 343) was sufficient for quantification, a second pair (m/e 414, 417) provided convenient corroborative information. The range of linearity extended from 5 ng to 1 μg of morphine per ml of urine. The sensitivity of the method was comparable to that of the radioimmunoassay and hemaglutination methods. Cross interferences are less

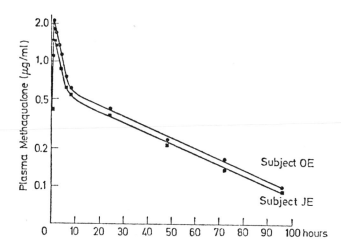

FIG. 9.   Plasma concentration curves of methaqualone after a single oral dose measured by SIM of ion current at m/e 250. Reproduced, with permission, from "Plasma Kinetics of Methaqualone in Man after Single Oral Doses" by Alvan et al., 1973, *European Journal of Clinical Pharmacology*, Volume 6. Copyright © 1973 by Springer-Verlag Berlin.

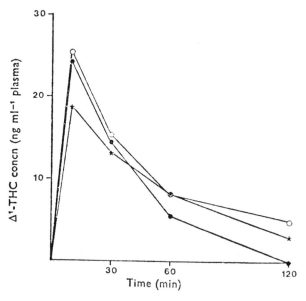

FIG. 10.   Plasma levels of Δ1-tetrahydrocannabinol (THC) in three volunteers after each having smoked 10mg of Δ1-THC in a tobacco cigarette. Data obtained with SIM by monitoring m/e 299. Reproduced, with permission, from "Quantitation of Δ1-Tetrahydrocannibinol in Plasma from Cannabis Smokers" by Agurell et al., 1973, *Journal of Pharmacy and Phamacology*, Volume 25. Copyright © 1973 by the Pharmaceutical Society of Great Britain.

likely with the SIM method, and a case was presented in which morphine was easily detected in the presence of codeine (Clarke and Foltz, 1974). Another method using electron ionization has also been accomplished (Ebbighausen et al., 1973). A quantitative assay for the measurement of codeine and codeine-d$_3$ as the internal standard was found to have a sensitivity of less than 5 ng/ml of plasma. Using only 0.5 ml of plasma and monitoring ions m/e 495 and 498 from the HFB derivatives, they measured 5 ng/ml of codeine in plasma 72 hours after a single oral dose of 45 mg. Morphine and morphine-d$_3$ could also be measured as their TFA derivatives with the same sensitivity as that of codeine.

Another analgesic, pentazocine, which is commonly used, has also been measured by selected ion monitoring (Agurell et al., 1974). Using cyclazocine as an internal standard, two fragment ions, of m/e 202 and 217 were monitored for pentazocine and m/e 230 for cyclazocine using electron ionization. The lower limit of sensitivity was 2 ng/ml; the precision of the method was 2 ng/ml ±12% standard deviation in the low range and 10 ng/ml ±7% for higher concentrations. The plasma half-life was shown to be 134 minutes after a single intravenous dose of 30 mg. The CSF levels reached 10 ng/ml after 30 minutes and climbed to about 15 ng/ml at 90-120 minutes. It has been reported that maximum analgesia after intravenous administration of pentazocine occurs after about 30 minutes (Berkowitz et al., 1969).

A method to identify and accurately measure non-labeled Δ$_1$-tetrahydrocannabinol (THC) in blood of cannabis smokers has been developed (Agurell et al., 1973). These investigators used the internal standard (THC-d$_2$) and monitored m/e 299 and 314 from THC and m/e 301 and 316 from THC-d$_2$ after electron ionization. The standard curve was made by plotting the ratio of 26 ng/ml within 15 minutes in 3 volunteers who smoked cigarettes containing 10 mg of THC (Figure 10).

When using selected ion monitoring, sample preparation seems to be a major problem in the development of assays of compounds from biological samples. Using relatively simple extraction procedures the lower limit of detection of a compound in the extract of a biological sample may be 100 to 500 picograms, which is much higher than the 5 to 10 pg limit which might be detected when pure standards are injected for analysis. Clearly, further purification before GC-MS will allow the measurement of lower levels, but this must be balanced with the time and the complexity of the procedures for the purification. The relative importance of sensitivity versus ease and time required for purification will be dictated by the requirements of the problem under investigation.

The previous examples which are cited are not intended to be a survey of the literature but to illustrate the versatility of utilizing the mass spectrometer as a qualitative and quantitative detector. Recent review articles provide comprehensive coverage of medicinal and biological applications (Falkner et al., 1974; Watson, 1973; Jenden and Cho, 1973; Frigerio and Castagnoli, 1974; Costa and Holmstedt, 1973; Burlingame et al., 1974).

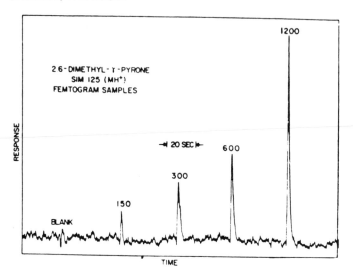

FIG. 11.   Response observed for femtogram samples of 2,6-dimethy-ɣ-pyrone injected in benzene solution using an atmospheric pressure ionization (API) mass spectrometer. Reproduced, with permission, from "Subpicogram Detection System for Gas Phase Analysis Based upon Atmospheric Pressure Ionization (API) Mass Spectrometry" by Carroll et al., 1974, *Analytical Chemistry,* Volume 46. Copyright © 1974 by the American Chemical Society.

CONCLUSION

Mass spectrometry has only recently been applied to the medical and biological area. Increasing demands for this kind of methodology should lead to the development of even more sensitive, but less complex and less expensive instruments. One relatively recent development is the atmospheric pressure ionization (API) mass spectrometer (Horning et al., 1973; Carroll et al., 1974). This development could be used either with direct probe samples, with very long capillary columns, and even with a high pressure liquid chromatograph in which the mass spectrometer could be a very sensitive detector. Briefly, this API instrument features an ion source operated at atmospheric pressure with ionization produced by means of the beta particles emitted by a [63]Ni foil. In operation, ions and neutral molecules from the reaction chamber enter the mass analyzer through a small aperture. In effect, the source is a reaction chamber which is monitored continuously. A typical experimental result for small samples is shown in Figure 11. Samples between 0 and 1200 femtograms of 2,6-dimethyl-g-pyrone were injected with 2 µl of benzene. The ion current at m/e 125 was continuously monitored as in SIM. Although the work is still in preliminary stages, this and other instrumental developments may extend the sensitivity for SIM for many compounds into the sub-femtogram range. Improvements in purification techniques for biological samples, coupled with new developments or newer designs should yield a powerful technique for selective, quantitative detection of specific compounds in many biological systems, both on a routine basis and in a research context.

The identification of various drugs often can be accomplished with the more general screening techniques (i.e., thin layer chromatography, spectrophotometric procedures). Also, the quantification of drugs often does not require the use of extremely sensitive methodology. If, however, only small sample sizes (i.e., 0.1-0.2 ml of blood) are available, the use of the very sensitive technique of gas chromatography may be required. The limited sample load of vapor phase analysis (30-50 samples a day), however, should be balanced by the particular needs of the investigator. Other methods for quantification are often available which will accommodate larger numbers of samples without forfeiting much sensitivity or selectivity (i.e., fluorescence, radio-immunoassays). However, the special techniques of vapor phase analysis are invaluable in re-examining those samples which give ambiguous results from other methods.

SUMMARY

Recent investigations of physiological systems have demonstrated that even minor chemical constituents can play a major role in mediating physiological responses. Recognizing this, the investigator seeks to isolate or selectively quantify the concentration of a specific drug or hormone that is available to target tissue. Today, as drugs are developed which are more and more potent, greater demands are made on analytical methodology for ever more sensitive yet specific techniques of quantification. The techniques of vapor phase analysis such as gas chromatography, especially in combination with mass spectrometry, offer great promise to investigative pharmacology/toxicology. Some of the potentials and limitations of vapor phase analysis will be described. More detailed descriptions of basic gas chromatography (McNair and Bonelli, 1969; Ettre and McFadden, 1969) and combined gas chromatography-mass spectrometry (McFadden, 1973) can be found elsewhere.

Notes

This work was supported by The Research Center for Clinical Pharmacology and Drug Toxicology (NIH-GM-14531). Eugene Heath is supported by a Research Fellowship (GM-53508-02), and J. Throck Watson by a Research Career Development Award GM 50290-02.

Requests for reprints should be addressed to Dr. Eugene Heath, Dep't. of Pharmacology, Vanderbilt University, Nashville, Tenn. 37232

References

Agurell, S., Gustafsson, B., Holmstedt, B., Leander, K., Lindgren, J. E., Nilsson, I., Sandberg, F., and Asberg, M. Quantitation of Δ1-tetrahydrocannabinol in plasma from cannabis smokers. *Journal of Pharmacy and Pharmacology*, 1973, 25. 554-558.

Agurell, S., Boreus, L. O., Gordon, E., Lindgren, J. E., Ehrnebo, M., and Lonroth, U. Plasma and cerebrospinal fluid concentrations of pentazocine in patients: assay by mass fragmentography. *Journal of Pharmacy and Pharmacology*, 1974, *26*. 1-8.

Alvan, G., Lindgren, J. E., Bogentoft, C., and Ericsson, O. Plasma kinetics of methaqualone in man after single oral doses. *European Journal of Clinical Pharmacology*, 1973, *6*. 187-190.

Berkowitz, B. S., Asling, J. H., Shnider, S. M., and Way, E. L. Relationship of pentazocine plasma levels to pharmacological activity in man. *Clinical Pharmacology and Therapeutics*, 1969, *10*. 320.

Boerner, U., Abbott, S., Eidson, J. C., Becker, C. E., Horio, H. T., and Loeffler, K. Direct mass spectrometric analysis of body of body fluids from acutely poisoned patients. *Clinical Chimica Acta*, 1973, *49*. 445-454.

Burlingame, A. L., Cox, R. E., and Derrick, P. J. Mass spectrometry. *Analytical Chemistry*, 1974, *5*. 248R-287R.

Carroll, D. I., Dzidic, I., Stillwell, R. N., Horning, M. G., and Horning, E. C. Subpicogram detection system for gas phase analysis based upon atmospheric pressure ionization (API) mass spectrometry. *Analytical Chemistry*, 1974, *46* (6). 706-710.

Clarke, P. A., and Foltz, R. L. Quantitative analysis of morphine in urine by gas chromatography-chemical ionization-mass spectrometry, with $(N-C^2H_3)$ morphine as an internal standard. *Clinical Chemistry*, 1974, *20* (4). 465-469.

Costa, E., and Holmstedt, B. (eds.). Gas chromatography-mass spectrometry in neurobiology. *Advances in Biochemical Psychopharmacology, 7*. New York: Raven Press, 1973.

Draffan, G. H., Clare, R. A., and Williams, F. M. Determination of barbiturates and their metabolites in small plasma samples by gas chromatography-mass spectrometry: amylobarbitone and 3-hydroxyamylobarbitone. *Journal of Chromatography*, 1973, *75*. 45-53.

Ebbighausen, W. O. R., Mowat, J. H., Vestergaard, P., and Kline, N. S. Stable isotope method for the assay of codeine and morphine by gas chromatography-mass spectrometry. A feasibility study. *Advances in Biochemical Psychopharmacology*, 1973, *7*. 135-146.

Ettre, L. S. and McFadden W. H. (eds.). *Ancillary Techniques of Gas Chromatography*, Wiley-Interscience, 1969.

Falkner, F. C., Sweetman, B. J., and Watson, J. T. Biomedical applications of selected ion monitoring. *Applied Spectroscopy Reviews*, E. Brame (ed.), Marcel Dekker (in press).

Forster, H. J., Kelley, J. A., Nau, H., and Biemann, K. Sequence determination of proteins and peptides by GC-MS-computer analysis of complex hydrolysis mixtures. *Techniques of Combined Gas Chromatography/Mass Spectrometry: Applications in Organic Analysis*, W. H. McFadden, ed., 1973. 358-367.

Frigerio, A. and Castagnoli, N. (eds.). *Mass Spectrometry in Biochemistry and Medicine*. New York: Raven Press, 1974.

Heath, E. C., Falkner, F. C., and Watson, J. T. Application of selected ion monitoring (SIM) to quantify metabolites of biogenic amines with GC-MS-computer system. *Proceedings of the Twenty-Second Annual Conference of Mass Spectrometry and Applied Topics*, 1974, pp 286-7.

Hites, R. A. and Biemann, K. Computer evaluation of continuously scanned mass spectra of gas chromatographic effluents. *Analytical Chemistry*, 1970, *42*. (8). 855-860.

Horning, E. C., Horning, M. G., Carroll, D. I., Dzidic, I., and Stillwell, R. N. New picogram detection system based on a mass spectrometer with an external ionization source at Atmospheric pressure. *Analytical Chemistry*, 1973a, *45* (6). 936-943.

Horning, M. G., Nowlin, J., Lertratanangkoon, K., Stillwell, R. N., Stillwell, W. G., and Hill, R. M. Use of stable isotopes in measuring low concentrations of drugs and drug metabolites by GC-MS-COM procedures. *Clinical Chemistry*, 1973b, *19* (8). 845-852.

Jenden, D. J., and Cho, A. K. Applications of integrated gas chromatography/mass spectrometry in pharmacology and toxicology. *Annual Review of Pharmacology*, 1973, *13*. 371-390.

Krauer, B., Draffan, G. H., Williams, F. M., Clare, R. A., Dollery, C. T., and Hawkins, D. F. Elimination kinetics of amobarbital in mothers and their newborn infants. *Clinical Pharmacology and Therapeutics*, 1973, *14* (3). 442-447.

McFadden, W. H., *Techniques of Combined Gas Chromatography/Mass Spectrometry*, Wiley-Interscience, 1973.

McNair, H. M. and Bonelli, E. J., *Basic Gas Chromatography*, Consolidated Printers, Berkeley, California, 1969.

Munson, B. Chemical ionization mass spectrometry. *Analytical Chemistry*, 1971, *43* (13). 28A-43A.

Palmer, L., Bertilsson, L., Collste, P., and Rawlins, M. Quantitative determination of carbamazepine in plasma by mass fragmentography. *Clinical Pharmacology and Therapeutics*, 1973, *14* (5). 827-832.

Pierce, A. E. *Silylation of Organic Compounds*, Pierce Chemical Company, 1968.

Sekerke, H. J., David, J., Janowsky, D. S. El-Yousef, M. K., and Manier, D. H. Assay for chlorpromazine using gas chromatography with electron capture detection. *Psychopharmacology Bulletin*, 1973, *9*. 23-30.

Smith, R. M. Forensic identification of opium by computerized gas chromatography/mass spectrometry. *Journal of Forensic Science*, 1973, *18*. 327-334.

Sweeley, C. C., Elliott, W. H. Fries, I., and Ryhage, R. Mass spectrometric determination of unresolved components in gas chromatographic effluents. *Analytical Chemistry*, 1966, *38*. 1549-1553.

Watson, J. T. Gas chromatography and mass spectroscopy. Chapter 5 in *Ancillary Techniques of Gas Chromatography*, Wiley Inter-science, 1969.

Watson, J. T. Application of new analytical techniques to pharmacology. *Annual Review of Pharmacology*, 1973, *13*. 391-407.

Weinkam, R. Applications of chemical ionization mass spectrometry to biomedical problems. *Summaries of the 2nd International Symposium on Mass Spectrometry in Biochemistry and Medicine*, 1974, *2*. 8 (abstract).

Wilson, D. J., Locker, D. J., Ritzen, R. A., Watson, J. T., and Schaffner, W. DDT concentrations in human milk. *American Journal of Diseases in Children*, 1973, *125*. 814-817.

Discussion

Q. *Dr. Braude:* Have you built a library of mass spectra of drug abuse?

A. *Dr. Watson:* We have not, but data banks of abused drugs are available in many facilities comparable to ours, and are available to virtually anyone who would wish to have such a library through the Mass Spectrometry Society. There are on the order of 300-500 mass spectra of drugs of abuse available.

Addictive Diseases: an International Journal 2 (1): 141-158 (1975)

Neonatal Abstinence Syndrome: Assessment and Management

LORETTA P. FINNEGAN
Department of Pediatrics,
University of Pennsylvania School
of Medicine;
Philadelphia General Hospital
Philadelphia, Pennsylvania

JAMES F. CONNAUGHTON, JR.
Department of Obstetrics and Gynecology,
University of Pennsylvania School
of Medicine;
Philadelphia General Hospital
Philadelphia, Pennsylvania

REUBEN E. KRON
Department of Psychiatry
University of Pennsylvania School
of Medicine
Eastern Pennsylvania Psychiatric Institute
Philadelphia, Pennsylvania

JOHN P. EMICH
Department of Obstetrics and Gynecology,
University of Pennsylvania School
of Medicine;
Philadelphia General Hospital,
Philadelphia, Pennsylvania.

During the past decade, narcotic addiction in the United States has reached epidemic proportions. A renewed interest in understanding its causes and in alleviating the suffering generated by drug dependency has come about in response to the rapid increase of this problem. The ratio of addiction in women of childbearing age has been steadily increasing, with the resultant birth of a large number of infants who must undergo the rigors of narcotic abstinence within the early neonatal period.

Many reports in the literature discuss the incidence of passive addiction in infants born to narcotic-addicted mothers, as well as the percentage of these infants who require drug therapy (Perlstein, M. A., 1947; Goodfriend, M. J., Shey, I. A., and Klein, M. D., 1956; Cobrinik, R. W., Hood, R. T., Jr., and Chusid, E., 1959; Hill, R. M., and Desmond, M. M., 1963; Rosenthal, T., Patrick, S. W., and Krug, D. C., 1964; Zelson, C., Rubio, E., and Wasserman, E., 1971; Nathenson, G., Golden, G. S., and Litt, I. F., 1971; Statzer, D. E., and

Wardell, J. N., 1972). Because there is no standard method for clinically evaluating these babies, nor is there a generally accepted approach to therapy, it is
difficult to compare the results reported by various investigators (Perlstein, M.
A., 1947; Goodfriend, M. J., Shey, I. A., and Klein, M. D., 1956; Cobrinik, R.
W., Hood, R. T., Jr., and Chusid, E., 1959; Hill, R. M., and Desmond, M. M.,
1963; Rosenthal, T., Patrick, S. W., and Krug, D. C., 1964; Zelson, C., Rubio,
E., and Wasserman, E., 1971; Nathenson, G., Golden, G. S., and Litt, I. F.,
1971; Statzer, D. E., and Wardell, J. N., 1972). However, it is well documented
that detection and treatment of infants undergoing the narcotic abstinence syndrome significantly reduces the mortality rate (Goodfriend, M. J., Shey, I. A.,
and Klein, M. D., 1956).

In response to the increasing number of infants born to narcotic-addicted
mothers at the Philadelphia General Hospital (PGH), the Departments of Obstetrics, Neonatology, and Psychiatry have embarked upon a collaborative
study of maternal narcotic addiction and passive addiction in the neonate. Although a number of investigators have studied the neonatal narcotic withdrawal
syndrome (Perlstein, M. A., 1947; Goodfriend, M. J., Shey, I. A., and Klein, M.
D., 1956; Cobrinik, R. W., Hood, R. T., Jr., and Chusid, E., 1959; Hill, R. M.,
and Desmond, M. M., 1963; Rosenthal, T., Patrick, S. W., and Krug, D. C.,
1964; Zelson, C., Rubio, E., and Wasserman, E., 1971) and various treatment
approaches have been reported (Hill, R. M., and Desmond, M. M., 1963; Zelson, C., Rubio, E., and Wasserman, E., 1971; Nathenson, G., Golden, G. S.,
and Litt, I. F., 1971; Finnegan, L. P., Connaughton, J. F., Emich, J. P., and
Wieland, W. F., 1973; Schiff, D., Chan, G., and Stern, L., 1971; Reddy, A. M.,
Harper, R. G., and Stern, G., 1971), the management of these infants is not yet
well defined.

From our own observations in the nursery, it appeared reasonable to assume that the greater the number and severity of withdrawal symptoms, the
higher the probability of morbidity or mortality to the afflicted infant. Therefore, by adding the individual symptom scores for a particular infant, an overall
abstinence score was generated to provide an estimate of the infant's clinical
status, information regarding progression or regression of the abstinence syndrome, and the adequacy of therapy.

This report describes our experience with the use of a clinically based scoring system that monitors the full spectrum of abstinence symptoms, and thus, is
used to regulate the therapeutic drug dosage level in the passively addicted infant.

MATERIALS AND METHODS

From January 1970 to June 1972, 121 passively addicted infants born to
known addicts at PGH were admitted to the high risk nursery for close observation and management, using methods described in the literature (Hill, R. M.,

and Desmond, M. M., 1963; Rosenthal, T., Patrick, S. W., and Krug, D. C., 1964; Zelson, C., Rubio, E., and Wasserman, E., 1971; Nathenson, G., Golden, G. S., and Litt, I. F., 1971; Reddy, A. M., Harper, R. G., and Stern, G. 1971; Kahn, E. J., Neumann, L. L., and Polk, G. A., 1969). Drug therapy commenced only after the withdrawal symptoms could no longer be managed by "conservative" measures such as swaddling the infant and administering demand feedings. (In our experience, approximately 85% of infants born to known narcotic-addicted mothers manifest clinical signs and symptoms of abstinence at sometime during the neonatal period.) The decision to administer drug therapy was based upon the examining pediatrician's observations along with the nursery nurse's report on the infant's symptomatology. The choice of a specific drug was left to the nursery physician assigned to the infant. The available drugs were those previously recommended as effective in neonatal abstinence (Hill, R. M., and Desmond, M. M., 1963; Zelson, C., Rubio, E., and Wasserman, E., 1971; Nathenson, G., Golden, G. S., and Litt, I. F., 1971; Kahn, E. J., Neumann, L. L., and Polk, G. A., 1969). Paregoric (Hill, R. M., and Desmond, M. M., 1963), phenobarbital (Kahn, E. J., Neumann, L. L., and Polk, G. A., 1969), chlorpromazine (Zelson, C., Rubio, E., and Wasserman, E., 1971; Kahn, E. J., Neumann, L. L., and Polk, G. A., 1969) or diazepam (Nathenson, G., Golden, G. S., and Litt, I. F., 1971) were initiated at the following dosage levels:

Paregoric—0.8 cc-2.0 cc in 6 divided doses p.o.

Phenobarbital—8-15 mg/Kg/day in 3 divided doses p.o. or I.M.

Chlorpromazine (Thorazine)—2.2 mg/Kg/day in 4 divided doses p.o. or I.M.

Diazepam (Valium)—1.0-2 mg q 8 hours p.o.

Subsequent dosage levels were titrated according to the symptomatic response of the infant, using methods described in the referenced publications.

In order to provide an improved method for assessment of the neonatal abstinence syndrome and to more carefully evaluate various therapeutic approaches, the comprehensive neonatal narcotic abstinence scoring system was devised. In constructing the abstinence scoring system, recognition of the literature was taken along with our own clinical experience (Finnegan, L. P., Connaughton, J. F., Emich, J. P., and Wieland, W. F., 1973; Kahn, E. J., Neumann, L. L., and Polk, G. A., 1969; Blinick, G., 1968; Rajegowda, B. K., Glass, L., Evans, H. E., Maso, G., Swartz, D. R., and LeBlanc, W., 1972). The major clinical signs and symptoms of neonatal narcotic withdrawal are related to increased levels of CNS excitation and include a group of readily observable behavioral characteristics, ranging from mild tremors to major seizures. From this gamut of symptoms and signs, we chose the 20 which are most commonly found during neonatal narcotic withdrawal (Perlstein, M. A., 1947; Goodfriend, M. J., Shey, I. A., and Klein, M. D., 1956; Cobrinik, R. W., Hood, R. T., Jr., and Chusid, E., 1959; Hill, R. M., and Desmond, M. M., 1963; Rosenthal, T.,

144 FINNEGAN, KRON, CONNAUGHTON, EMICH

Patrick, S. W., and Krug, D. C., 1964; Zelson, C., Rubio, E., and Wasserman, E., 1971). We then ranked these symptoms into groups. Those having the least pathological significance were arbitrarily given a score of "1"; those with the greatest potential for clinically adverse effects were scored as "5," while the others were given intermediate point values.

All PGH nursery nurses were trained in the application of the scoring system. Training included a detailed explanation of the scoring system and a practical experience in which representative infants undergoing various degrees of narcotic withdrawal were rated by supervised nursing personnel. After the training period, pairs of nurses were randomly selected to independently rate the same group of passively addicted infants. Four infants were independently scored at prescribed intervals by four different pairs of nurses from the various nursing shifts in order to demonstrate the reproducibility of the abstinence scoring method applied by a variety of nursing personnel within the Newborn Nurseries. The abstinence scoring was performed by each member of the pair within a 15-minute period so as to minimize the variance introduced by random changes in the infant's level of arousal. Tests for inter-rater reliability were performed.

The scoring system was then applied throughout the first five days of life to *all* infants born to drug-dependent mothers, and thereafter only to those evidencing withdrawal. Scoring was accomplished at birth and once every hour thereafter during the first 24 hours. The total score for each hour was added and entered at the bottom on the scoring sheet (Fig. 1). In the second 24 hours, the same signs and symptoms were evaluated but the score was entered every two hours on the scoring sheet (Fig. 2).

After 48 hours, the infants were scored every four hours at times corresponding to their nursery feedings (Fig. 3). It should be emphasized that the complete evaluation of all the listed behavioral and physiological signs was repeated at *each* of the prescribed intervals, and the item scores were totaled. The infants were scored every four hours until two days after drug therapy had been discontinued.

The infant with a score of "7" or less was not treated with drugs for the abstinence syndrome because, in our experience, he would recover rapidly with swaddling and demand feedings. Infants whose score was "8" or above were treated pharmacologically. Currently, we are investigating the relative effectiveness of sedatives (such as phenobarbital) and opiates (such as paregoric) in treating the abstinence syndrome. In our study, alternate infants received either phenobarbital or paregoric according to a specified dosage schedule, which is regulated according to the abstinence score and the weight of the infant.

Table I describes the dosage schedule of phenobarbital employed in this study according to the abstinence score. An infant with a score of 8 to 10 was given 3 mg/lb/day in 3 divided doses. The initial dosage determined by the schedule was not changed unless the abstinence score indicated the baby was not

FIGURE 1

NEONATAL ABSTINENCE SCORE

(FIRST 24 HOURS OF LIFE)

NAME _____

DATE _____

DAILY AVERAGE SCORE _____

AGE IN HOURS

SIGNS AND SYMPTOMS	SCORE	BIRTH	1	2	3	4	5	6	7	8	9	10	11	12	13	14	15	16	17	18	19	20	21	22	23	24
High Pitched Cry	2																									
Continuous High Pitched Cry	3																									
Sleeps Less Than 1 Hour After Feeding	3																									
Sleeps Less Than 2 Hours After Feeding	2																									
Sleeps Less Than 3 Hours After Feeding	1																									
Hyperactive Moro Reflex	2																									
Markedly Hyperactive Moro Reflex	3																									
Mild Tremors When Disturbed	1																									
Marked Tremors When Disturbed	2																									
Mild Tremors When Undisturbed	3																									
Marked Tremors When Undisturbed	4																									
Increased Muscle Tone	2																									
Generalized Convulsion	5																									
Frantic Sucking of Fists	1																									
Poor Feeding	2																									
Regurgitation	2																									
Projectile Vomiting	3																									
Loose Stools	2																									
Watery Stools	3																									
Dehydration	2																									
Frequent Yawning	1																									
Sneezing	1																									
Nasal Stuffiness	1																									
Sweating	1																									
Mottling	1																									
Fever-Less Than 101O	1																									
Fever-Greater Than 101O	2																									
Respiratory Rate Over 60/min.	1																									
Respiratory Rate > 60 With Retractions	2																									
Excoriation of Nose	1																									
Excoriation of Knees	1																									
Excoriation of Toes	1																									
Total Hourly Score																											

FIGURE 2

NEONATAL ABSTINENCE SCORE

(SECOND 24 HOURS OF LIFE)

NAME _____

DATE _____

DAILY AVERAGE SCORE _____

AGE IN HOURS

SIGNS AND SYMPTOMS	SCORE	26	28	30	32	34	36	38	40	42	44	46	48	COMMENTS
High Pitched Cry	2													
Continuous High Pitched Cry	3													
Sleeps Less Than 1 Hour After Feeding	3													
Sleeps Less Than 2 Hours After Feeding	2													
Sleeps Less Than 3 Hours After Feeding	1													
Hyperactive Moro Reflex	2													
Markedly Hyperactive Moro Reflex	3													
Mild Tremors When Disturbed	1													
Marked Tremors When Disturbed	2													
Mild Tremors When Undisturbed	3													
Marked Tremors When Undisturbed	4													
Increased Muscle Tone	2													
Generalized Convulsion	5													
Frantic Sucking of Fists	1													
Poor Feeding	2													
Regurgitation	2													
Projectile Vomiting	3													
Loose Stools	2													
Watery Stools	3													
Dehydration	2													
Frequent Yawning	1													
Sneezing	1													
Nasal Stuffiness	1													
Sweating	1													
Mottling	1													
Fever-Less Than 101°	1													
Fever-Greater Than 101°	2													
Respiratory Rate Over 60/min	1													
Respiratory Rate > 60 With Retractions	2													
Excoriation of Nose	1													
Excoriation of Knees	1													
Excoriation of Toes	1													
Total Hourly Score (Sum over 2 Hours)														

FIGURE 3

NEONATAL ABSTINENCE SCORE

(DAILY SCORE AFTER 48 HOURS)

NAME _____

DATE _____

SIGNS AND SYMPTOMS	SCORE	TIME DATE 2 6 10 2 6 10	COMMENTS	TIME DATE 2 6 10 2 6 10	COMMENTS
High Pitched Cry	2				
Continuous High Pitched Cry	3				
Sleeps Less Than 1 Hour After Feeding	3				
Sleeps Less Than 2 Hours After Feeding	2				
Sleeps Less Than 3 Hours After Feeding	1				
Hyperactive Moro Reflex	2				
Markedly Hyperactive Moro Reflex	3				
Mild Tremors When Disturbed	1				
Marked Tremors When Disturbed	2				
Mild Tremors When Undisturbed	3				
Marked Tremors When Undisturbed	4				
Increased Muscle Tone	2				
Generalized Convulsion	5				
Frantic Sucking of Fists	1				
Poor Feeding	2				
Regurgitation	2				
Projectile Vomiting	3				
Loose Stools	2				
Watery Stools	3				
Dehydration					
Frequent Yawning	1				
Sneezing	1				
Nasal Stuffiness	1				
Sweating	1				
Mottling	1				
Fever-Less Than 101°	1				
Fever-Greater Than 101°	2				
Respiratory Rate Over 60/min.	1				
Respiratory Rate >60 With Retractions	2				
Excoriation of Nose	1				
Excoriation of Knees	1				
Excoriation of Toes	1				
Total Hourly Score (Sum Over 4 Hours)					

TABLE I
Phenobarbital Dosage Schedule According to Abstinence Score

SCORE	PHENOBARBITAL DOSAGE
Score of 8-10	3 mg/lb/day In 3 divided doses
Score of 11-13	4 mg/lb/day In 3 divided doses
Score of 14-16	5 mg/lb/day In 3 divided doses
Score of 17 or above	6 mg/lb/day In 3 divided doses

TABLE II
Amount of Paregoric per Dose as Administered 4 Times Daily According to Abstinence Score

	SCORE				
WEIGHT IN POUNDS	<8	8-10	11-13	14-16	>17
2-2 lbs.15 oz.	0.04cc	0.06cc	0.13cc	0.25cc	0.31cc
3-3 lbs.15 oz.	0.07cc	0.10cc	0.20cc	0.40cc	0.50cc
4-4 lbs.15 oz.	0.10cc	0.14cc	0.27cc	0.55cc	0.69cc
5-5 lbs.15 oz.	0.12cc	0.18cc	0.35cc	0.70cc	0.98cc
6-6 lbs.15 oz.	0.13cc	0.20cc	0.40cc	0.80cc	1.00cc
7-7 lbs.15 oz.	0.15cc	0.23cc	0.47cc	0.95cc	1.18cc
8-8 lbs.15 oz.	0.18cc	0.27cc	0.55cc	1.10cc	1.37cc
9-9 lbs.15 oz.	0.20cc	0.30cc	0.60cc	1.20cc	1.50cc

being controlled by that dose. If the abstinence score of an infant receiving treatment increased to the next level (i.e., 10 to 12), the drug dosage was also increased to the next level (i.e., 4 mg/lb/day). If the infant's score decreased, e.g., from 15 to 12, the drug dosage was lowered to the next level (i.e., 4 mg/lb/day) provided he had been at the previous dosage level for at least two days. If a high score dropped precipitously in response to therapy (i.e., from 16 to 8), the drug dosage was not immediately reduced but rather was lowered gradually over a two-day period in order to prevent an exacerbation of abstinence symptoms. When the score had remained less than "8" for two days, the dosage was reduced to 2 mg/lb/day in 3 divided doses for two days before therapy was discontinued.

Table II describes the dosage level of paregoric used in our study. This amount of paregoric was given four times daily according to the abstinence score. The dosage schedule is similar to the phenobarbital schedule in relating the abstinence score to the variable doses; however, paregoric is prescribed in cc's per pound rather than milligrams per pound. When the abstinence score first fell below "8" in the paregoric-treated infant, the dosage was continued as listed in the first column of the table (<8) in 4 divided doses for two days, and then drug therapy was discontinued.

Large fluctuations may occur in the hourly total scores, especially during the first day of life. Therefore, running averages were used to smooth out the first-day variability. During the first 24 hours, three consecutive hourly totals were averaged to obtain the score. If the average was greater than "8," the infant was treated. If the average was below "8," drug therapy was withheld. On the second day, when scores were recorded every two hours, two successive scores of "8" or above were required before therapy was instituted.

After 48 hours, the infant was scored every four hours. Obviously, if one waits for two scores of more than "8" to occur, the infant may experience abstinence symptoms in the treatable range for an eight-hour period. Therefore, when a score of greater than "8" is recorded after 48 hours, a re-evaluation is performed two hours after the high score. On the basis of these two scores, a decision regarding institution of therapy should be made.

In order to justify the scoring system, four groups of infants were defined for comparison. The first included 37 infants who were born of drug-dependent mothers prior to the development and application of the clinical scoring system (Group 1)[(evaluations of withdrawal symptoms were made by pediatricians and nurses by means of standard clinical methods of observation and recording used in the Newborn Nursery at PGH) (Finnegan, L.P., and MacNew, B.A., 1974)]. The second (Group 2) included the first 37 infants born after the scoring system was devised. Both groups showed a nearly identical distribution in birth weights and in incidence of low birth weight (<2500 grams). The mean birth weight was 2740 grams in Group 1 and 2743 grams in Group 2. The similarities of these two groups are also notable in reference to the clinical severity of abstinence. Group 1 had mild to moderate withdrawal in 74% of cases, whereas in Group 2, 81% had mild to moderate symptomatology. Severe symptoms were seen in 16% of Group 1 and in 14% of Group 2.

The type of drug treatment given each group was compared. It should be noted that in Group 1, three drugs (phenobarbital, paregoric and diazepam) were used as well as combinations of phenobarbital with the other two. In Group 2, only phenobarbital and paregoric were used. The possible effects of the different pharmacologic treatment regimens on Groups 1 and 2 must be considered in any evaluation of the scoring system.

Further validity of the abstinence score was attempted by analyzing data from objective measures of newborn behavior obtained concurrently with the scoring system data. Two studies of nutritive sucking behavior (Kron, R. E., Litt, M., and Finnegan, L. P., 1973; Kron, R.E., and Finnegan, L. P., 1974) were carried out on infants born to mothers enrolled in the Methadone Maintenance Clinic associated with PGH. The behavioral effects of neonatal narcotic abstinence and of various pharmacologic preparations for the abstinence syndrome were monitored by measuring how vigorously the infant sucked milk formula from a special nipple. Sucking rates, sucking pressures, amounts of nutrient consumed, and the percentage of time that the infant sucked during the test feedings were recorded using suitable instrumentation. Behavior reflects CNS activity, and therefore measures of sucking behavior provide quantitative estimates of the infant's level of CNS excitation or depression. Prior reports (Kron, R. E., Stein, M., and Goddard, K. E., 1966; Kron, R. E., Stein, M., Goddard, K. E., and Phoenix, M. D., 1967) have described the usefulness of sucking measures in studying drug effects upon the neonate.

The first sucking study (Kron, R. E., Litt, M., and Finnegan, L. P., 1973) was carried out on 26 newborn infants (Group 3) undergoing withdrawal after *in utero* exposure to maternal methadone addiction. The study was aimed at discovering differences in the behavioral effects produced by pharmacologic agents routinely used in the treatment of the neonatal abstinence syndrome. Group 3 is comparable to Group 1 described above, in that treatment for abstinence was prescribed and monitored by standard clinical approaches (Finnegan, L. P., and MacNew, B. A., 1974) which did not include the use of the abstinence scoring system.

After the development of the abstinence scoring system, a second sucking study (Kron, R. E., and Finnegan, L. P., 1974) was carried out on 38 infants (Group 4) born to methadone-addicted mothers. The goal of this study was to test the comparative efficacy of phenobarbital (a sedative) and paregoric (an opiate) in relieving neonatal abstinence symptoms. Assignment of infants to each drug was made on a strict alternating basis in order to obviate bias in selection of the test population and to ensure adequate numbers in each treatment subgroup.

RESULTS

The assessment of nursing personnel to administer the scoring system revealed an inter-rater reliability coefficient in the four pairs which ranged between 0.75-0.96, with a mean of 0.82. All the reliability coefficients were significant ($P < .005$).

In the group of infants who were *not* assessed by the scoring system (Group 1), less were managed without drug treatment, whereas significantly more of the group utilizing the abstinence score (Group 2) were managed without drug treat-

TABLE III
Mean Sucking Parameters for Groups 3 and 4 According to Treatment Group

TREATMENT		Group 3			Group 4	
	N	Rate, sucks/min.*	Sucking time %**	N	Rate, sucks/min.*	Sucking time %**
Paregoric	4	31.1	22.1	12	29.0	24.2
Phenobarbital	17	19.9	15.6	13	24.1	22.5
No Treatment	5	23.8	14.5	13	24.5	19.0

*Rate = $\dfrac{\text{Total number of sucks}}{\text{Total time available in min.}}$

**% Sucking time = $\dfrac{\text{Total time of active sucking}}{\text{Total time available}} \times 100$

ment (30% versus 46%). The average number of treatment days in Group 1 was greater in contrast to Group 2 (8 versus 6 days). Because fewer infants who were evaluated with the abstinence scoring system received treatment, the average number of hospital days was reduced by nearly 25%.

The sucking data generated by Group 3 indicated that infants who received sedation with phenobarbital or Valium were much more depressed in sucking behavior than those who were treated with paregoric (Table III). Indeed, the paregoric-treated infants showed better sucking performance than those infants who were considered by the nursery pediatrician to require no pharmacologic treatment whatsoever for withdrawal. As with Group 1, the particular treatment drug for abstinence and the dosage schedule were prescribed using standard clinical methods. In addition, the dosage level was determined on the basis of the neonatologist's clinical impression of the infant's arousal state. There was a strong tendency on the part of the nursery staff to treat most of the infants with phenobarbital.

Representative sucking data, including sucking rate and percent of time the infant engaged in active sucking, from Groups 3 and 4, are summarized in Table III. Groups 3 and 4 were further divided into subgroups in order to explore the effects of paregoric, phenobarbital, and "no therapy" in infants undergoing narcotic withdrawal. In both Groups 3 and 4, the paregoric-treated infants sucked at higher rates and sucked a greater percentage of time than those included in the other two subgroups. Reference to Table III indicates that sucking measures for the paregoric subgroups agree closely in those studies which were carried out "before" as well as "after" introduction of the abstinence scoring system. However, the phenobarbital group (though remaining depressed in sucking relative to paregoric-treated infants) increased 20% in sucking measures between the "before" and "after" studies, while the "no treatment" group also increased a comparable amount.

DISCUSSION

The neonatal abstinence score has been defined in order to monitor the passively addicted infant in a more comprehensive and objective way than has previously been described. The results of the inter-rater reliability tests have shown that the method can be taught to nursery personnel, and the level of agreement among raters represents more than two-thirds of the variance in the scores. In order to further improve the reliability of these measures, we plan to carry out multifactorial analyses designed to pinpoint ambiguous and redundant items which may contribute to the error variance. However, even as it is now formulated, the neonatal abstinence score is highly reliable.

It was evident that the infants tended to be poorly regulated by standard clinical methods of observation and recording used in the PGH Newborn Nurseries. It was especially difficult to titrate the dosage of diazepam and phenobarbital, both of which tended to overly sedate the infant. There appeared to be little latitude in the application of these sedative drugs. Concomitant objective measures of feeding behavior (Kron, R. E., Litt, M., and Finnegan, L. P., 1973) confirmed that infants treated with sedatives were significantly less responsive than were those treated with paregoric, an opiate with only minimal sedating side effects.

By relating the dosage schedule of each pharmacologic agent with the abstinence scores, we were able to make more precise clincial estimates of the withdrawal syndrome and to test the comparative usefulness of recommended drug treatments for neonates undergoing abstinence. The scoring method was also useful in following the progression or diminution of symptomatology before, during, and after drug therapy was instituted.

As validation procedures were carried out, it was evident that, *a priori*, the symptom checklist is a valid representation of the abstinence syndrome in the newborn, since it includes all clinically significant symptoms and signs previously described in the literature (Perlstein, M. A., 1947; Goodfriend, M. J., Shey, I. A., and Klein, M. D., 1956; Cobrinik, R. W., Hood, R. T., Jr., and Chusid, E., 1959; Hill, R. M., and Desmond, M. M., 1963; Rosenthal, T., Patrick, S. W., and Krug, D. C., 1964; Zelson, C., Rubio, E., and Wasserman E., 1971), and it is in agreement with our own observations on a large series of neonates born to addict mothers at PGH (currently over 200). The question that must be answered is whether application of such a schema can improve upon standard clinical approaches (Finnegan, L. P., and MacNew, B. A., 1974), and thereby sharpen clinical judgment. For example, can the scoring system lead to better application of therapy or help in evaluating clinical change with greater precision? We have attempted two experimental approaches to validation of the method: first, by comparing a group of infants treated by means of standard, clinical approaches (Group 1) with a second group whose pharmacologic treatment for abstinence was regulated by means of the abstinence scoring system (Group 2). Also, two other groups of infants were studied by means of an objective behaviorial measure which has been found in previous investigations to be capable of monitoring the level of CNS excitation or depression generated by pharmacologic agents administered to the mother during labor. Measures of sucking behavior were carried out on infants undergoing narcotic withdrawal: the first series (Group 3) shows drug therapy regulated by standard clinical procedures, and the second (Group 4) represents treatment given according to the abstinence scoring system. In each case, there were differences between the paired groups that suggested the superiority of the scoring system over the usual clinical judgment. The results suggest that paregoric is a better treatment than phenobarbital for narcotic addiction; however, the improvement in sucking measures for the phenobarbital-treated subgroup in Group 4 as compared to Group 3 reflects the effect of the abstinence score used to prescribe medication for Group 4. Since phenobarbital is a powerful CNS depressant, whereas paregoric is not, imprecision in prescribing dosage levels may depress the sucking measures of the phenobarbital subgroup much more than those of the paregoric subgroup. In Group 4, phenobarbital was prescribed in accordance with the abstinence score, which tended to minimize inadvertent overdosage and thereby improve the sucking measures within the phenobarbital group. The more objective criteria for determining whether treatment was to be given (or not) also tended to raise the relative size and mean sucking scores of the "no treatment" group.

Methods for scoring the narcotic abstinence syndrome have already been described in animals (Goldstein, D. B., and Pal, N., 1970; Goldstein, D. B., and Pal, N., 1971) and in the human adult (Himmelsbach, C. K., 1942). However, a practical method for objectively scoring the abstinence syndrome in the human newborn has been lacking.

Recently, several classification systems for the neonatal abstinence syndrome were proposed (Finnegan, L. P., Connaughton, J. F., Emich, J. P., and Wieland, W. F., 1973; Blinick, G., 1968; Kahn, E. J., Neumann, L. L., and Polk, G. A., 1969; Rajegowda, B. K., Glass, L., Evans, H. E., Maso, G., Swartz, D. P., and LeBlanc, W., 1972). Disadvantages to these methods include the focus on only a few of the abstinence symptoms, a lack of precision in distinguishing levels of abstinence, and the subjectivity involved in grading withdrawal severity. Besides questions regarding validity of such classification systems, in most nurseries, pediatricians with varying levels of experience must evaluate and treat infants undergoing narcotic withdrawal. Therefore, a precise method for observing and scoring the clinical manifestations of abstinence, and upon which therapeutic decisions can be based, is an important contribution to the care of the passively addicted infant.

This report has described a clinically based scoring system which monitors the full spectrum of abstinence symptoms found in the passively addicted infant. At PGH, this new method has proven useful for: (1) rating the severity of narcotic abstinence, (2) regulating drug dosage level during therapy, and (3) comparing the relative efficacy of various pharmacologic agents in the management of the abstinence syndrome. Moreover, it provides a basis for evolving uniform criteria for the evaluation and treatment of the passively addicted neonate. Such standard criteria are necessary if the results from different centers are to be meaningfully compared.

SUMMARY

A scoring system for the neonatal abstinence syndrome has been devised and implemented as both a clinical and investigative tool. The score monitors the passively addicted infant in a more comprehensive and objective fashion, and facilitates a more precise evaluation of the clinical status of the infant undergoing withdrawal. In addition, the scoring system has been applied in research designed to test the comparative usefulness of various pharmacologic agents currently recommended for the neonatal abstinence syndrome, and has been found useful in following the progression and diminution of withdrawal symptomatology before, during, and after therapy. Furthermore, the scoring system provides a basis for developing uniform criteria for the assessment and treatment of the neonate born to the addicted mother.

Notes

This effort was supported in part by Research Grant IROI DA00325-01 from the National Institute for Mental Health, Research Grant HD 06009 from the National Institute for Child Health and Human Development, and Research Grant #1674 from Commonwealth of Pennsylvania.

* This paper was presented in part at the International Symposium on Perinatal Pharmacology in Milan, Italy, June 1974

Requests for reprints should be addressed to Loretta P. Finnegan, M.D., Philadelphia General Hospital, Division of Nurseries, 700 Civic Center Boulevard, Philadelphia, Pennsylvania 19104.

The studies described herein were performed within the Newborn Nurseries of the Philadelphia General Hospital and the laboratories of the Departments of Psychiatry and Pediatrics of the University of Pennsylvania School of Medicine.

We wish to acknowledge the cooperation of Drs. Jacob Schut and Harvey Weiner of the West Philadelphia Mental Health Consortium Methadone Clinic. We are also grateful to the staff of the Newborn Nurseries of the Philadelphia General Hospital for their cooperation and patience in collecting the abstinence score data. In addition, we extend our thanks to Dr. Evelyn Delmelle for her assistance in analyzing the data, to Mrs. Marianne D. Phoenix, R.N., for her aid in collecting and analyzing the sucking data, and to Ms. Janice McGill for the editing and preparation of this essay.

References

Blinick, G. Menstrual function and pregnancy in narcotic addicts treated with methadone. *Nature*, 1968, 219 (5150). 180.

Cobrinik, R. W., Hood, R. T., Jr., and Chusid, E. The effect of maternal narcotic addiction on the newborn infant. *Pediatrics*, 1959, 35 (2). 288-304.

Finnegan, L. P., Connaughton, J. F., Emich, J. P., and Wieland, W. F. Comprehensive care of the pregnant addict and its effect on maternal and infant outcome. *Contemporary Drug Problems*, 1973, I (4). 795-809.

Finnegan, L. P., and MacNew, B.A. Care of the addicted infant. *American Journal of Nursing*, 1974, 74 (4). 685-693.

Goldstein, D. B., and Pal, N. Physical dependence to ethanol in mice. *Pharmacologist*, 1970, 12 (2). 276.

Goldstein, D. B., and Pal, N. Alcohol dependence produced in mice by inhalation of ethanol: grading the withdrawal reaction. *Science*, 1971, 172 (3980). 288-290.

Goodfriend, M. J., Shey, I. A., and Klein, M.D. The effect of maternal narcotic addiction on the newborn. *American Journal of Obstetrics and Gynecology*, 1956, 71 (1). 29-36.

Hill, R. M., and Desmond, M. M. Management of the narcotic withdrawal syndrome in the neonate. *Pediatric Clinics of North America*, 1963, 10 (1). 67-86.

Himmelsbach, C. K. Studies on the addiction liability of "Demerol" (D-140). *Journal of Pharmacology and Experimental Therapeutics*, 1942, 75 (1). 64-68.

Kahn, E. J., Neumann, L. L., and Polk, G. A. The course of heroin withdrawal syndrome in newborn infants treated with phenobarbital or chlorpromazine. *The Journal of Pediatrics,* 1969, 75 (3). 495-500.

Kron, R. E., and Finnegan, L. P. Effect of maternal narcotic addiction on sucking behavior of neonates. *Proceedings of the Committee on Problems of Drug Dependence of the National Research Council,* 1974, 731-735.

Kron, R. E., Litt, M., and Finnegan, L. P. Behavior of infants born to narcotic addicted mothers. *Proceedings of the Committee on Problems of Drug Dependence of the National Research Council,* 1973, 270-281,

Kron, R. E., Stein, M., and Goddard, K. E. Newborn sucking behavior affected by obstetric sedation. *Pediatrics,* 1966, 37 (6). 1012-1016.

Kron, R. E., Stein, M., Goodard, K. E., and Phoenix, M.D. Effect of nutrient upon the sucking behavior of newborn infants. *Psychosomatic Medicine,* 1967, 29 (1). 24-32.

Nathenson, G., Golden, G. S., and Litt, I. F. Diazepam in neonatal narcotic withdrawal syndrome. *Pediatrics,* 1971, 48 (4). 523-527.

Perlstein, M. A. Congenital morphinism: a rare cause of convulsions in the newborn. *Journal of the American Medical Association,* 1947, 135 (10). 633.

Rajegowda, B. K., Glass, L., Evans, H. E., Maso, G., Swartz, D. P., and LeBlanc, W. Methadone withdrawal in newborn infants. *The Journal of Pediatrics,* 1972, 81 (3). 532-534.

Reddy, A. M., Harper, R. G., and Stern, G. Observations on heroin and methadone withdrawal in the newborn. *Pediatrics,* 1971, 48 (3). 353-358.

Rosenthal, T., Patrick, S. W., and Krug, D. C. Congenital neonatal narcotic addiction: a natural history. *American Journal of Public Health,* 1964, 54 (8). 1252-1262.

Schiff, D., Chan, G., and Stern, L. Fixed drug combinations and the displacement of bilirubin from albumin. *Pediatrics,* 1971, 48 (1). 139-141.

Statzer, D. E., and Wardell, J. N. Heroin addiction in pregnancy. *American Journal of Obstetrics and Gynecology,* 1972, 113 (2). 273-278.

Zelson, C., Rubio, E., and Wasserman, E. Neonatal narcotic addiction: 10 year observation. *Pediatrics,* 1971, 48 (2). 179-189.

DISCUSSION

Q. *Dr. Kahn*: I think you and your colleagues should be commended for trying to get this into some type of quantitative measure to evaluate efficacy of therapy. I would like to broaden the discussion just a little bit. I have never really understood the pharmacologic rationale, in any event, of using other than narcotics to treat neonatal withdrawal. We all know from animal and human studies that you can suppress withdrawal syndrome very nicely by using a narcotic and replacing the drug. This extends to other drug classes as well. Have you ever used anything like methadone? The reason I ask the question is that we know paregoric is tincture of opium—camphorated—and camphor is a stimulant. In your analysis, do you see phenobarbital and diazepam as being more of a depressant? Do you think the better, more active newborn is the result of having camphor in paregoric? Could methadone accomplish the same thing?

A. *Dr. Finnegan: First of all, let me say that whenever I discuss this, I always get the same question. In answer to the first part—"Why do we use phenobarbital?"—Pharmacologically, this does not seem appropriate, but as pediatricians, in newborn nurseries we have used phenobarbital for many years, and have felt very comfortable with this drug in any infant who has CNS irritation. This is the* reason for such wide usage of this drug in newborn nurseries for infants in withdrawal. As far as the paregoric is concerned, there is a definite risk here concerning use of the camphor. The reason we chose these two drugs is that this is what pediatricians are using, and we felt that to use something different, such as a pure tincture of opium, would not really identify with what pediatricians are presently using. I think that our next step in this, then, is to go on to a drug such as methadone and a pure tincture of opium, and perhaps include some of the other drugs that are being used, such as the tranquilizers.

Q. *Dr. Neumann:* I have a question about the scoring system itself. Do you have a quantitative evaluation of each item? Is it a yes or no answer to each observation?

A. *Dr. Finnegan: No.*

Q. *Dr. Neumann:* I wonder if that is not a limitation. If a single symptom is more or less severe, does it get scored the same?

A. *Dr. Finnegan: No. for example, in Figure 1, tremors get different values according to whether they occur when the child is disturbed, or when he is not disturbed. If they do occur under those two conditions, are they mild or are they severe? So there are four different ways that you can classify tremors. Similarly, for high-pitched crying, is it present intermittently or is it continuously there?*

Q. *Dr. Kandall:* Do you have any data on the prognostic implications of the scoring system? Have you compiled anything to prognosticate whether babies with higher scores in the beginning will have worse outcomes in the long term?

A. *Dr. Finnegan: You are talking about long-term follow-up, I assume. The only way we have looked at this is according to a classification of mild, moderate, severe, and no withdrawal; and not actually correlating the scoring system per se. For example, the definition for us is very similar to what Dr. Connaughton presented this morning. That is, "no withdrawal" is a "Class I"—child born to an addicted mother with no withdrawal symptomatology. The second class is what we call mild withdrawal—withdrawal that does not necessitate therapy. Class III—moderate withdrawal necessitating therapy for 2 weeks, Class IV— severe withdrawal necessitating therapy for 2 weeks. Of course, these infants were not treated according to the scoring system, since I am talking about patients that were viewed prior to its initiation. Fifty infants, three quarters of which had Class II or III, had normal neurological examinations, and comparable developmental examinations (evaluated by Gesell's schedule) to controls. They did seem to be significantly smaller in height and weight in comparison to our control infants. (These infants were seen in follow-up between 6 and 41 months of age.)*

Q. *Dr. Davis:* How do you apply the scoring criteria, provided the home situation is a factor?

A. *Dr. Finnegan: The scoring system is applied until two days after we stop the therapy and we have found, in general, that the babies are ready to go home after that; and do not need further therapy. In other words, we stop the therapy* *according to the scoring system as we reduce the dosage. Two days after the drug is stopped, we continue to score the baby; and if the scores do not rise above eight, we send the baby home. Usually they are down to a score of one, two, or three, which means the baby, just as Dr. Desmond described, frequently has a few tremors, and is a little irritable, but certainly does not need hospital care. We counsel the mother as far as doing the various things that Dr. Desmond describes, such as swaddling, demand feeding the child, and things of this sort.*

Q. *Dr. Davis:* Have you found return of the withdrawal symptoms?

A. *Dr. Finnegan: Yes, in a few babies, and I am talking now of less than five babies in over two hundred which we have seen. In these, symptoms have returned and have been fairly severe. Half of these were before the scoring system was used and a couple of those were admitted to the hospital. One of those, I might add, had meningitis and the other was probably having withdrawal.*

Q. *Dr. Glass:* I would like to make one brief comment about the effect of phenobarbital on respiratory performance of these infants. We found in our series that phenobarbital in a dose of about seven or eight mg per kilo opium per day, primarily orally, did not affect the respiratory rate. In spite of this therapeutic dose, the abstinence-induced tachypnea did not occur, and a median of about 70 respirations per minute persisted throughout the first week of life, in spite of phenobarbital treatment during this period.

Q. *Dr. Ostrea:* I would like to know when you do your scoring—is there a specific time of day? And suppose you get a score of eight? Do you, once it reaches that magic number of eight, automatically treat, or does she have to have an eight for three observations?

A. *Dr. Finnegan: When we first started the scoring system, we found that scores varied greatly over a short period of time. To eliminate this problem, on the first day we determine the necessity for treatment based on three scores. Babies are scored every hour in the first day of life, so that when they have three scores that are eight, or averaged to be above eight, we would then treat them. On the second day, we used two scores. After that, if they should have a late withdrawal, we again observe them every two hours for two scores, because they can have a transient high score. This happens with infants on whom, for example, the resident has just done a septic work-up, and the nurse subsequently does the scoring, not knowing that the septic work-up has been done. Obviously, if you took any baby at that time, he would be quite irritable, and perhaps would not fare well. This is why we look at the variables, so that we do not inadvertently treat a child who does not need it. It is amazing that some babies need so few days of treatment. We did not realize this before, because we did not observe them as frequently in this fashion.*

Addictive Diseases: an International Journal 2 (1): 159-168 (1975)

Acute Management of Neonatal Addiction

CARL ZELSON
*Department of Pediatrics,
New York Medical College at
Metropolitan Hospital Center,
New York, New York*

Because of the rapid increase in the incidence of drug addiction among the adult population in the area surrounding our hospital during the past fifteen years, we have had the opportunity of observing and caring for a large number of passively addicted infants born to drug-addicted mothers.

During the five years prior to the onset of our study—1955 to 1959—there were only 22 infants born to drug-addicted mothers at our institution. In 1960 we noted a very marked increase in the number of births of these infants. Twenty-six infants were born to drug-addicted mothers during that year (one out of every 164 births).

In each of the succeeding years, the number of such births has increased at our hospital in spite of a progressive drop in the birth rate. In 1972 one in every 27 births was to a drug-addicted mother, more than a sixfold increase. In 1973, for the first time in 14 years, there was a decrease in the proportion of drug-addicted infants born; in 1974, one in every 29 births was to a drug-addicted mother. The progression of increase has been noted in many large municipal hospitals throughout the country.

During the early years of our study, heroin was the drug most frequently used. In recent years, maternal ingestion of methadone has become the more frequent drug used, obtained either in a "methadone maintenance program" or bought on the street. The abstinence syndrome, in our experience, occurs with equal frequency in both groups of infants. We found, as have others (Reddy, et al, 1971; Rajegowda et al, 1972; and Zelson et al, 1973) that the abstinence syndrome in the neonates born to methadone-addicted mothers is more severe and more difficult to control than the withdrawal in infants born to heroin-addicted mothers.

Between 70 to 90% of all infants born to mothers addicted to heroin or methadone will manifest signs of withdrawal. Some infants may show only very mild signs, whereas others may show severe signs. Why some infants do not develop signs of withdrawal is not known. Severity, but not frequency of withdrawal, does not necessarily relate to dosage intake or to serum levels of methadone (Inturissi, 1974; and Rosen et al, 1974). We have observed mothers who had a history of heavy and long-term usage of heroin, but whose infants showed no signs of withdrawal. We have also observed infants in withdrawal who were born to mothers taking only minimal amounts of heroin. We have, on several occasions, observed mothers who developed withdrawal signs, but their offspring showed no clinical evidence of withdrawal. We have observed infants who, in spite of the presence of morphine, quinine, or methadone in their urine, did not manifest any evidence of clinical withdrawal. At the present time we cannot explain these facts. It has been stated, however, and generally accepted, I believe, that chronic exposure to the addictive drugs produces physiologic changes that result in altered cellular reactivity. How this relates to the clinical signs is not known. Cochin and Kornetsky, (1968) have demonstrated in animals that behavioral changes, drug-seeking tendencies, and tolerance persist long after detoxification. Another indication that some physiologic change has occurred is demonstrated by our studies of sleep patterns that were done in over 90 of these infants. We have found that the sleep patterns of every infant born to drug-addicted mothers is abnormal, even though some of these infants showed no clinical evidence of withdrawal.

The clinical picture of the abstinence syndrome in the newborn infant is, I am sure, familiar to all of you. This condition, once seen, can be easily recognized thereafter. It is imperative that all personnel involved with the care of the neonate should be familiar with the condition and be able to recognize it when it occurs. Conditions that might present with similar clinical findings such as intracranial injury, tetany, hypoglycemia, and meningitis must be ruled out in the differential diagnosis. Drug addiction is not a simple problem. In the adult, addiction is characterized by psychologic dependence, tolerance, and physical dependence, and in treating the condiion, all three factors must be taken into consideration. In the newborn infant, however, we are dealing only with physical dependence and this may be the reason that the clinical response to treatment is so good.

The infants will usually manifest signs of withdrawal within the first 48 hours of life; a few will have their onset of signs as late as 96 hours of age, and on occasion, particularly infants of methadone addicts may manifest signs of withdrawal later. We have observed several infants born to methadone-addicted mothers who presented with mild signs of withdrawal within the first 48 hours of life, but who seven to 10 days later, suddenly developed severe signs of withdrawal. We have seen no infants who first manifested signs of withdrawal beyond 10 days of age.

Approximately one-third of the infants showing signs of withdrawal can be managed conservatively and will require no treatment. The remainder of these infants will show increasing severity and increasing number of signs of withdrawal, and should be treated. What criteria should we use as an indication for the need for treatment? As of now, no clear-cut objective scoring system has been widely accepted to indicate the level of severity at which treatment should be initiated. Each investigator has his or her own criteria for mild, moderate, and severe withdrawal, and who, on the basis of their experience rather than any specific "score of severity," will decide when to treat. Since the criteria for treatment by each investigator are different, data reported by the various groups until now cannot be compared. Several scoring systems have been suggested, but in our opinion, these have not been objective enough for use for group comparison.

As part of the entire problem in treating neonatal narcotic addiction, a good deal of effort must go into the treatment of the mother, with medical support and treatment, psychological help, and complete and honest information as to the effect of her addiction on herself and her infant. She must be handled with patience and consideration. The investigative group must continue to keep contact with the mother with supportive help after her discharge from the hospital.

At the present time, the treatment of acute narcotic withdrawal in the infant is basically quite simple, and, on the surface, the reults are excellent. I do not, however, believe at this time that the relief and correction of clinical signs of withdrawal is the answer to the problem of addiction. We are only relieving the external evidence of the condition. Further study and prolonged follow-up may eventually help us correct the condition completely.

All infants born to drug-addicted mothers should be admitted to an intensive care area for careful observation. The infant should be maintained, preferably, in an incubator, and undressed except for a diaper. In this manner the infant can be watched more carefully and the onset of signs of withdrawal can be recognized early. The infant should be evaluated at four-hour intervals. If signs of withdrawal become evident, evaluation should be repeated at one- to two-hour intervals. Blood specimens should be obtained for levels of electrolytes, blood sugar, blood gases and pH to rule out such conditions as hypocalcemia, hypoglycemia, and any abnormality of the homeostatic mechanisms. Where indicated, blood cultures to rule out sepsis should be done.

Urine should be collected as soon after birth as possible and examined for the presence of morphine sulfate, quinine, and methadone, and other commonly abused drugs.

TREATMENT

Once the diagnosis of the withdrawal syndrome is made and the condition is clearly delineated from other causes that could possibly produce a similar clinical condition, treatment must be considered. In institutions where few such infants are seen, I would suggest starting treatment rather than waiting for possible progression of the signs of withdrawal. In institutions familiar and experienced with this problem, observation should be continued until the criteria that have been set as indication for therapy are fulfilled. Since as many as 30% of the infants who manifest signs of withdrawal show only mild signs and will recover spontaneously within a short period of time, these infants will certainly not require treatment. However, once treatment is started, medication must be given in sufficient dosage so that conditions can be controlled quickly. Numerous drugs have been recommended, but there still is no one drug that is specific.

Narcotics, sedatives, and tranquilizers have been the drugs of choice. Each observer uses the drug with which he is most familiar. Thus far, there have been no controlled comparative studies of these various drugs on the basis of identical criteria. Drugs most frequently used are: 1) paregoric given in doses of 3 to 8 drops at 3- or 4-hour intervals with increasing or decreasing dosage as the clinical picture indicates; 2) phenobarbital is given in the dosage of 5-8 mgs/kg/24hrs, by mouth or injection, divided into 3 daily doses; 3) Valium has recently been recommended and is being used in doses of ½ to 1 mg given at 6- to 8-hour intervals; 4) chlorpromazine in doses of 2.2 mgs/kg/24 hours given orally or by injection in 4 divided doses daily.

Paregoric, I believe, should not be used except under special conditions. We must remember that in the infant, after months of intrauterine exposure to a narcotic drug, some type of an abnormal physiologic change has occurred, probably at the cell level. With the use of paregoric, there is a continuation and perhaps an accentuation of the abnormal physiologic change. Frequently, large doses of paregoric must be given to control the signs of withdrawal. This, in turn, can produce marked constipation and, at times, deep depression of the infant. Treatment for the complete control of signs of withdrawal may extend over a long period of time. We use this drug only when diarrhea is part of the withdrawal syndrome.

Phenobarbital is also effective in controlling the signs of withdrawal. Although it is used with great frequency, we have had no extensive experience with this drug. Since phenobarbital may have a depressing effect on the respiratory center, respiratory depression can occur; laryngospasm has been reported with its use. Furthermore, it will not stop the vomiting that so commonly occurs among these infants. We use phenobarbital only when seizure activity occurs during the withdrawal syndrome.

Valium is the most recent of the drugs advocated for use in treating the neonatal abstinence syndrome. This drug was originally introduced for the treatment of anxiety, skeletal muscle spasm, for combating alcoholism and for the control of status epilepticus. We have had no experience with this drug when used for the neonatal narcotic abstinence syndrome. It has been reported that the side effects are minimal and that the period of treatment necessary to control the syndrome is comparatively short—5 to 7 days at the most. However, it has been shown that, in large doses, this drug can produce apnea, bradycardia, thrombophlebitis, hypotension and cardiac arrest. It is not recommended for use when jaundice is present since the solvent contains 5% sodium benzoate, a chemical which competes with bilirubin for the albumin binding sites, and thus may possibly increase the hyperbilirubinemia and the complications which go with this condition. It has been recommended that when given intravenously, it should be followed by a saline flush of the vein. Further experience with this drug must be obtained before it can be recommended for the routine use in the treatment of the withdrawal syndrome. We have used Valium intravenously to control convulsive seizures in the newborn.

Chlorpromazine has been our drug of choice for therapy. This drug has been shown to have sedative, hypnotic and anticonvulsant properties with little or no untoward reactions. It has a stabilizing effect on the autonomic system and a relaxant effect of the smooth muscles. All of these actions are opposite to the effects resulting from the use of morphine and heroin. In the adult, the patient is more amenable to psychotherapy. We have used chlorpromazine in the treatment of about 300 newborn infants born to narcotic-addicted mothers who manifested moderate to severe signs of withdrawal. The response at our hands has been excellent. The infants relax and fall into quiet sleep. They sleep from feeding to feeding and can be easily aroused; tremors are controlled unless the infant is disturbed; they feed well, and vomiting, if present, is controlled. No ill effects have been seen. Jaundice has not occurred as a complication. Sisson et. al., (1974) in a study of sleep patterns done on infants of drug-addicted mothers (addicted to both heroin and methadone) before and during treatment with chlorpromazine, have shown that the abnormal sleep patterns present in these infants before treatment were completely corrected by this drug.

With each of the drugs used, when signs of withdrawal are under control, the same dosage level should be maintained for a period of 1 to 3 days before a gradual tapering off of the dose is started. Should signs of withdrawal recur during the tapering, the dose must be increased to the previous level and maintained until it is evident that a decrease in the dose can be started again. It is difficult to determine how long a period of therapy will be needed. If clinical control is evident, the infant is slowly weaned off the drug, usually over a period of 5 to 7 days. We have found that about 50% of the infants will be treated for 10 to 20 days, 25% of the infants will be treated for less than 10 days, and 25% of the infants will be treated up to 40 days before complete control can be obtained.

Feeding difficulties, respiratory distress, aspiration pneumonia and other infections or dehydration and acidosis may occur among these infants. These complications must be watched for and treated with accepted routines as quickly as possible and with all necessary modalities.

In conclusion, we consider that adequate management requires:

1. Good cooperation between Obstetrics, Pediatrics and the Social Service Department.
2. Signs of withdrawal should be recognizable by nurses and doctors in the nursery.
3. Treatment, when necessary, should be started early and that dosage should be adequate to control signs.
4. Fluids should be adequate to prevent dehydration.
5. Infants should be watched carefully so that complications can be recognized and treated early.

Adequate treatment is indicated by:

1. Decrease or complete control of clinical signs.
2. Ability of infant to sleep from feeding to feeding.
3. Infant must show no untoward reaction to the drug used.
4. Infant must take feedings well with no vomiting or diarrhea.

Notes

Requests for reprints should be addressed to Carl Zelson, M.D., 71 Bennett's Farm Road, Ridgefield, Connecticut 06877.

This paper was supported by research grant MC-R-360049-02-00 from the Maternal and Child Health and Crippled Children's Services, U.S. Dept. of Health, Education and Welfare.

References

Inturissi, Personal Communication.

Rajegowda, B.K., Glass, L., Evans, H.E. et al. Methadone withdrawal in newborn infants. *Journal of Pediatrics*, 1972, *81*, 532-534.

Reddy, A.M., Harper, R.G., and Stern, G. Observations on heroin and methadone withdrawal in the newborn, *Pediatrics*, 1971, *48*, 353-358.

Rosen, T.S., and Pippenger, C.E. Neonatal withdrawal syndrome: correlation with plasma methadone concentration and maternal methadone dosage, *Pediatric Research Obst*, 1974, *8*, No. 4, p. 92.

Sisson, T.R.C., Wickler, M., Pieng, T., and Rao, I.P. Effect of narcotic withdrawal on neonatal sleep patterns, *Pediatric Research*, 1974, *8*, abstract, p. 177.

Wikler, A. (ed). *Addictive States*, Baltimore, Williams and Wilkins, 1968, Chapter 20.

Zelson, C., Lee, S.J., and Caslino, M. Neonatal narcotic addiction: comparative effects of maternal intake of heroin and methadone, *New England Journal of Medicine*, 1973, *289*, 1216-1220.

DISCUSSION

Q. *Dr. Harbison:* It has been suggested that the severity of withdrawal is dependent on the last dosage that the mother received and the time at which she received it. When you compare adverse reactions or severity of withdrawal in methadone and heroin babies, were the dosages the babies received comparable? You reported methadone babies had more severe withdrawal, but they may have been exposed to higher dosages of drugs. Were the dosages comparable?

A. *Dr. Zelson: No, I do not think so.*

Q. *Dr. Harbison:* So that is not really a valid comparison?

A. *Dr. Zelson: Actually not from that point of view, but I can say this. We found that the signs of withdrawal in methadone babies did not relate to the actual dosage. We found that, for instance, babies who were born of mothers who were on levels below 50 mg had fewer signs of withdrawal, and groups above 100 mg also had fewer signs of withdrawal; and that most of the babies that had problems were babies born to mothers who were on levels of between 50 and 100 mg. The actual dose that the heroin mothers took, of course, is very difficult to estimate. We have to judge on the basis of the number of bags taken, and we never know what the bags contained. Therefore, we cannot give you a differential on that.*

Q. *Dr. Harbison:* You said that none of the infants had withdrawal signs for longer than 10 days.

A. *Dr. Zelson: No, none of the babies developed signs beyond the tenth day in our experience.*

Q. *Dr. Harbison:* With the use of the chlorpromazine, with the reports of increased susceptibility of the newborn to the extrapyramidal symptoms, how can you differentially diagnose the extrapyramidal symptoms that might be produced by the chlorpromazine versus the increased muscular activity and rigidity that might be a sign or symptom of the withdrawal syndrome?

A. *Dr. Zelson: First of all, we have never found extrapyramidal symptoms in the babies that we treated with chlorpromazine. The doses are comparatively small. The patients that have been reported with extrapyramidal symptoms were those whose mothers were given chlorpromazine or phenothiazine. The babies born to these mothers did develop extrapyramidal signs.*

Q. *Dr. Braude:* You mentioned that the sleep pattern of every infant born to drug-addicted mothers is abnormal. How abnormal is it—is it an increase in REM sleep?

A. *Dr. Zelson: It is definitely an increase in REM sleep. As a matter of fact, REM sleep in babies born to methadone mothers was even worse. The first case that we had was a baby that had been born to a methadone mother. That baby had no quiet sleep at all. The entire sleep pattern was all REM.*

Q. *Dr. Harper:* In your studies where you have reported that those babies born to methadone—maintained mothers had more severe withdrawal, has multiple drug abuse been ruled out on the basis of the urine studies, or on the basis of blood studies?

A. *Dr. Zelson: Well, 53 percent of our babies' urines were positive either for morphine, quinine, or methadone. We had a few who had barbiturates in their urine.*

Q. *Dr. Harper:* If you had such a high percentage that had more than just methadone in their urine, how can you implicate methadone as the causative drug that produced more severe withdrawal?

A. *Dr. Zelson: I am not saying that each one was present; I am saying that one of the three was definitely present in that high a percentage.*

Q. *Dr. Harper:* Why is it that you do not feel that what you are really seeing is the result of multiple drug abuse rather than just methadone?

A. *Dr. Zelson: Firstly, we did not know the dosage of the various drugs that were being taken; and secondly, the signs of withdrawal with phenobarbital do not manifest themselves in the early days of life. These usually do not start until the third, fourth, or fifth day of life. Many times the baby is sent home, and the signs of withdrawal from phenobarbital will become evident when the baby is at home. I do not believe that the phenobarbital relates to withdrawal in the early days.*

A. *Dr. Kron: We have some data that might be helpful to explicating Dr. Zelson's findings. We have been using measures of sucking behavior comparing both street addicts and methadone patients, as well as different types of methadone patients; those who have been attending methadone clinics for long periods of time, for years and longer, those who entered the program late in their pregnancy, and those entering rather early in their pregnancy. We have found a significant correlation between the sucking behavior of infants born to these three groups of addicts, and the length of time they have been on methadone. There also is a correlation between sucking behavior and the dosage of methadone prescribed. Now, it is quite clear that there are confounding factors, mainly the dosages of varieties of mixtures that addicts do take. However, there is such a clear correlation between the length of time in the program and the dosage of methadone that this must be taken into account as at least one of the contributing factors to altered behavior as observed in the neonatal period. We have also found differences in the sucking behavior of infants born to street addicts, as I said, and methadone addicts.*

Of course, here is the confounding influence of the variety of drugs that the addicts may be taking, both methadone and the street addicts. They account for the differential sucking behavior, as well as the fact that the methadone addict is being assured of a steady dose of a very potent pharmacologic agent, while the street addict is taking "pot luck," never sure of what the dosage is of those bags of heroin she is purchasing on the street. Similarly, she does not know the particular capsules or pills that she also is acquiring. So, we do have these data that do support some of Dr. Zelson's contentions and we will talk about that tomorrow. But we do have some question also regarding some other assertions that Dr. Zelson has made about the greater efficacy of one treatment approach versus another. In our experience in Philadelphia, using measures of early adaptive behavior, such as sucking behavior, plus a variety of other measures which are involved in the technique which we will describe tomorrow, the Brazelton

Neonatal Assessment, we have found that all of the drugs that we have used, except for the opiates, do have a significant depressant effect upon adapted behavior. Now, it may be that this depressant effect is interpreted by the clinician, as Dr. Zelson suggested, that he was pleased to see the babies sleeping from feeding to feeding. Now, indeed, this may represent an improved form of response from the point of view of the clinician or the person working in the nursery. The babies are quieter. However, it is a link in our experience with a decrease in certain adaptive functions, which may be necessary for normal development during the neonatal period, including adaptation to spontaneous nutritive sucking.

A. *Dr. Zelson: I have been very much impressed by your work on the "sucking" reflex. Unfortunately, we have been unable to do any of this until now. And I agree with you that this would be very helpful. The only other thing that I would like to say is, that, certainly in our experience, we are not convinced that the dose that is given in a methadone-maintenance program is the dose that the women are taking. Because after a great deal of discussion with these patients, many of them admit that they have been buying methadone on the street and using it in conjunction with what they are getting in the maintenance program. I know work has been done to show that the clinical signs of withdrawal certainly are not related to the serum levels of methadone, as shown by a number of observers.*

Q. *Dr. Hug:* Just to belabor a point a bit, you did say that none of the drugs have proven to be specific, but going along a bit with the comments from Dr. Kron, I think that there is adequate data in animals to show that rather specific depression of abstinence syndrome can be accomplished with any of the narcotics. If you are to do it with the barbiturates or tranquilizers, you usually require quite large doses and you suppress all activity. Now, my point is that you made one specific comment that interested me, and that was that with chlorpromazine you find relatively normal sleep patterns. By implication, I gather, with paregoric treatment you do not?

A. *Dr. Zelson: I did not do these studies; they were done by Dr. Sisson in Philadelphia.*

Q. *Dr. Hug:* Has he tested paregoric?

A. *Dr. Zelson: No, I do not think so.*

Q. *Dr. Hug:* Because, again, I bring up the issue of the camphor being present. I am at a disadvantage and I cannot remember. One time I sat down and calculated the dose of camphor you can get with this, and it is considerable. Obviously, we do not know the sensitivity of the newborn as compared to some of the other species or even man, in terms of sensitivity of this particular stimulant. But I think there is good, solid evidence to support a rationale for using narcotic to suppress abstinence syndrome, and then tapering the narcotic. I shall be very interested to hear your comments tomorrow. Dr. Kron just handed me the paregoric recipe, and there are 380 mg of camphor in a 100 milliliters. Now all I have to do is to figure that out. That is three mg per milliliter and get that down into drops, I guess. Thank you.

A. *Dr. Zelson: I am sure that paregoric is effective, and when we first started our study we did use paregoric. I am not convinced and I feel very uncomfortable giving a narcotic to a newborn over a prolonged period of time. Because what you are doing is accentuating the exposure that the babies have in utero to the narcotic. Whether it is going to increase the problem or not, I cannot say. All I know is that you do have a definite cellular change; there is no question about it. The metabolic change, whether it is at the cell level or whether it is somewhere in the brain, I cannot say. All I can tell you is that if a drug addict is given a "cold turkey," and he has not been able to get to it for months or years; if he starts taking drugs again within a period of one to two weeks, he can tolerate the level that he had been tolerating maybe even ten years ago. So that there is definite evidence that it is bad to give a narcotic. The other thing is that we have a number of studies in which we show that there are certain abnormalities that are present in the babies who are given methadone, rather than heroin. Sweating response is marked in the heroin addict; and is not as marked in the methadone baby. The sleep patterns are absolutely different. We have now found that even the renal function is different between methadone-and heroin-treatment babies. Sodium excretion in the methadone baby is markedly increased; in a heroin baby, sodium excretion is perfectly normal. So that continuing to give the drug is, I think, absolutely wrong.*

Q. *Dr. Kron:* Just a brief rebuttal, and that is, that I think somebody asked, "What are our objectives in treating these babies?" I think the first objective is to stabilize them as far as physical dependence is concerned, so that he can handle the other stresses of the newborn period. And again from human studies, I think the stabilization is best achieved with the narcotic. True, you are going to perpetuate his physical dependence, maybe reestablish some degree of tolerance, but at that point, a slow, gradual withdrawal can be accomplished, and I think, again with a minimum of stress to the infant.

Q. *Dr. Davis:* Valium has been the drug used almost exclusively for the withdrawal symptom at our hospital. In about 140 babies within the last two and one-half years, it has been used without untoward effect, and in lower doses as Dr. Nathenson has explained.

A. *Dr. Zelson: I can tell you that sleep patterns are not changed by treatment. The sleep patterns continue abnormally even after the baby has gone through withdrawal, has been treated, and seemed perfectly all right. The sleep patterns remain abnormal.*

Addictive Diseases: an International Journal 2 (1): 169-178 (1975)
© 1975 by Spectrum Publications, Inc.

Disposition of Methadone and its Relationship to Severity of Withdrawal in the Newborn

TOVE S. ROSEN
CHARLES E. PIPPENGER
Deparments of Pediatrics and Neurology
Columbia University,
College of Physicians and Surgeons
New York, New York

INTRODUCTION

In recent years an increasing number of infants born to drug-addicted mothers have been seen in our hospitals (Reddy, 1971; Zelson, 1971; Zelson, 1973; Stone, 1971; and Rajegowda, 1972). Whereas in the past most of these infants were born to heroin-addicted mothers, at present more are born to mothers who take methadone either alone or in combination with heroin or other drugs (Zelson, 1973). These mothers seem to have better prenatal care and nutrition than heroin addicts (Blatman, 1970; Newman, 1974; Cohen, 1973), but when one compares the effects of heroin and methadone on the newborn there appears to be no improvement in neonatal morbidity (Reddy, 1971; Zelson, 1973; Rajegowda, 1972; Cohen, 1973). Because of this we have begun a study of the pharmacokinetics of methadone in the newborn. For this purpose, a gas chromatographic micro-assay was developed by modifying the method of Inturrisi and Verebely (1972). We then investigated 1) the placental transfer of methadone from the mother to her newborn; 2) the relationship of neonatal plasma methadone concentration to withdrawal symptomatology; and 3) the relationship between maternal methadone dose and severity of neonatal withdrawal.

METHODS

During the period from July 1973 to July 1974 every mother entering the labor-delivery suite who was on methadone maintenance was entered into our study. Careful histories were obtained from the mother regarding drug use. Maternal blood was drawn into an EDTA or heparin anticoagulated tube as close to delivery as possible. A maternal urine sample was also collected at this time for drug screening. At delivery, 5 cc of cord blood was obtained. On the day of birth and/or day one of life .75-1 cc of neonatal blood was collected by heel stick into an EDTA anticoagulated tube. Subsequent samples were drawn daily for 5 days thereafter. The blood was centrifuged and the plasma was extracted. Twenty-four-hour collections of urine were obtained for three days starting on the day of birth. A record of urine volume was kept. The plasma and urine were frozen for subsequent methadone analysis. To screen for multiple drug abuse, maternal and/or neonatal urine samples were screened using the EMIT (Enzyme Immunoassay) system (Rubenstein, 1972). Infants were examined daily by the same neonatologist, and any signs of withdrawal (graded from absent to severe) and other pertinent findings were noted.

Plasma and urine methadone concentrations were analyzed by our modification of the gas chromatographic method of Inturrisi and Verebely (1972) using .2 ml of plasma or a 1 ml aliquot of urine. The method is as follows:

Chemicals and Reagents

Crystalline L-methadone was used to prepare all standards. The metabolites of methadone, 2 ethylene 1,5 dimethyl-3,3 diphenyl pyrrolidine as the perchlorate salt (Metabolite 1) and 2 ethyl 5 methyl-3,3 diphenyl pyrrolidine as the hydrochloride (Metabolite 2) were supplied by Dr. H. R. Sullivan of Lilly Research Laboratories. The internal standard, β-diethylaminoethyldiphenylpropylacetate (SKF 525A) was supplied by Smith, Kline, and French Laboratories. Glass distilled N-butyl chloride (Burdick and Jackson), spectrograde chloroform and n-hexane (Fisher) were utilized for extraction. All other solvents were reagent grade.

Stock Solutions

Methadone was dissolved in an appropriate volume of ethyl acetate to prepare a 4 ng/ml solution. The internal standard (SKF 525A) stock solution contained 20 ng/ml of ethyl acetate. Both were kept refrigerated at 4°C.

Sample preparation from plasma or whole blood

Into a 15 ml centrifuge tube previously siliconized with dichloromethylsilicone (Pierce Chemical Co.) 0.2 ml plasma was added, followed by 0.05 ml SKF 525A stock solution, 0.5 ml Delory and King's carbonate-bicarbonate buffer (Biochemical J., 39: 245, 1945) as a 1 M solution at pH = 9.8, and 1 drop of octyl alcohol. This was extracted with 5 ml N-butyl chloride by shaking for 5 minutes and centrifuging for 5 minutes at 2600 rpm. The N-butyl chloride layer (upper phase) was carefully transferred to another set of siliconized tubes. This was extracted with 3 ml 0.25 N HC1 by shaking for 10 minutes and centrifuging for 5 minutes (2600 rpm). The upper layer was discarded. The lower layer was washed with 2 ml n-hexane by shaking for 4 minutes and centrifuging for 4 minutes (2600 rpm). Again the upper layer was discarded. Three drops 60% NaOH was added to the lower layer to alkalinize it to pH 11. The mixture was extracted with 5 ml chloroform by shaking for 5 minutes and centrifuging for 5 minutes at 3200 rpm. The upper layer was discarded and the chloroform layer evaporated to dryness in a multiple flash evaporator (Buchler Instruments, Evapomix). The dried sample was dissolved in 40 μl ethyl acetate and a 3 μl aliquot was injected into the gas chromatograph.

Standards were prepared by addition of 3, 5, 10, 15, 20, 30, 40, and 50 μl of L-methadone stock solution, and 0.05 ml SKF 525A stock solution to 0.2 ml blank plasma. The standards were extracted as above and injected into the gas chromatograph.

Gas liquid chromatographic analysis

Gas chromatographic analysis was performed on a Hewlett-Packard 7610 gas chromatograph equipped with dual flame ionization detectors.

A 6 ft x 2 mm ID glass column packed with 3% OV 225 on Gas Chrome Q80-100 mesh (Applied Science) was utilized throughout the study. The carrier gas was nitrogen at a flow rate of 30 ml/min. The air flow was 300-350 ml/min. Hydrogen flow was 40 ml/min. The injector port temperature was 235°C, oven temperature was 220°C, and detector temperature 300°C. The detector sensitivity was 2 x 10 for plasma samples and 8 x 10 for urine samples.

Urine sample preparation and gas chromatographic analysis

To 1 ml of urine was added 0.1 ml SKF-525A standard and 1 drop 60% NaOH. The mixture was extracted with 6 ml chloroform by shaking for 5 minutes and centrifuging for 5 minutes at 3200 rpm. The upper layer was discarded. The lower layer was evaporated to dryness and 40 μl ethyl acetate added. A 2 μl aliquot was injected into the gas chromatograph for analysis. Urine standards were prepared by addition of 50, 100, 150, 200 and 250 μl L-methadone stock solution to 1 ml urine, 0.1 ml SKF-525A stock was added and the mixture carried through the extraction procedure as described above.

Quantitation and calibration curves

A standard calibration curve was obtained by plotting the ratio or peak height of methadone or metabolite to that of the internal standard against the known concentration (μg/ml) of methadone or metabolite. Each standard curve

TABLE I:
Maternal Methadone Dose, Gest. Age, Birth Wt., Apgar Score (31 Patients)

	RANGE	MEAN ± SE
Maternal Methadone dose mg/day (29 pts)	10-100	38.1±3.9
Gestational Age (weeks)	34-43	39±0.4
Birth Weight (gms)	27 full term 2130-3920* 4 premature 1830, 2510 1730, 1800	3087±75
Apgar Score (1,2,5 min)	$\frac{1}{1-9}$ $\frac{2}{1-9}$ $\frac{5}{7-10}$	$7.\overline{5+0.4}$ $7.\overline{6+0.5}$ $8.\overline{9+0.2}$

Birth Asphyxia - 3

*3 were SGA (11.1% of total)

was constructed from determinations of at least 5 points. Standards were carried through each extraction procedure. Quantitation of patient samples was performed on the basis of peak height ratio.

The recovery of methadone was determined by adding a known quantity of methadone and SKF-525A to blank plasma or urine and extracting as described above. The same quantity of methadone and SKF-525A in stock solution was prepared (but not extracted) and was evaporated to dryness, resuspended in ethyl acetate, and assayed by GLC. Utilizing these procedures, methadone recovery from plasma was 88-94%; SKF-525A recovery was 70-75%, methadone and SKF recoveries from urine were 90-95%.

RESULTS

Table I is a summary of the maternal methadone dose and immediate newborn histories for 31 patients. In 28 instances, the mothers were taking methadone throughout their pregnancy and in 2 instances they had been detoxified from methadone in the third trimester. The maternal methadone dose was 10-100 mg/day (mean 38).

The gestational age of the infants was 34-43 weeks (mean 39). Twenty-seven of the infants were full-term, and had birth weights of 2130-3920 gms (mean 3087). Three of these infants were small for gestational age. The other four infants (including a set of fraternal twins) were premature and weighed 1730-2510 gms. The mean Apgar scores were 7.5 (1 min.), 7.6 (2 min.), and 8.9 (5 min). Three infants experienced birth asphyxia.

The withdrawal symptoms and signs experienced by the neonates are summarized in Table II. The symptoms most commonly noted were hypertonicity,

TABLE II:
Withdrawal Signs in 31 Infants Born to Methadone-Maintained Ex-Addicts*

Signs	Mild	Mod.	Severe	% Total Group
Tremor	4	15	6	86
Hypertonicity	4	15	6	86
Irritability	4	15	5	86
Myoclonic jerks	1	4	6	42
Seizures	0	1	5	23
High Pitched cry	0	6	0	23
Vomiting	1	5	0	23
Diarrhea	0	4	0	15
Fever	0	4	1	19
Respiratory distress	3	5	0	31
Total no. pts.	5	14	5	86%

* Of the 31 patients, 25 had symptoms and 6 (2 of whom were born to detoxified mothers) had no symptoms.

irritability, and tremors. In all, 86% of the infants underwent withdrawal. Of the symptomatic patients, 17% experienced mild withdrawal, 48% moderate and 21% severe. In order to rule out concurrent maternal abuse of other drugs contributing to withdrawal, urinary drug screening using the EMIT system (Rubenstein, 1972) was performed on maternal and/or neonatal urine samples. Four (16%) of the 25 symptomatic patients had urines positive for opiates; one of these patients experienced severe, two moderate and one mild withdrawal. The urine of the same patient who experienced severe withdrawal also was positive for barbiturates. None of the urine samples was positive for amphetamine or cocaine derivatives.

For 26 of our patients we attempted to correlate maternal methadone dose with neonatal withdrawal symptomatology. As shown in Figure 1, the dose of methadone taken by the mother did not appear to influence the severity of neonatal withdrawal. In infants with severe withdrawal the maternal dose ranged from 10-100 mg/day. In the moderate group the maternal dose was 10-65 mg/day; in those with absent to mild withdrawal the dose was 20-60 mg/day. Hence, in this group of patients there was no way of predicting the likelihood of occurrence or severity of withdrawal on the basis of maternal methadone dose.

Figure 2 shows the plasma and urine methadone concentrations for 27 of

CORRELATION BETWEEN MATERNAL METHADONE DOSE AND SEVERITY OF NEONATAL WITHDRAWAL

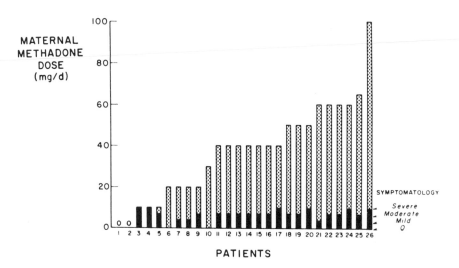

FIG. 1.   Correlations between maternal methadone dose and severity of neonatal withdrawal. Results from 26 patients, 2 of whom (1 and 2) were detoxified in the third trimester. The left vertical axis and the stippled bar graph refer to stated maternal methadone dose in mg/day. The right vertical axis and filled bar graph refer to severity of neonatal symptomatology. For patients 3 and 4 the filled and stippled bars are of equal height. The longitudinal axis refers to the patients. See text for discussion.

our patients. The other 4 patients were not included because blood and/or urine collections were not complete for the test period. The plasma half life for methadone in the 27 neonates was 26 hours. By day 5 of neonatal life plasma methadone levels were no longer detectable. The urine methadone concentrations were consistently higher than the plasma levels over the 72-hour period studied. A major factor noted with respect to the relationship of plasma methadone concentration to the withdrawal syndrome was that at plasma concentrations greater than .06 μg/ml withdrawal did not occur. When levels fell below this value, withdrawal occurred within 12-24 hours.

DISCUSSION

The purpose of this study was to investigate the placental transfer of methadone from the mother to her newborn, and the relationship of maternal methadone dose and neonatal plasma methadone concentration to neonatal withdrawal. We know clinically that methadone crosses the placenta because 80-90% of the infants born to methadone-maintained mothers have been reported to devel-

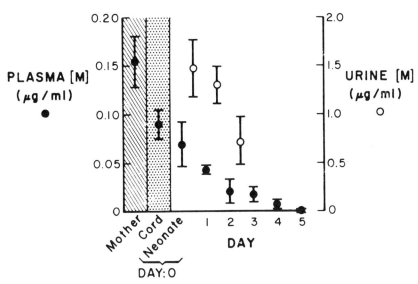

FIG. 2.   Plasma and urine methadone concentrations (Mean ± S.E.) in 27 patients. The left vertical axis and filled circles refer to plasma methadone concentration in μg/ml. The right vertical axis and open circles refer to the urine methadone concentration in μg/ml. Note that the scale for the right axis is 10 x greater than that for the left. The longitudinal axis includes day 0 values for maternal, cord and neonatal plasma, day 1-5 values for neonatal plasma, and day 1-3 values for neonatal urine. The latter were collected as 24-hour samples and the Mean ± S.E. for 0-24, 21-28 and 48-72 hours of life is presented. See text for discussion.

op withdrawal (Zelson, 1973; Rajegowda, 1972). Amniotic fluid studies done by Inturrisi and Blinick (1973) also indicate that methadone crosses the placenta commencing during early pregnancy.

Our present studies of neonatal plasma methadone concentrations provide further evidence that methadone crosses the placenta. The fact that we found methadone levels in neonatal plasma to be much lower than the maternal plasma levels, may indicate that methadone transport to the fetus is limited by placental factors. This is supported by the studies of Peters (1972) comparing the distribution of methadone in non-pregnant, pregnant, and fetal rats. The fetus had a considerably lower total body concentration of methadone on a weight basis than the mother rat.

When we compared the severity of neonatal withdrawal with the maternal methadone dose there appeared to be no consistent relationship between the two. This may be due to differences in maternal drug metabolism resulting in widely disparate plasma levels in the individual mothers. Such an interpretation is supported by the studies of Kreek (1973). She measured the plasma levels in men and non-pregnant women who were taking methadone 100 mg/day. There was marked variability in both plasma and urine drug levels when individual patients taking the same dose were compared. If this same individual variability in methadone withdrawal is true for the pregnant patient it would result in different quantities of methadone being made available for transfer across the placenta. Similarly, individual variability of methadone metabolism in the neonate might further modify the neonatal plasma drug levels and withdrawal symptomatology.

The neonatal plasma methadone concentrations declined gradually over the first few days of life, and by day 5, we were unable to detect plasma concentrations. It is likely that with a more sensitive method and an extended collection period, methadone might be detected in plasma for longer periods. Despite the limitations of the method at the lower drug concentrations (25 ng/ml) a consistent and dramatic observation was that in those infants who experienced withdrawal their symptoms did not begin when the plasma methadone level was above approximately 60 ng/ml. When the plasma concentration dropped below this value the neonates became symptomatic in 12-24 hours. It appears that when the plasma methadone concentration is above this level there is enough tissue-bound methadone to prevent withdrawal, but as soon as the plasma level falls below this point, the infant is no longer protected. Why some infants undergo withdrawal with varying severity and others do not develop withdrawal is being further investigated. As previously mentioned, this may be due to individual variability in metabolism and excretion of methadone as illustrated for the adult (Kreek, 1973).

SUMMARY

We studied the placental transfer of methadone, the relationship of neonatal plasma methadone concentrations to withdrawal symptomatology, and the relationship between maternal methadone dose and severity of neonatal withdrawal in 31 methadone-maintained mothers and their neonates. Methadone concentrations in maternal, cord and neonatal plasma were measured using a gas chromatographic micromethod. Neonatal plasma was assayed on days 0-5 of life. Urine methadone levels were measured for the first 3 days of neonatal life, using a similar assay. Twenty-five of the neonates experienced mild to severe withdrawal symptoms. There was no consistent relationship between the maternal methadone dose and the severity of neonatal symptoms. However, when neonatal withdrawal did occur, it began after plasma methadone levels fell below .06 μg/ml. The neonatal plasma methadone levels were consistently lower than those of the mother. Maternal methadone is transferred across the placenta and can induce significant withdrawal symptomatology in the newborn.

Notes

This study was supported in part by Grant HRC U-2349 awarded by the New York City Health Research Council.

Requests for reprints should be addressed to Tove S. Rosen, M.D. Department of Pediatrics, Columbia University, College of Physicians & Surgeons, 630 West 168 Street, New York, New York 10032.

The authors wish to thank Drs. Brian F. Hoffman, Frederick G. Hofmann and L. Stanley James for their advice and encouragement in the performance of these studies. We also wish to thank Mr. Donald Sichler for his expert technical assistance.

References

Blatman, S. Infants born to heroin addicts maintained on methadone. Neonatal observations and follow-up. *Proceedings of the 3rd National Conference of Methadone Treatment,* N.I.M.H., 1970, 32-85.

Cohen, S.N., and Newman, L.L. Methadone maintenance during pregnancy. *American Journal of Diseases in Childhood,* 1973, *726,* 445-6.

Inturrisi, C.E., and Blinick, E.E. The quantitation of methadone in human amniotic fluid. *Research Communication of Chemistry Pathology Pharmacology,* 1973, *6*:353-356 (abstract).

Inturrisi, C.E., and Verebely, K. A gas liquid chromatographic method for the quantitative determination of methadone in human plasma and urine. *Journal of Chromatography,* 1972, *65*: 361-369.

Kreek, M.J. Plasma and Urine Levels of Methadone in Man. *New York State Journal of Medicine,* 1973, *73*: 2773-2777.

Newman, R. Pregnancies of Methadone Patients. *New York State Journal of Medicine,* 1974, *74*: 52-54.

Peters, M.A., Turnbow, M., and Buchnauer, D. The distribution of methadone in the nonpregnant, pregnant and fetal rat after acute methadone treatment. *Journal of Pharmacology and Experimental Therapeutics,* 1972, *181*: 273-278.

Rajegowda, B.K., Glass, L., Evans, H.E., Swartz, D.P., and Leblanc, W. Methadone withdrawal in newborn infants. *Journal of Pediatrics,* 1972, *81*: 532-534.

Reddy, M.A., Harper, R., and Stein, G. Observations on heroin and methadone withdrawal in the newborn. *Pediatrics,* 1971, *18*: 353-358.

Rubenstein, K.E., Schneider, R.S., and Ullman, E.F. Homogenous Enzyme Immuno assay "A New Immuno Chemical Technique". *Biochemical and Biophysical Research Communication,* 1972, *47:* 846-51.

Stone, M.L., Salerno, L.S., Green, M., and Zelson, C. Narcotic Addiction in pregnancy. *American Journal of Obstetrics and Gynecology,* 1971, *109*: 716-723.

Zelson, C., Lee, S.S., and Caralino, M. Neonatal Narcotic Addiction. *New England Journal of Medicine,* 1973, *289*: 1216-1220.

Zelson, C., Rubio, E., and Wasserman, E. Neonatal Narcotic Addiction—10-Year Observation. *Pediatrics,* 1971, *18*: 178-189.

DISCUSSION

Q. *Dr. Nathenson:* Dr. Rosen, was the urinalysis for methadone in newborn infants done by the gas chromatographic techniques?

A. *Dr. Rosen: They were done by the EMIT system at first because it is a much* *quicker and easier screening system. Our subsequent analysis, was done by gas chromatography.*

Q. *Dr. Nathenson:* We have some preliminary data on urinary excretion of methadone using an immunological system and our small data sample seems to agree that the level of drug that we can find in the urine does not correlate with the severity of symptoms, but may correlate when it reaches a low point, where the onset of withdrawal occurs later on. We do not have large numbers, however. We have utilized this test for as long as three weeks now in some patients, and are able to identify the presence of methadone that long, and perhaps longer in some babies.

A. *Dr. Rosen: We have done spot samples on urines on days 5, 7, 9, and 13 on about 10 patients now, and I have picked up methadone on day 10 in two of them: but the others were all negative. We have to extend the collection much further.*

Q. *Dr. Kron:* You suggested in one of the slides that you did not find a relationship between the dosage of methadone and the level of symptomatology. However, at the 20 mg per day level, I think you have evidence of a non-linear trend that those babies as a group did better. They had either moderate or mild symptoms, so you really have hidden in the data a U-shaped curve. Some babies were even getting very low levels of methadone. They may actually be taking other medication. Maybe 20 mg is just the right amount for your group.

A. *Dr. Rosen: We looked for barbiturates, morphine, and amphetamines. They may be taking Thorazine, phenothiazines, or Valium which we do not look for. But two of our babies whose mothers were on only 10 mg (maternal levels were very low with urines positive only for methadone). These two babies both had seizures and were very sick. The mothers had been on 10 mg for at least two months prior to delivery. There also were some mothers who were on 30 and 50 mg methadone per day whose infants were completely asymptomatic.*

Addictive Diseases: an International Journal 2 (1): 179-185 (1975)

Phenobarbital Disposition in the Neonate

L.K. GARRETTSON
Department of Pharmacy and Pharmaceutics
Department of Pediatrics
Virginia Commonwealth University

INTRODUCTION

Phenobarbital has several uses in newborn infants. These include use as an anticonvulsant, and enzyme inducer for the therapy of hyperbilirubinemia, and as a sedative for infants displaying drug withdrawal symptomatology or colic. Infants may receive the drug prenatally from mothers who receive the drug for seizures or sedation. An understanding of the disposition of the drug in the infant may be expected to improve management by optimizing dose and dosing interval for improved effect and diminished side effects.

Infants requiring phenobarbital are often available for prolonged study, especially if prematurely born. This permitted urine collections up to 3 weeks after a single dose of phenobarbital. The analysis of phenobarbital eliminations in urine is reported in this paper and compared with serum elimination.

MATERIAL AND METHOD

Infants were cared for in the premature high-risk nursery of the Children's Hospital of Buffalo. Total care, particularly the need for phenobarbital therapy, was not under the direction of the investigator. A single dose of phenobarbital was used for hyperbilirubinemia as preliminary studies showed resulting serum levels remained high for several days. As hyperbilirubinemia is a self-limiting condition, a single dose of phenobarbital was judged sufficient.

Serum samples were collected from heel punctures and assayed by a standard double extraction method (Butler 1954) reducing all volumes by a factor of 10.

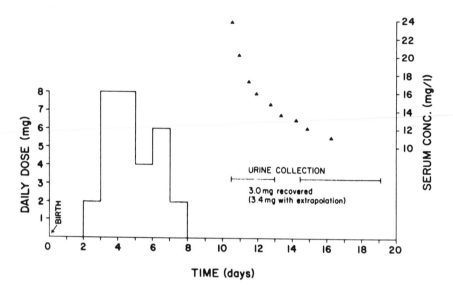

FIG. 1.   Course of Phenobarbital Therapy in a 2000 gm. Infant
The bar graph shows daily dose in mg. Serum concentration is plotted on the right. The horizontal bar shows the 2 periods of urine collection. For duration of the observed and extrapolated amounts excreted, see text.

Urine was collected from infants using a stainless steel frame with nylon mesh screen on which the infant was nursed. Urine was assayed for phenobarbital and p-hydroxyphenobarbital after ether extraction, by gas chromatography (Martin, 1966).

RESULTS

The course of phenobarbital therapy and resulting serum concentrations in one infant are shown in Figure 1. Therapy was instituted to control signs of narcotic withdrawal. Total dose administered was 30 mg given orally as powder dissolved in glucose water. Each dose contained 2 mg of drug. Decline of serum concentration followed neither first nor zero order rates, i.e., data plotted on Cartesian and semilog coordinates did not form a straight line.

Cummulative exertion of phenobarbital and p-hydroxyphenobarbital from the same infant is shown in Figure 2. The excretion rate of p-hydroxyphenobarbital appeared constant as indicated by the linear plot of metabolite accumulation. The correction for the period of urine loss was made by extending the line through the earliest period of continuous collections. The correction for phenobarbital loss was by visual fit. The urinary recovery of phenobarbital and metabolite was estimated by addition of the total urinary excretion as indicated by the 2 extrapolated curves. This value was 3.4 mg.

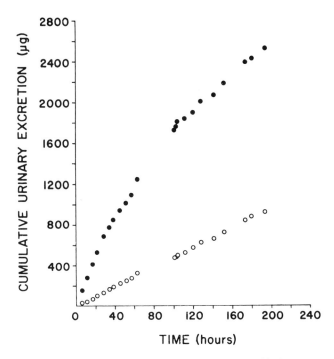

FIG. 2   Urinary Recovery of Phenobarbital and p-Hydroxyphenobarbital.
Urine was collected during time indicated in Fig. 1.
Closed circles represent phenobarbital and open circles represent p-hydroxyphenobarbital.

During the time of urine collection, serum concentration fell by approximately 50%. If total body drug was reflected in the serum concentration, the amount remaining to be excreted at the beginning of the urine collection would have been 6.8 mg. The amount excreted before the urine collection may be crudely estimated by using the most rapid rate of excretion for both phenobarbital and metabolite. Using this estimate, a total of 7 mg is estimated to have been excreted before collection began. Thus, a total of 14 mg is estimated to have been excreted by the end of the collection. This is less than half of the administered dose.

The serum and urine findings in a 2100 gm. small-for-dates infant who received a single dose of phenobarbital for seizures on the 7th day of life is presented in Figure 3. The infant had a low serum calcium, which was corrected. Phenobarbital therapy was not continued once hypocalcemia was diagnosed and treated.

Excretion of p-hydroxyphenobarbital was constant from the time of administration. There was no apparent decline in excretion rate as serum concentration of drug declined. In contrast, renal excretion of unchanged drug changed in rate, and this rate slowed with decline of serum concentration.

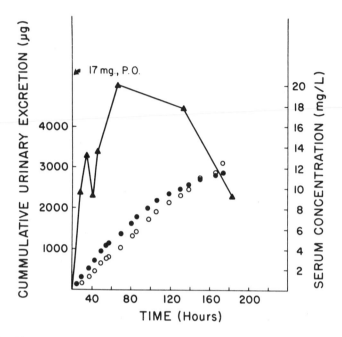

FIG. 3.   Phenobarbital Disposition in an Infant with Birth Weight of 2100 gm.
A dose of 17 mg (8 mg./kg.) was administered in glucose on the 7th day of life. Total recovery 35% of the dose.
Closed circles represent phenobarbital and open circles represent p-hydroxyphenobarbital. The solid line represents serum concentration and the ordinate is on the right.

Serum concentration of drug rose irregularly over a 2-day period. The serum concentration was in the same range one week after the single dose as it had been at 2 days.

The slow rise and sustained plateau suggest prolonged absorption of drug coupled with a slower rate of excretion.

Similar patterns were observed in 5 other infants who were premature and treated for hyperbilirubinemia. Maxium recovery, in one infant where collection was extended for 3 weeks, was 40% of the single dose administered. In all infants, serum concentration rose over a 2-day period and declined slowly. Change in serum concentration was not reflected in altered rates of drug or metabolite excretion.

DISCUSSION

Elimination of phenobarbital in the premature and newborn is slow, as has been indicated by others. Serum elimination fell within the 77 to 404 hour figures found by Jalling, et al. (1973). This study showed that elimination when serum concentrations are low may be even slower than published values.

Study of urine elimination rates of drug and metabolite has shown a discrepancy with serum elimination rate. This was an unexpected finding, but coincides with similar findings in the adult (Ravn-Jonsen, 1969). In all cases, the rate of elimination determined by urine analysis was slower than the rate determined by serum analysis. Adult studies suggest that initial distribution is prolonged, and the discrepancy between rates derived from serum and urine studies may be due to slow rates into and out of deep compartments (Garrettson, unpublished).

In none of the seven infants had urine recovery approached completion. The recovery was 40% or below. In adults, up to 75% of a single dose has been recovered. The low recovery may have been the result of incomplete absorption, but elucidation awaits further study. A cyclohexadienyl metabolite of phenobarbital, 5-(3,4-dihydroxy-1,5-cyclohexadien-1-yl)-5-ethylbarbituric acid, found in small amounts, in adult humans (Harvey, 1972), was not assayed in this study. Quantitative studies of the elimination of this metabolite have not been published.

The apparent saturation of phenobarbital metabolism seen by the constant elimination rate of p-hydroxyphenobarbital excretion casts doubt on the findings that phenobarbital elimination in the infant is by simple first order kinetics. While full-term infants have apparent first order serum decay rates, full definition of the kinetic pattern elimination must await corroboration from urine data. Speculation on the mechanism of this apparently saturated process cannot be made at this time.

The very slow rate of elimination suggests that current practices of dosing two or three times a day, or even daily, may be unnecessary. However, frequent small doses may be absorbed more rapidly. Total dose, on multiple dose regimens, needs to be monitored by frequently performed serum levels particularly if administration is to proceed for more than a week. The transition time when the slow rate of phenobarbital elimination in the newborn changes to a much faster rate found in some one-month-old infants (Heinze, 1971) and children (Garrettson, 1970) has not been defined.

SUMMARY

The disposition of phenobarbital in premature infants was assessed by repeated measurement of the serum concentration of unmetabolized drug and the urinary excretion of both phenobarbital and its metabolite, p-hydroxyphenobarbital. Serum elimination rates did not adequately reflect the elimination of total body phenobarbital. A prolonged distributive phase is postulated. The elimination rate of p-hydroxyphenobarbital was constant, suggesting capacity limited kinetics. Slow elimination in serum concentrations which remained in the therapeutic range for several days suggests that short courses of therapy may have prolonged effect in the newborn premature infant.

Notes

Supported by Grant GM-17696 from General Medical Sciences.

Requests for reprints should be addressed to L.K. Garretson, M.D., Box 666, MCV Station, Virginia Commonwealth University, Richmond, VA 23298.

The skillful technical assistance of OK Kyung Kim is gratefully acknowledged. Dr. David Weintraub, Director of Nurseries, Children's Hospital of Buffalo, cared for the infants and gave valuable support and advice.

References

Butler, T.C., Mahaffee, C., and Waddell, W. Phenobarbital studies of elimination accumulation tolerances and dosage schedules. *Journal of Pharmacology and Experimental Therapeutics,* 1954, *111.* 425-435.

Martin, H.F., and Driscoll, J.L. Gas chromatographic identification and determination of barbiturates. *Analytical Chemistry,* 1966, *38.* 345-346.

Jalling, B., Boreus, L.O., Kallberg, N., and Agurell, S. Disappearance from the newborn of circulating prenatally administered phenobarbital. *European Journal of Clinical Pharmacology,* 1973, *6.* 234-238.

Ravn-Jonsen, A., Lunding, M., and Secher, O. Excretion of phenobarbital in urine after intake of large doses. *Acta Pharmacologica (Kobenhavn).* 1969, *27.* 193-201.

Heinze, E., and Kampffmeyer, H.G. Biological half-life of phenobarbital in human babies. *Klinische Wochenschrift,* 1971, *49.* 1146-1147.

Garrettson, L.K., and Dayton, P.G. Disappearance of phenobarbital and diphenyldantoin from serum of children. *Clinical Pharmacology and Therapeutics,* 1960, *11.* 674-679.

Harvey, D.J., Glazener, L., Stratton, C., Nowlin, J., Hill, R.M., and Horning, M.G. Detection of a 5-(3, 4-dehydroxy-1, 5-cyclohexadien-l-yl)-metabolite of phenobarbital and mephobarbital in rat, guinea pig, and human. *Research Communications in Chemical Pathology and Pharmacology,* 1972, *3* (3). 557-564.

Discussion

Q. *Dr. Kron:* We have some behavioral data which may be of interest, or correlatable with your findings in a study of infants born to mothers who have received secobarbital (200 mg doses), within three hours prior to delivery. These babies were quite depressed in the sucking behavior on the first day of life. These babies underwent recovery which lasted throughout their in-hospital period. They went home in four days, but, by the fourth day, they had not as yet come up to half the level in their sucking response that was evidence on the first day (of babies born to mothers who had no obstetric sedation). This puzzled us in terms of the alleged short action (supposed) of the secobarbital. Indeed, the Eli-Lilly Co., in its blurbs to the medical profession (obstetricians in particular), suggests that this is a particularly safe obstetrical drug. Now, our findings with sucking suggest that it surely has a significant effect on adaptive behavior; however, I wonder to what degree this might be correlated with the serum level, or whether it might give some indication as to where the storage, if any, is occurring?

A. *Dr. Garretson: Thank you very much. The kind of measurement that you*

have done with sucking is the kind of measurement that is going to be required for pharmacokinetic analysis of the drugs that we deal with. The simple reason is that we have talked about serum level today, and yet, not any of the drugs that we have discussed are active in the serum. And the rate of distribution of the drug outside the serum, and into both active and inactive compartments, is what is important. We know of drugs which do not adequately reach their distribution equilibrium, get redistributed as they are supposed to in the body for over a month. The very first study I ever did in pharmacokinetics was with Dr. Wayland Hayes, who is with us this morning; it was on a pesticide, which is such a drug. Thiopental reaches an equilibrium 12 hours or more after it is given. In the infant we have no thought; we have no idea about what these rates of redistribution are, and it is entirely reasonable that they are changing by the fact that the compartments into which the baby can redistribute drugs will be changing as fluids change, and as he adds fat to his body. Many of these infants I was studying, prematures, are essentially fatless individuals when they are born. The bizzare result of having the serum level fall dramatically, and very little come out in the urine, and yet have low-serum concentrations, suggests to me the need to be doing what you are doing. In conjunction with this, we should be looking at an active place in the body for a "drug analysis," and you have to do this by drug effect. I think it is very important and thank you for your point because it gave me a chance to expand on that further.

Q. Dr. Braude: I think it is very important, Dr. Garretson, to measure urinary excretions, and not only blood levels. Recently, or at least in the last year, we have found the same thing with marijuana. For instance, with canabinoids, after a single dose, there is excretion of metabolites up to easily 8 to 10 days. These are considerations that we must make more and more in looking at the effects of drugs of abuse.

A. Dr. Garretson: *It is very difficult to get a four-week collection on a newborn baby.*

Addictive Diseases: an International Journal 2 (1): 187-199 (1975)

A Study of Factors That Influence the Severity of Neonatal Narcotic Withdrawal

ENRIQUE M. OSTREA, JR.
CLEOFE J. CHAVEZ
MILTON E. STRAUSS
Wayne State University
Departments of Pediatrics and Psychology
Hutzel Hospital and Children's Hospital of Michigan
Detroit, Michigan

A STUDY OF FACTORS THAT INFLUENCE THE SEVERITY OF NEONATAL NARCOTIC WITHDRAWAL

Many reports in the literature have attempted to delineate the factors which may influence the severity of neonatal narcotic withdrawal (Zelson et al., 1971; Goodfriend et al., 1956; Blinick, 1968; Zelson et al., 1973; Reddy et al., 1971; Rajegowda et al., 1972; and Annunziato, 1971). Since a majority of these reports were retrospective studies, different or contradictory conclusions have been reached partly because of inadequate controls in the study, too much reliance placed on maternal history in correlating her drug habit to the severity of neonatal withdrawal or the lack of a uniform set of criteria to evaluate the severity of withdrawal. It has been our experience and perhaps by most people involved in maternal drug abuse programs that mothers who are on a methadone program do not usually abandon their heroin intake. When we compared the amount of total morphine recovered in the urine or serum of mothers and their infants at delivery, the mothers on the Hutzel methadone program did not differ from the walk-ins insofar as recovered total morphine levels are concerned (Table I): 1.85 mgs% vs. 0.67 mgs% in maternal urine; 1.31 mgs% vs. 0.90 mgs%

TABLE I
Total Morphine (mg%) in the Urine or Serum of Mothers and Their Infants at Delivery: Hutzel Program vs. Walk-in

Source	Hutzel	Walk-in
1. Maternal urine	1.85 ± 2.83 (33)	0.67 ± 1.99 (12)*
2. Infant's urine **	1.31 ± 1.94 (55)	0.90 ± 1.25 (22)*
3. Cord blood	0.26 ± 1.56 (41)	0.40 ± 1.25 (13)*

* Difference is not statistically significant.

** Initial two voiding samples.

NOTE: Sample size is indicated in parentheses.

TABLE II
Correlation Between Maternal History of Drug Use and Morphine Level in the Infant's Urine

	Total Morphine (mgs%)
1. Mother denies use of heroin for at least 1 month before delivery.	1.02 ± 1.24 (61)*
2. Mother denies use of heroin for at least 3 months before delivery.	0.99 ± 1.30 (45)*
3. Mother admits to the use of morphine for at least 1 month before delivery	1.13 ± 0.96 (74)*

* Difference is not statistically significant, $P < 0.35$

in infant's urine and 0.26 mgs% vs. 0.40 mgs% in cord serum. Furthermore, maternal history is unreliable in assessing her drug habit. Table II shows the correlation between maternal history of drug use and morphine level in the infant's urine. Whether the mother denies the use of heroin, one or three months before delivery, or whether she admits to its use at least one month before delivery, the amount of recovered total morphine in the infant's initial urine is statistically the same.

About 5-10% of mothers who deliver at our hospital are drug dependent and 70% of them attend our maternity methadone clinic. So we had the opportunity to prospectively study the possible materna, neonatal and/or environmental factors which may affect the severity of neonatal withdrawal with the use of

TABLE III
Characteristics of Study Population (N = 198)

A. Infant:

1. Birth weight (g)   2885.5 ± 464.5

    a) Clinic   2949.5 ± 462.8 (131)

    b) Non-Clinic   2764.6 ± 383.6 (57)*

2. Length (cm)   48.7 ±   2.4

3. Gestational Age (wks)   39.2 ±   1.1

4. APGAR (1 minute)   7.5 ±   1.0

5. APGAR (5 minutes)   8.7 ±   0.6

6. Sex: Male   107 (54%)

          Female   91 (46%)

7. Race: Black   184 (93%)

           White   13 (7%)

B. Maternal:

1. Age (years)   23.0 ±   3.5

2. Gravidity   3.0 ±   1.6

* Statistically significant difference, P < 0.01

more objective parameters such as clinic records and quantitative measurement of drug levels in the urine and serum of the mother and her infant at birth (Feldstein et al., 1956). The study period was from December 1972 to December 1973 and involved a total of 198 mothers and their infants. We excluded at the outset any baby likely to develop neonatal problems other than those clearly due to narcotic withdrawal, and this group consisted primarily of the premature infants and those with complications during delivery.

The characteristics of the infants and their mothers in the study population (N = 198) are seen in Table III. The infants had a mean birthweight of 2886 grams, length of 49 centimeters and gestational age of 39 weeks. If one compared the birthweight to gestational age, these infants were above the 10th percentile. It is interesting to note that the infants of clinic mothers had a significantly greater birthweight than the non-clinic or walk-ins (2950 vs. 2765 grams,

TABLE IV
The Signs and Symptoms of Neonatal Narcotic Withdrawal

		Frequency
1.	Fist sucking	80%
2.	Irritability	78%
3.	Tremors	71%
4.	Sneezing	65%
5.	High-pitch cry	45%
6.	Hypertonicity	41%
7.	Stuffy nose	26%
8.	Spitting and drooling	23%
9.	Sore buttocks	22%
10.	Sweating	19%
11.	Diarrhea	18%
12.	Vomiting	8%
13.	Yawning	8%
14.	Convulsion	0%

$p < 0.01$). This may reflect the better care mothers receive at the prenatal clinic or may also reflect a possible effect of methadone on the fetal weight. The 1 and 5 minute APGAR scores were all above seven. There was about an equal sex distribution in the group, although the majority of the infants were black. The mean maternal age was 23 years and mean gravidity of 3. The latter indicates that the drug dependent mother is not infertile as previously thought to be (Gaulden et al., 1964).

The signs and symptoms of neonatal narcotic withdrawal in decreasing order of frequency are shown in Table IV. The central nervous system manifestations in the form of fist sucking, irritability, tremors, sneezing, high-pitch cry and hypertonicity were the most common, followed by stuffy nose and gastrointestinal manifestations such as spitting, drooling, sore buttocks, diarrhea and vomiting. Outside of tremors, we did not observe any overt convulsion.

It is not enough to document the presence of withdrawal symptoms. What is more important is to determine their severity so that a fixed indication for treatment is established and better studies can be made on the possible long-

TABLE V
Assessment of the Severity of Neonatal Narcotic Withdrawal

	Mild	Moderate	Severe
Vomiting	<50% of each feeding	>50% or more of feeding for 3 successive feedings	>50% and assoc. with electrolyte imbalance
Diarrhea	Watery stools not > 4 times per day	Watery stools 5-6 times per day for 3 days	>7 x per day or if associated with electrolyte imbalance
Weight Loss	<10% of birth weight	11-15% of birthweight	>15%
Irritability	Minimal	Marked but relieved by cuddling or feeding	Unrelieved by cuddling or feeding
Tremors or Twitching	Mild tremors when stimulated	Marked tremors when stimulated or twitching	Convulsions
Tachypnea	60-80/minute	80-100/minute	>100/minute with associated respiratory alkalosis

term side effects of maternal addiction on the infant. We therefore devised our own scoring system to evaluate the severity of narcotic withdrawal (Table V). Essentially, it was selecting major signs and symptoms of narcotic withdrawal—major in the sense that if they remained unchecked, they could be life-threatening. These were: vomiting, diarrhea, weight loss, irritability, tremors or twitching, and tachypnea. Severity was assessed either as mild, moderate or severe according to the table. With a checklist, each infant was observed three times daily for a minimum of five (5) days. The severity of withdrawal was always decided by the same individual (C.C.).

NEONATAL AND MATERNAL FACTORS

Based on this set of criteria, the withdrawal rating on 95 infants is shown in Table VI. Sixty-seven percent had mild withdrawal; 27% had moderate and 6% had severe withdrawal. We then examined the various infant and maternal factors and correlated them to the severity of withdrawals. Table VII shows the factors which *did not* correlate with the severity of neonatal narcotic withdrawal

TABLE VI
The Severity of Withdrawal of 95 Infants of Drug-Dependent Mothers

Withdrawal	Total	Frequency
1. Mild	64	67%
2. Moderate	26	27%
3. Severe	5	6%
T O T A L	95	100%

($p \leq 0.05$). Infant factors such as gestational age, 1 and 5 minute APGAR, sex and race did not correlate with withdrawal severity. Among maternal factors, maternal age, parity, duration of heroin addiction and duration of methadone intake were also not significantly different in those whose babies developed mild or moderate to severe symptoms. These findings are consistent with the recent observations of Lipsitz and Blatman (1974). The treatment program did not also influence the severity of withdrawal, although it appears that the walk-in mothers seem to have a higher percentage of their babies developing only mild withdrawal. The total morphine levels measured in the infant's urine, maternal urine and cord did not correlate with severity. This observation is opposite to the report of Zelson et al. (1971) which states that more severe neonatal narcotic withdrawal is observed if the mother has had a very recent intake of heroin prior to delivery. However, their conclusion was based on the information obtained from maternal history and not from any quantitative measurement of morphine in either the mother or her infant. The serum calcium and glucose levels were normal and were not statistically different in those who developed either mild or moderate to severe withdrawal.

Table VIII shows the factors which correlated significantly to the severity of neonatal narcotic withdrawal ($p \leq 0.025$). Foremost in these was the methadone dose of the mother. Expressed in milligrams per day as the initial, final or average dose,* the daily methadone dose of the mother significantly correlated to the severity of withdrawal in the infant ($p \leq 0.005 - 0.025$). As previously mentioned, there was no significant difference in the withdrawal severity based on the treatment program in general, i.e., methadone program vs. walk-in (see Table VII, C.). However, if one divided the methadone clinic mothers into two groups based on the daily methadone intake, a statistically higher incidence of moderate to severe withdrawal is seen in babies whose mothers were on more than 20 mg of methadone per day as compared to walk-ins ($x_2 = 7.045$; p

*The average dose was calculated by taking the total methadone the mother took during her clinic attendance, divided by the number of days she attended clinic.

TABLE VII
Factors Which Did Not Correlate with the Severity of Neonatal Narcotic
Withdrawal (P > 0.05)

	Up to Mild	Moderate to Severe
A. Infant Factors:		
1. Gest. Age (wks)	39.1 ± 1.4 (63)	39.5 ± 0.7 (31)
2. APGAR (1 minute)	7.4 ± 1.0 (55)	7.4 ± 1.0 (30)
3. APGAR (5 minutes)	8.7 ± 0.6 (55)	8.6 ± 0.8 (30)
4. Sex: Male/Female	38/26	12/19
5. Race: Black/White	60/4	17/3
B. Maternal Factors:		
1. Age (years)	23.1 ± 4.2 (62)	22.1 ± 6.7 (30)
2. Parity	2.5 ± 1.2 (62)	2.9 ± 1.4 (30)
3. Duration of heroin addiction (mos.)	33.9 ± 30.3 (62)	34.4 ± 21.1 (30)
4. Duration of methadone	13.9 ± 7.8 (26)	11.6 ± 5.8 (20)
C. Treatment Program		
1. Methadone Program	38	24
2. Walk-in	20	6
D. Total Morphine Level (mgs%)		
1. Infant's urine	0.97 ± 1.53 (53)	1.12 ± 1.09 (29)
2. Maternal urine	1.37 ± 2.35 (30)	2.29 ± 4.33 (17)
3. Cord blood	0.16 ± 0.75 (37)	1.15 ± 4.99 (17)
E. Serum Chemistry		
1. Calcium (mgs%)	9.54 ± 0.73 (53)	9.72 ± 0.70 (28)
2. Sugar (mgs%)	64.59 ± 17.94 (54)	59.46 ± 12.99 (28)

≤ 0.01), and no significant difference in withdrawal rating in babies whose mothers were on less than 20 mg per day compared to walk-ins ($x_2 = 0.352$; $p \leq 0.352$). Thus, although recent reports have documented that methadone can produce serious withdrawal in the infant of a drug-addict mother (Zelson et al., 1973; Reddy et al., 1971; Rajegowda et al., 1972; and Annunziato, 1971), this report indicates that the severity of the withdrawal is a dose-related response.

For reasons we cannot explain, gravidity is significantly higher in those mothers whose babies developed moderate to severe withdrawal. The birth-weight of their babies was also significantly higher (3076 vs. 2884 gm), an obser-

TABLE VIII
Factors Which Correlated with the Severity of Neonatal Narcotic Withdrawal
(P >0.025)

Methadone Dose of Mother (mgs/day)	Up to Mild			Moderate to Severe			"P" Value
a) Initial dose	20.19 ±	8.18	(26)	28.17 ±	16.29	(26)	0.025
b) Final dose	11.9 ±	6.94	(26)	18.7 ±	11.68	(20)	0.025
c) Average dose/day	15.2 ±	6.05	(26)	23.4 ±	11.72	(20)	0.005
Maternal Gravidity	2.7 ±	1.3	(63)	3.6 ±	1.4	(31)	0.005
Birthweight (grams)	2844.1 ±	471.1	(64)	3075.6 ±	415.0	(31)	0.010
Length	48.5 ±	2.2	(61)	49.5 ±	2.0	(28)	0.025
Postnatal Weight Loss	4.1 ±	2.3	(59)	7.8 ±	3.6	(31)	0.005
Days of Hospital Stay (Infants)	6.5 ±	1.4	(56)	10.4 ±	7.1	(25)	0.005

vation which has been documented by others (Zelson et al, 1973). For obvious reasons, infants with moderate to severe withdrawal have a greater postnatal weight loss (7.8 vs. 4.1%) and longer hospital stay (10.4 vs. 6.5 days) than the infants with mild withdrawal.

ENVIRONMENTAL FACTORS

We have also been interested in determining how much nursery environment, i.e., noise, illumination, room temperature, etc., affects the severity of neonatal narcotic withdrawal. Does an infant require a special quiet and dimly lit room during his period of withdrawal, much like the way one would treat a case of tetanus? We therefore randomly assigned our drug-addicted infants to either a regular or study nursery. The study nursery was a secluded, quiet (maximum of 60-70 decibels) and dimly lighted room. The infants in the study nursery were bundled and placed in non-motorized Armstrong incubators and fed every three hours. The infants (control) in the regular nursery were bundled in open bassinets and exposed to the usual nursery noise* and illumination and were fed every four hours. The infants in the two groups were matched in terms of birthweight, length, gestational age, APGAR scores, sex, race, maternal age, gravidity, average maternal methadone dose per day, and morphine levels in urine or serum (Table IX).

The clinical signs and symptoms of the infants in the control and experimental groups are shown in Table X. The frequency of central nervous system,

---

*In the absence of any crying infant or beeping monitoring equipment in the regular nursery, the noise level in that nursery was essentially the same as that in the study nursery (60-70 decibels).

TABLE IX
Effects of the Environment on the Severity of Neonatal Narcotic Withdrawal:
Characteristics of Control and Experimental Groups*

	Control (N=97)	Experimental (N=101)
A. Infant:		
1. Birthweight (grams)	2910.8 ± 462.8	2861.1 ± 447.3
2. Length (cm)	48.8 ± 2.1	48.6 ± 2.7
3. Gestational Age (wks)	39.3 ± 1.2	39.2 ± 0.96
4. APGAR (1 minute)	7.4 ± 1.0	7.6 ± 1.1
5. APGAR (5 minutes)	8.7 ± 0.7	8.7 ± 0.6
6. Sex: Male/Female	51/46	56/45
7. Race: Black/White	89/07	95/06
B. Maternal:		
1. Age (yrs)	23.4 ± 3.5	22.6 ± 3.4
2. Gravidity	3.0 ± 1.5	2.9 ± 1.7
C. Morphine Level (mgs%)		
1. Maternal urine	1.567 ± 2.639 (48)	1.061 ± 2.103 (50)
2. Infant's urine	1.134 ± 1.706 (85)	0.929 ± 1.072 (90)
3. Cord blood	0.271 ± 1.420 (59)	0.322 ± 1.569 (62)
D. Average Methadone Dose (mgs/d)	18.76 ± 11.72 (46)	17.52 ± 7.00 (55)

* The difference between the control and experimental group was not statistically
significant. ($P < 0.10$)

vasomotor and gastrointestinal manifestations were essentially the same in both
groups. The incidence of mild, moderate, or severe withdrawal was not significantly different in the control vs. study group ($x_2 = 0.99$; $p < 0.50$). The withdrawal rating, obtained by assigning a score of 1 to mild, 2 to moderate, and 3 to
severe, and then getting their mean were the same in both groups. Despite more
frequent feedings in the experimental group, the weight loss was essentially identical in both groups. The bilirubin values were also identical, despite the curtail-
ment of light in the experimental group. These bilirubin values, however, were
lower than the average third-day bilirubin of normal-term infants. This observation is consistent with the findings of other workers that infants born to drug-addicted mothers have a lower incidence of hyperbilirubinemia (Nathenson et. al.,
1972).

TABLE X
The Clinical Course of Neonatal Narcotic Addiction: *Comparison Between the Control and Experimental Groups*

A. Signs and Symptoms:	Control	Experimental
1. Fist sucking	80%	81%
2. Irritability	78%	66%
3. Tremors	71%	87%
4. Sneezing	65%	95%
5. High pitch cry	45%	66%
6. Hypertonicity	41%	53%
7. Stuffy nose	26%	45%
8. Spitting & drooling	23%	27%
9. Sore buttocks	22%	12%
10. Sweating	19%	28%
11. Diarrhea	18%	12%
12. Twitching	11%	4%
13. Vomiting	8%	20%
14. Yawning	8%	13%
15. Convulsion	0%	0%
B. Withdrawal rating	1.371 ± 0.583 (97)	1.317 ± 0.528 (101)*
C. Weight Loss	5.50 ± 3.24 (93)	5.22 ± 2.92 (101)*
D. Laboratory data:		
1. Bilirubin (total) mgs%	6.12 ± 3.46 (80)	5.99 ± 3.79 (90)*
2. Bilirubin (direct)	0.42 ± 0.24 (80)	0.39 ± 0.23 (90)*
3. Calcium	9.61 ± 0.72 (81)	9.56 ± 0.84 (93)*
4. Glucose	62.84 ± 16.52 (82)	66.19 ± 16.23 (94)*

* Difference is not statistically significant, ($P \geq 0.10$).

SUMMARY:

1. History is unreliable in assessing maternal drug habit. Morphine was detected in significant amounts in maternal and fetal urine regardless of whether the mother was on a methadone program or whether she denied any use of heroin during the last trimester of pregnancy.

2. Infants born to drug-addicted mothers were, in general, of birthweight normal and appropriate for gestational age (i.e., > 10th percentile). The infants born to mothers on a methadone clinic program had a higher birthweight compared to those whose mothers were not on any methadone program.
3. In order of frequency, the signs and symptoms of withdrawal were: central nervous system manifestations—fist sucking, irritability, tremors, sneezing, high-pitch cry, hypertonia; vasomotor in the form of stuffy nose; and gastrointestinal in the form of sweating, diarrhea, vomiting and yawning. Convulsions were not noted. No death occurred.
4. The severity of neonatal narcotic withdrawal did *not* correlate with the infant's gestational age, APGAR, sex or race; nor with maternal age, parity, duration of heroin addiction or duration of methadone intake. Also, it did not correlate with the total morphine level measured either in infant's or mother's urine or in cord blood. The serum levels of calcium and glucose were normal and identical in either mild or severe withdrawal.
5. The severity of neonatal withdrawal correlated significantly with the methadone dose per day of the mother (in initial, final or average dose). A maternal methadone dose of more than 20 mg per day was associated with a higher incidence of moderate to severe withdrawal in their babies. As a corollary, it was also noted that infants whose mothers were on a high methadone dose (i.e.,>20 mg per day) had a greater postnatal weight loss despite a significantly higher birthweight initially, and stayed in the hospital longer.
6. Finally, the modification of the environment to reduce external stimuli to the infant born to a drug-dependent mother, does not prevent or diminish the severity of neonatal narcotic withdrawal. Thus, there is no need to manage these infants in a special nursery.

Notes

*Supported in part by a grant from the Michigan Bureau of Maternal and Child Health and by NIMH Grant No. 1 RO3 DA00696-D1.

The authors wish to acknowledge Cheryl A. Gwisdalla, B.A., and the nursery nurses for their invaluable assistance in making this paper possible.

References

Annunziato, D. Neonatal addiction to methadone. *Pediatrics,* 47:787, 1971.
Blinick, G. Menstrual function and pregnancy in narcotic addicts treated with methadone. *Nature* (Lond), 219:180, 1968.
Feldstein, M., and Klendshoj, N.C. Rapid spectrophotometric method for the determination of morphine in urine. *J. Forens. Sci.,* 1:47, 1956.
Gaulden, E.C., Littlefield, D.C., Putoff, O.E., and Seivert, A.L. Menstrual abnormalities associated with heroin addiction. *Amer. J. Obstet. Gynec.,* 90:155, 1964.
Goodfriend, M.J., Shey, I.A., and Klein, M.D. The effects of maternal narcotic addiction on the newborn. *Amer. J. Obstet. Gynec.,* 71:29, 1956.

Lipsitz, P.J., and Blatman, S. Newborn infants of mothers on methadone maintenance. *New York State J. Med.,* 994, 1974.

Nathenson, G., Cohen, M.I., Litt, I.F., and McNamara, H. The effect of maternal heroin addiction on neonatal jaundice. *J. Pediat.,* 81:899, 1972.

Rajegowda, B.K., Glass, L., Evans, H.E., et al. Methadone withdrawal in newborn infants. *J. Pediat.,* 81:532, 1972.

Reddy, A.M., Harper, R.G., and Stern, G. Observations on heroin and methadone withdrawal in the newborn. *Pediatrics,* 48:353, 1971.

Zelson, C., Lee, S.J., and Caslino, M. Neonatal narcotic addiction. Comparative effects of maternal intake of heroin and methadone. *New Engl. J. Med.,* 289:1216, 1973.

Zelson, C., Rubio, E., and Wasserman, E. Neonatal narcotic addiction: 10 year observation. *Pediatrics,* 48:178, 1971.

DISCUSSION

Q. *Dr. Kandall:* One striking observation is about the lack of any seizures in almost 200 patients. We have been recording an incidence, including myoclonic jerks, of 22 percent in methadone babies, and about 7 percent in heroin babies. It is very striking to notice the absence.

A. *Dr. Ostrea: We try our best to distinguish which are just simple tremors and which are actually myoclonic jerks, especially if they are isolated (or unilateral). Of course what we would definitely call a seizure would be a generalized form with eye rolling, but we have never seen this in our series.*

Q. *Dr. Kron:* The findings you have of the relationship between methadone dose and severity of withdrawal are very interesting to us because we have had similar findings of correlations between methadone dose, and in the severity or changes in the adaptive behavior, in our study groups in Philadelphia. However, there has been one confounding factor, namely, that in our group the dosage of methadone seems to be correlated also with the length of time that the patients have been in the methadone program. Those who have been on the methadone program longer tend to have received larger doses of methadone. I wonder if there is such a correlation with your own group.

A. *Dr. Ostrea: We did not find the correlation but I have to qualify that statement. If you notice, the duration of methadone intake in our program has not been more than 15 weeks. In other words, despite the fact that we wanted to get these mothers early, they usually came during the last trimester of pregnancy. I do not know if your data would extend farther than that.*

Q. *Dr. Kron:* We have some people who have been on methadone programs for three years.

A. *Dr. Ostrea: We did not have any in our studies for that long; we usually got them at the first trimester.*

Q. *Dr. Kron:* The other question is related to our seeing essentially only one-half of the picture. You pointed out that you were not going to discuss therapy, but abstinence symptoms are an interaction phenomena, once therapy is instituted. You see the results, whatever the nature, of the withdrawal being undergone by the infant, plus the effect superimposed of the drugs being provided by the physician. I wonder to what degree the treatments were standardized, so that we were looking at data which tended to represent more of what the infant was bringing into the interaction, and to what degree some of this represented a variance introduced by different therapeutic approaches.

A. *Dr. Ostrea: By therapy I meant specifically the use of drugs to abate the withdrawal symptoms. We have major criteria (because we consider this life-threatening) that would automatically be treated. Firstly, we noted that if we treated these babies naturally, they stayed at the hospital much, much longer, an average of two to three weeks, as compared to one who was not treated. And, as I said, our findings show that there was no mortality with this form of approach. Also, while we were still studying the effect of the controlled environment vs. the noncontrolled environment, we found that you could go ahead and treat the baby, since we knew we were not causing the baby to die. In fact, the future study will involve treating a group of babies the moment they have signs and symptoms, and another group which will treat only if they had severe withdrawal. Offhand, I can tell you that if we do the regimen that we have, that is, if we only treat them when they have severe withdrawal, it seems to do good. They live and they get off the withdrawal fast enough, but the long-term side effects I do not know; it needs a longitudinal study.*

Q. *Dr. Kron:* In other words, most of the subjects that you discussed were not receiving drug therapy, but with only one treatment in the regular nursery.

A. *Dr. Ostrea: No, in either nursery they would be treated if they had severe withdrawal, or one of the criteria, and in these 198 babies which we had, we only treated 11.*

Q. *Dr. Finnegan:* I just wanted to comment about the convulsions. Of the 206 babies that we have had, we only had three that have had seizures. One was the baby that I think I mentioned earlier, who had meningitis. A second baby was one whose mother absolutely denied use of any drugs within the four months prior to delivery. She had been an occasional user of heroin and we found no morphine, quinine, methadone, or any of the drugs of abuse. We analyze for about 16 drugs in mothers' urine and babies' urine, and we found nothing there at all to relate to these seizures. We related them to some form of fetal asphyxia that we had never defined. A third infant was very early in our study; and this baby was born to a mother who was on heroin, a very high dosage (a very large number of bags), and, again, I do not know why. That is our experience, which is in contrast to yours.

Q. *Dr. Davis:* I should like to say that our findings of 130+ babies were strikingly similar to Dr. Glass', in that we did find instances of myoclonic jerks which were considerably higher in the methadone vs. the heroin babies, and in the range of nearly 20 percent vs. about 4 percent.

Addictive Diseases: an International Journal 2 (1): 201-208 (1975)

Drug Impediments to Mothering Behavior

H. P. COPPOLILLO, M.D.
Department of Psychiatry and Pediatrics
Division of Child Psychiatry,
Vanderbilt University Medical Center
Nashville, Tennessee

There can be no doubt that the causes of drug abuse in general are complex and can be viewed in a number of frames of reference. Who can doubt that social blight creates an optimal terrain in which addiction thrives? No doubt the "friendly neighborhood pusher" has helped to nurture this terrain, and certainly a society that is as committed to problem solving by drug ingestion as ours (Coppolillo, 1972; Burack, 1970) sets the unspoken ethic in the milieu of the drug abuser. Despite all this, it is in the last analysis the personal vulnerability of the individual which determines whether or not they will become addicted. That there is social and economic blight and that drug pushers exist in society are preconditions that may even be necessary for drug abuse to occur (though I strongly doubt their necessity), but to say that they are sufficient or ultimate causes of drug abuse is like saying that oxygen in the air caused the arsonist's fire. For our purposes, I should like to argue that the *necessary* and *sufficient* cause for vulnerability to addiction is in the psychological pathology of the individual, and that this pathology originated from developmental problems. I would then submit a model to describe the impediments to mothering which occur in female addicts which render subsequent generations vulnerable to addiction in their turn. In order to present this model it will be necessary to review some basic notions of personality development and mother-child transactions.

The best evidence we have currently indicates that at birth the child's autonomous equipment for survival consists of some reflexes, his physiologic homeostatic mechanisms, and sensory capacity to perceive external and especially internal stimuli. The child's repository of memories is essentially empty and the executive functions of his personality have not yet developed and it has therefore no way to help itself. To thrive, the child must have immediately available an adult who can respond to the signals and signs he emits when he is prey to need tensions. This adult person who perceives these signs then undertakes what we call mothering functions by drawing on their empathy, factual knowledge, and memories to gratify the infant's needs and wants. In the early days of life, the child then sinks back into a state of quiescence and a cycle of transaction is completed (Spitz, 1965).

From the point of view of the child, what is essential in early infancy is relief from need tensions. In a primitive way he learns that having something put into him or done to him is associated with the disappearance of bad feelings. Slowly and gradually the person associated with this ministration is recognized and invested with positive feelings. In time the relationship with this nurturing person becomes as important and in some instances more important than the nurturance itself. Evidence of this can be found in the phenomenon of the eight-month anxiety (Spitz, 1965) and the studies on hospitalism (Spitz, 1945). This developmental step the child takes from cherishing comforts to an investment in the human purveyors of comfort is of enormous importance, since it is the template upon which the capacity for all future relationships rests.

Psychological examination of the addict reveals that it is precisely in the area of weak commitments to object relatedness and in the exploitation of the humans who surround him for immediate, concrete gratification, usually in the that the pathology is most prominent.

Let us leave the area of addiction for a moment to return to the issue of mothering. Where does a mother glean the sensitivity, strength, and intuitive wisdom to mother her child? Benedek has explored the psychobiology of mothering (Benedek, 1952; Benedek, 1956; Benedek, 1956; and Benedek, 1959) and has demonstrated that when the mother tends her newborn she is both unconsciously reliving the gratification she experienced with her own mother and is experiencing the pleasure of successfully living up to an ego ideal of motherliness.

The arduous task of adapting her life to the needs of her newborn is rendered more manageable and easier by the fact that in a well-related and comfortable family, the father can become very maternal and supportive during the latter stages of her pregnancy and the early months of the child's infancy.

Finally, in tending her child, mother is stimulated to motherliness and is gratified by seeing her child thrive. Graphically this state of balance and achievement of a successful symbiosis can be represented by Fig. 1. Mother's capacity for concern and for investment of care-taking energies (A) toward the child takes its origin from the past and develops from her experiences with her own mother (B). In her current life, she receives succor from father (or other intimates) (C) and gratifying feedback from her own infant (D).

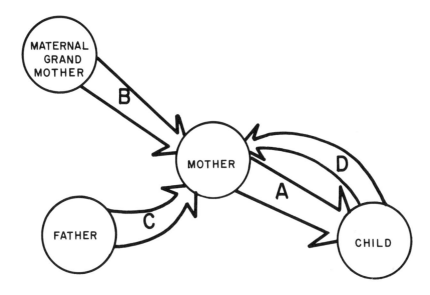

These latter transactions between mother and infant concern us most directly and might be scrutinized more closely by employing an ethological model.

We can conceive of the child as having a repertoire of activities which act as stimuli to the mothering person. This repertoire consists of his cries, reflexes, his very size and helplessness, his movements, etc. In the ideal situation, which seldom, if ever, exists, each signal the child emits reaches a mother who is sensitized and responsive. The maternal responses, which can range from a biologic reaction such as lactation at the sound of certain kinds of crying to a psychological experience of tenderness, gratify the child and allow him to return to a state of serene quiescence. This transaction leaves behind a series of pleasantly experienced memory traces in both mother and child which prepares them both for a more vigorous and secure undertaking the next time need tensions arise in their symbiotic system (Fig. 2A). A store of these memory traces in the child lays the groundwork for development of those attitudes that have been variously called hope (French, 1952), confidence (Benedek, 1938), and optimism (Erickson, 1963). These traits in the child gratify and stimulate the mother more effectively and the development of what Spitz calls dialogue (1965) is on its way, based on the firm footing of mutually gratifying experiences.

A perfect dialogue exists only in theory, of course. Actually, while most of the signals emitted by the child elicit gratifying responses from the mother, a small but important number of them do not. Who has not experienced directly or known of situations in which a father arriving home in the evening is greeted by the mother saying, "Thank God, you're home. Johnny's been a bear-cat all afternoon. I just don't know what he wants." She is reporting that the baby's

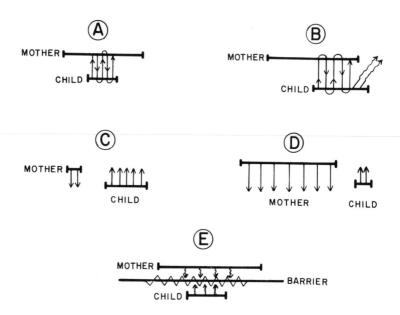

signals have been indecipherable and have left both her and the child in a state of chronic need tension. These periods are important because if they are not too numerous or too prolonged for the child, they increase his tolerance for frustration and introduce that sometimes painful awareness we call reality (Fig. 2B).

Needless to say, the situation is not always felicitously successful. There are instances in which, as Spitz (1965) puts it, "derailment of dialogue" occurs.

One group of such instances are those in which a child's perfectly competent and valid signals find no resonance in the environment because factors in the mother (physical illness, depression, temperament, drug-induced stupor) impede an appropriate response (2C). As an example, think only of the number of young mothers discharged from psychiatric facilities on massive doses of tranquilizing drugs, who attempt to care for young children in practically a zombie-like state.

Conversely, there are times when a mother's readiness to respond remains distressingly fallow because of the infant's inability to stimulate her or to respond to her ministrations (Fig. 2C). An example of this condition can be found in Brazelton's important description of how an over-sedated newborn's lethargy distresses and precipitates self-doubt in the mother. Other descriptions of the child's part in the "derailment of dialogue" are offered by Thomas, Chess, and Birch (1963) in their studies on temperament (Fig. 2D).

Finally, there are situations in which this bonding process between mother and child is impeded by barriers which have been imposed by external agencies. Spitz's (1945) work on hospitalism speaks of one aspect of this subject. Klaus and his co-workers studying an experiment in nature, in which mother and child had to be separated during the neonatal period, suggested that the incidence of child abuse, "failure to thrive" and abandonment in these non-contact situations was significantly higher than in control groups where mother and child were allowed early and undisturbed communion. These studies support the thesis that there is a phase in the mother-child interaction that is critical for the development of a successful symbiosis. The mother and child must be available to each other during this critical period, and the development of the bonding process can be damaged by *intrapersonal* difficulties in either partner, as well as *interpersonal* barriers (such as plate glass windows, intrusive grandmothers, obstructive medical personnel, books with poorly conceived and articulated concepts and poorly tested edicts on how to mother, etc.) that interfere with the bonding process.

To return now to the situation of addiction in the nursery, we can see that there is jeopardy at several levels.

First off, if we accept that the damage which rendered the future addict vulnerable occurred early in her development (that is, when she moved from a style of wanting only immediate material supplies to relieve need tensions to a stage in which she became firmly committed to cherishing the person relieving these need tensions), we can see how little motherliness the female addict acquired from her own mother. She has little in the way of conscious or unconscious experiences of mothering to fall back on.

Furthermore, since the addict's style is to seek only material gratification from her object relationships, she is enormously vulnerable in pregnancy and postpartum when the support that is needed is largely emotional or psychological. Too, the amount of psychological gratification that she can glean from viewing, holding or fondling her baby is minimal because of her essentially materialistic orientation.

Finally, we must add that the infant's withdrawal symptoms render it less than an adequate stimulator to the mothering activities. It would appear then that what suffers in the condition of addiction in mother and newborn is the necessary symbiosis by which the infant's psychological and biological survival is assured. This model has been proposed to study and explain another condition which occurs in infancy and early childhood. The condition is child abuse and and neglect, and indeed there are many points of similarity in the two situations (Coppolillo, 1974). One of the most prominent differences is that in the case of the addict the stress of pregnancy, delivery, and nurturing induces the mother to revert to the characteristic style of handling stress: withdrawal through narcotic-induced stupor. The abusive mother, for reasons not yet discovered, has no such refuge and lashes out to eliminate the imagined source of stress and irritation (Balikov): her own child!

Turning now to notions of management, it is clear that here, as in any other clinical situation, no rule can substitute for clinical judgment. Before formal intervention begins, decisions must be made about what will be optimal. Is the mother going to be able to keep the baby with support and therapy? Does she want to keep it? Is she going to require hospitalization for her habit or is she under criminal indictment? Has the baby sustained any irreversible damage? Will it thrive in the environment the mother can provide? While it may not be possible to answer these questions immediately, the asking of them sensitizes the staff to the interpersonal and intrapsychic variables that must be considered.

If it is decided that the mother and child will be together, even if it is for a limited period, then the mother and her infant should have early and repeated contact. A staff member with whom the mother has a relationship should initiate repeated, relatively brief contacts in which the status of the child is described and reassurance about him is offered. The therapist would be well advised to avoid issues involving personal and social value judgments regarding addiction at this time. The reassurance ought to be along the lines of predicting that with the disappearance of withdrawal symptoms, the child will feed more vigorously and respond to maternal ministrations with serenity rather than irritability.

If it appears that the child will have to be placed, the medical staff would do well to remember that one of our vulnerabilities in medicine is that we become so fascinated by pathology that we ignore the requisites of normal growth and development. Although in the throes of withdrawal symptoms, the infant will still need the human contact which will permit bonding to occur. Periods of holding and fondling by staff members for the child while still in the nursery should be planned.

In closing, we might review our therapeutic armamentariums for the psychological cure of the adult addiction syndrome and recognize that our track record is not good. Let us remember, too, that the long span of time between the damaging experience and the onset of addiction tends to deflect our attention from the childhood of the future addict. With these issues in mind we may one day conclude that our best attack on drug addiction will be the prevention of psychological vulnerability in the individual and not just massive programs of social reform.

References

Balikov, H. Personal communication.

Benedek, T. Adaptation to reality in early infancy. *Psychoanalytic Quarterly*. 1938, 7: 200-215.

Benedek, T. *Psychosexual Functions in Women*. New York, Ronald Press, 1952.

Benedek, T. Toward the biology of the depressive constellation. *Journal of the American Psychoanalytic Association*, 1956, IV: 389-427.

Benedek, T. Psychobiological aspects of mothering. *American Journal of Orthopsychiatry*. 1956, 272-278.

Benedek, T. Parenthood as a developmental phase. A contribution to Libido Theory. *Journal of the American Psychoanalytic Association*. 1959, 7: 389-417.

Burack, R. *The New Handbook of Prescription Drugs*. Rev. ed. New York, Pantheon, Division of Random House, 1970.

Coppolillo, H. The age of aquarius. Youth and drugs. *Journal of Occupational Medicine*. 1972, 14: 373-376.

Coppolillo, H. A Conceptual model for the study of some abusing parents. Paper presented at the Eighth International Congress of Child Psychiatry, Philadelphia, July 1974. Submitted for publication.

Erickson, E. *Childhood and Society.* New York, W.W. Norton and Company, 1963.

French, T.M. *The Integration of Behavior.* Chicago, The University of Chicago Press, 1952.

Spitz, R. Hospitalism. *The Psychoanalytic Study of the Child.* New York, International Universities Press, 1945.

Spitz, R. *The First Year of Life.* New York, International Universities Press, 1965.

Thomas, A., Chess, S., and Birch, H. *Behavioral Individuality in Early Childhood.* New York, New York University Press, 1963.

DISCUSSION

Q. *Dr. Davis:* Well, first of all, I wish to commend Dr. Coppolillo on his presentation because it was the kind of presentation I was waiting for. The missing link between the kinds of things that most physicians have been interested in, especially the obstetrical, pediatrics, even social workers' role in the treatment of these children, is forgetting perhaps the biggest and most important dimension, which is the mother. Studying the child's development, and as a neurologist interested in the effect of the narcotics on the child's alternate development, I feel that bypassing this very important role is really a dangerous omission. I would further like to point out that this is very important. You have already spoken about some of the items that I was planning to talk about tomorrow. The correlation between the symptoms and the role of the mother in the management is so important that I wish to perhaps suggest to the neonatalogists and point out the absence of infections, as the result of having the mothers in the nurseries more often. The babies should not be kept shielded in these glass cages, which are rather frightening to the mothers also. This should be reserved only for the children who have symptoms serious enough to warrant ICU's. There should be a movement toward having rooming-in, even for the first few days. This should take place at least for a number of hours every day so that maternal attachment can take place. I believe it is going to reduce the number of problems that we have seen clinically, and I have some evidence to show that this exists.

Q. *Dr. Merritt:* Is there any evidence that the abnormal activity of the baby who has had tremors, and all of the symptomatology and signs, will prevent adequate bonding by the mother?

A. *Dr. Coppolillo: I think hard, conclusive evidence is hard to come by in human beings. There is, however, cumulative evidence that anxiety in mothers can prevent or interfere with bonding. A mother who is guilt-ridden and ashamed would find it comforting to surrender those functions which only she can undertake to physicians and nurses. Yes, there is evidence from newborns with central nervous system disease, with perinatal injury and from premature newborns that any deviance in the child is accompanied by great maternal anxiety which interferes with the bonding process. I would recommend Marshall Klaus's work to you with enthusiasm.*

Q. *Dr. Davis:* I wonder what kind of psychopathology you thought you were referring to when you said it was psychopathology itself that gave rise to drug addiction?

A. *Dr. Coppolillo: In drug addicts that are studied, there are adaptive patterns that are monotonously similar and could be considered pathological. While studying responses to the M.M.P.I. in addicts at Lexington, for example, they found such a consistent massive response to the psychopathic deviant scale that subdividing it into three sub-scales was necessary to differentiate the population. I believe the pathology that is most destructive in addicted people is the inability to engage in and enjoy an object relationship. I believe this is one of the reasons why we as psychiatrists do poorly with these patients and group approaches like Synanon do better. They do not leave it to the addict to initiate the relationship, but rather intrude and force the relationship on them.*

Dr. Davis: Yes, I agree that generally, in the addicted population, that there is a great need to produce some ability to internalize, and to create good object relations. One thing that we have seen in our mothers is that, and this corresponds some to the kind of family history that Leon Wormser has delineated in the addicts he has seen in intensive psychotherapy—on many occasions the mother is quite able to vicariously enjoy the care that the infant is getting, unless it is thwarted by severe withdrawal in the infant, where again she is not able to enjoy that response. But when the withdrawal symptom is well controlled in the infant, the mother is much better able to mother.

Addictive Diseases: an International Journal 2 (2): 209-211 (1975)
© 1975 by Spectrum Publications, Inc.

GENERAL DISCUSSION

Dr. Davis: I would like to encourage clinicians and investigators in the area to make reports adopting World Health Organization terminology for terms relating to addiction and drug dependence. I think we, unwittingly sometimes, perpetuate untoward attitudes by referring, for example, to neonates as addicts. The World Health Organization recommends using the definition of addiction to be "one who compulsively seeks after and uses drugs," as opposed to one who is physically dependent upon a drug or chemical compound, as opposed to or in conjunction with, a person who is psychologically dependent on a chemical compound. I think that, probably, the use of the term "addiction" also can inhibit the proper application of pharmacological principles on house staff, on residents, and so forth. I am a bit sensitive about the use of the term "addiction" where it is not, in fact, applied properly.

Dr. Braude: Can we return to that question of seizures which have been reported by some of you in those babies born to addicted mothers as part of the withdrawal syndrome? I wonder what is happening, and why some investigators do see them and others do not.

Dr. Hug: Maybe I am just repeating what everyone knows. That is, in the human, particularly, seizures are not part of the abstinence syndrome in the adult. When it is seen, it is clear evidence that the adult is taking some other drug, usually alcohol, which is easier to detect sometimes, or one of the barbiturates, or other depressants; diazepam and that whole category of drugs. So that the first inclination, certainly among people dealing with physically dependent, adult individuals, is that they are on a mixture of drugs. I also might add that even in animals, in the primate monkey, rhesus monkey, etc., seizures are not a part of withdrawal from morphine.

Dr. Harper: We have seen seizures in methadone-maintained mothers, but these mothers certainly could have been taking other drugs. The point that I want to make is that, in the infants of these mothers, the seizures were very prolonged, very severe, and extremely difficult to control. Frequently, although we used quite high doses of either phenobarbital or Valium, in an attempt to control the seizures, the only thing that would control it was if we gave an opiate, such as methadone or morphine. I never had seizures that were so difficult to control under any other circumstances in the newborn.

Dr. Harbison: Thank you. I think we also have to remember that the central nervous system of the newborn is not fully developed in the cerebellar function, and so forth. This takes several weeks, which could explain the differences in the symptoms seen.

Dr. Abrams: I just wanted to make the comment that in these two days we have not heard much about congenital anomalies of the newborn infants, and I presume that it is because nobody has seen much, and it is generally accepted in the literature that these anomalies (congenital abnormalities) are not common in the drug-addicted infant. However, we might be deluding ourselves, we may be under a false sense of complacency, because we know that there are—somebody quoted—nine cases. I would not call these congenital anomalies, but perhaps neonatal problems, in morbidity and mortality, that we have not focused attention on. Nine cases of sudden death have occurred in the early infancy period—I think Jacobson and Bernen reported—amongst LSD-taking mothers. There were about eight children with neurotube defects, meningomyelocele, and such, that would seem a high incidence. We have seen in the patients we are following, amongst a group of 70, three with enlarged heads, which were transient—in other words, were resembling arrested hydrocephalus, —and two or three with foot deformities, in the form of talipes equinovarus and hydroceles. I am just wondering whether perhaps the incidence of these minor abnormalities and other illnesses is a little higher than in the general population. Maybe these studies have not been done yet and I think we should look into that a little more carefully.

Dr. Braude: In which infants did you see these congenital abnormalities?

Dr. Abrams: Infants who were exposed to methadone-taking mothers.

Q. *Dr. Nathenson:* We, too, have seen two instances, in 200 patients, of club deformity, talipes equinovarus, and we do not know whether that means anything. It seems to be the only congenital "anomaly" that has turned up in our group of babies. Now that you mentioned one other type, has anyone else seen that?

A. *Dr. Zelson: Yes.*

Q. *Dr. Nathenson:* How frequently, Dr. Zelson?

A. *Dr. Zelson: In the incidence of one in a hundred, which we would have in this group, is about a tenfold incidence over the general population, if two cases mean anything statistically. In 625 babies, we have had seven or eight babies that had inguinal hernias in the immediate newborn period. We had one baby who had a clubfoot, and a few babies that had minor, extra digits and things of that sort, but actually, the total percentage is less than 3 percent.*

Q. *Dr. Nathenson:* Were these hernias in white babies or black; or was there a difference?

A. *Dr. Zelson: I do not think there was a difference. I might as well mention the problem of convulsive seizures. We have seen, definitely, convulsive seizures as a symptom, as one of the manifestations of withdrawal. In the methadone group, we had approximately 10.5% of the babies having convulsive seizures. In the heroin group we had only about 4.4% of convulsive seizures. There is no question in my mind that these are real seizures, and the seizures that we saw, Dr. Rita Harper, the methadone babies were very much more severe than the babies on the herion.*

Dr. Hug: I think this makes a good point, and one that some of us, including myself, are often guilty of, and that is, we tend to generalize. We study much about morphine in a species and then translate that to others. Certainly this brings to mind something else; and that is with Demerol, I think that many of you may be aware of the fact that Demerol is metabolized, particularly when given orally to normeparadinic acid, which is a convulsive agent in its own right. As far as methadone studies are concerned, I am not up on the literature, but I do not know how much it has been looked at, for example, in terms of seizures, in animal species or in man, for that matter. That is not the kind of study you do on man. So I think maybe we do have to segregate our thinking and be rather specific about which compounds we are talking about. My earlier remarks, for example, were based almost exclusively on morphine.

Addictive Diseases: an International Journal 2 (2): 213-226 (1975)

Neurological Aspects of Perinatal Narcotic Addiction and Methadone Treatment

MIRYAM M. DAVIS
Department of Neurology
Children's Hospital, Washington, D.C.;
Narcotics Treatment Administration,
Perinatal Treatment Program, NTA,
Washington, D.C.

BETTY SHANKS
Department of Neurology
Children's Hospital, Washington, D.C.

INTRODUCTION

For infants born to heroin-addicted mothers, life begins and unfolds under the most precarious conditions. The high-risk factors complicating these mothers' pregnancies are by no means limited to direct drug pathology. Many other factors can derogate the outcome. Among these are protein malnutrition, neglected health, and guilt, depression, and self-destructive behavior—all of these being by-products of the addict's life-style (Blinick et al, 1969; Cobrinick et al, 1959; Zelson et al, 1971; Zelson, 1972; Rosenthal et al, 1964; Statzer et al, 1972; and Chappel et al, 1972).

Contrary to widespread belief, the pathology is not corrected by "legal methadone replacement," still the main ingredient of most treatment programs. Worse yet, pregnancy adds its own inimitable measure of stress (Zelsson, Personal Communication Aug. 73). And the unkindest cut of all, as Dr. Coppolillo illustrated, is a gross detriment to the quality of mothering. This is further dampened by postpartum separation from the newborn and the ultimate receipt home of a purportedly normal but in fact irritable and demanding infant by an ill-equipped mother.

The complexity of these factors has been well explored. Desmond reported extensively on the effects of various maternal psychoactive drugs on the off-spring, on their disruptive effect on the mother-infant interaction, and on their deleterious effect on crucial early development (Hill et al, 1963; Desmond et al, 1969). Kron showed depressed sucking responses, and Brackbill found changes in avoidance response to conditioned stimuli persisting in one-month newborns after drugged deliveries (Kron, 1966; Kront, et al, 1973; Kront et al, 1966; and Bowes et al, 1970). Likewise, Brazelton extensively explored and implicated ob-stetrical tranquilizers and analgesics as a cause of transient feeding and adaptive behavioral changes which *delayed* early weight gain and affected mother-child interaction during a period considered critical for imprinting processes (Brazel-ton, 1961; and Brazelton, 1970).

In such context, it becomes imperative to investigate the *basic issue* of changes induced in the fetal brain by maternal narcotics (methadone included) and their impact on the child's ultimate development. Elucidation requires so-phisticated studies designed to minimize the confounding effects of associated high-risk factors on long-term neurological and behavioral outcome (Birch, et al, 1970; Rosenwaike, 1971; Drillien, 1970; and Winick, 1970). Epidemiological work must thoroughly clarify the relative effect of improved maternal health, nutrition, and motivation, and patient self-selection in achieving any gains de-scribed under the greatly varying methadone programs. Pediatric studies, while expanding in size, duration, and scope, are still too limited to allay fears of pos-sible damage to the vulnerable growing brain (Harper et al, 1974; Davis et al, 1973; Davis, 1974; and Blatman, 1972, 1973).

We have thus implied the main approach and objectives of our current research project. The basic contributions of the study are to be as follows: (a) the systematic investigation of neurological and behavioral characteristics, their evolution and prognostic significance; (b) the application of electrophysiological measurements (e.g., sleep studies and computer-averaged EEG responses to sensory stimulation) as a possibly sensitive indicator of early cerebral dysfunc-tion (27-43) (Dustman et al, 1969; Barnet et al, 1965; Barnet et al, 1967; Barnet et al, 1971; Barnet, 1971; Engel et al, 1963; Engel, 1965; Ohlrich et al, 1972; Lewis et al, 1970; Khazan et al, 1967; Kay et al, 1969;Hartman, 1967; Oswald, et al; Way et al, 1968; Feinberg et al, 1969; Ertl et al, 1969; and Schulman, 1969).

This presentation will be introductory and restricted to neurological obser-vations and therapeutic application, which still await pathogenic elucidation. These will be further elaborated and complemented by Dr. Lodge, an early co-investigator, now conducting similar studies in San Francisco since 1972, who will present preliminary data on her behavioral and EEG studies.

SUBJECTS

The sample consisted of 130 infants born to narcotic-addicted mothers, both untreated and treated with methadone in various dosages and modalities ranging from high to low and slow detoxification. Ninety-two percent of our subjects were black and most qualified for Medicaid. Twins and newborns with serious complications were excluded. The following procedures were carried out:

Neurological examinations were conducted utilizing techniques and scoring criteria established by Prechtel and Beintema (1964, revised 1968); R. Paine, and the P.R.B. Collaborative Study Protocol (Prechtel et al, 1964; and Paine et al, 1962). Examinations were standardized for their timing (usually late morning, 2 to 2½ hours postprandial) and environmental factors. The first examination was conducted 24 to 48 hours after birth, repeated at least 3 and up to 16 times during hospitalization. The mothers were encouraged to observe the second to third day and discharge examinations.

Brazelton's Neonatal Behavioral Neurological Assessment Scale was utilized (Brazelton, 1973). This is a sensitive index of the newborn's behavioral characteristics and ability to control and organize his responses to the environment. We were possibly the first to explore its usefulness in this context (1970, 1972). The test grades (on a scale of nine) 26 behavioral responses to stimuli, and 16 reflexes. It was conducted initially after 24 hours and repeated at least twice during the hospitalization.

The *Bayley Scales of Infant Development* were administered to a subsample of 21 infants and young children ranging in age from 2 months through 25 months, all exposed to methadone in utero. Their developmental status (mental and psychomotor) will be described primarily in relation to the average expected for children of the same chronological age according to published norms (Bayley, 1969)

FINDINGS

Consistent with known reports, these babies show high incidence of low birthweight, but good Apgar scores (Blinick, et al, 1969; Blatman, 1973; Chappel, 1972; Davis, et al, 1973; Davis, 1974). Our statistics on major withdrawal are similar to those reported by Harper et al (Harper, 1974). The spectrum and severity of symptoms tended to correlate with size of maternal narcotic intake (Davis, 1973; 1974).

"Classical" Neurological Findings Findings are those of CNS hyperexcitability, with irritability, tremors, and hypertonicity, impaired nutritive sucking, vomiting, severe sleep deficit, hyperthermia and tachypnea, this leading to failure to thrive in the most severe. Autonomic dysfunction varies from vasomotor lability and diaphoresis to the less frequent diarrhea.

Almost universal in the early weeks, and deserving some comment is the lability of "states," with frequent shifts through the various stages of sleep and wakefulness, often precipitated by environmental or, possibly, internal stimuli. Sleep is disturbed in quality and in quantity at the expense of the decreased quiet, or non-REM sleep.

Similarly universal is the increased oral drive; non-nutritive sucking is tireless, sometimes frantic. When unfulfilled, it leads to mounting agitation, persistent crying, tremulous hyperactivity, and exhaustion. Proper positioning is essential for enhancing the neonate's own "hand to mouth" facility. While hard to achieve on supine, it is greatly enhanced in prone, and better even by swaddling infants with their extremities flexed and hands placed before their mouths. The use of a pacifier (easier to prop in this position) is the most effective complement to soothe the baby.

When unaware of the significance of non-nutritive sucking and the proper means of handling it, mothers receiving their newly-arrived babies interpret and treat this as a sign of insatiable hunger. Feedings are frequently offered, but a few sucks can soothe only for short periods. After 20 or 30 minutes of restless sleep they cry again, and the cycle is repeated for days until diarrhea, vomiting, and exhaustion supervene. Maternal frustration and the return of the baby to the hospital thus follows, with the so-called rebound, or sub-acute withdrawal. Incidentally, proper training of mothers on the use of pacifiers and proper spacing of feedings dramatically reduced this complication.

Hyperactivity, an important sign of irritability, seems to be one of the most persistent findings, and may endure through the early school age. It is worthwhile to point out its characteristic. There is an exaggerated relationship of these motor behavior changes with changes of body posture. When the infant is supine and unrestrained, movements assume a jerky, purposeless, "en masse" character, apparently perpetuated by unchecked proprioceptive stimuli.

The effect of turning the infant into the prone position is dramatic. Motor behavior becomes organized and, at times, self-controlled: (a) crawling movements which may lead to his displacement along the crib; (b) lifting chin and moving head from side to side, elevating chest and leaning on elbows and forehead; and (c) use of hand-mouth facility to quiet self. Control of hyperactivity is further improved by swaddling in the "fetal" position. Early infantile automatisms and postural reflexes are intact but usually exaggerated. This applies to the Moro, traction response, weight bearing, placing, stepping, crawling, and Landau reflexes. They are also often accelerated in their maturational sequencing. This is well illustrated by the evolution of the tonic neck reflexes. In our subjects this is prematurely superseded by body-righting responses and thence followed by premature "turning over" as early as one to two weeks. In the normal, 6-12 weeks are necessary for this to develop. Increasingly complex motor milestones such as crawling, weight bearing, and standing are frequently acce-

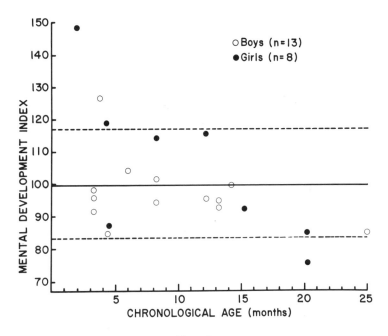

Figure 1

lerated, but the rate of this advance appears to slacken with the increasing complexity of the milestone.

As for the much-discussed incidence and implications of myoclonic jerks and seizures, we are prepared for general statements only, at this time. They appear to be greater in methadone than in heroin withdrawal, and associate least frequently with the smallest drug exposure. Their prevalence suggests a probable dose-effect relationship.

Brazelton Neurobehavioral Findings These findings are generally consistent with those described in an earlier study in which we participated (Soule et al, 1973). The Brazelton test was valuable in quantitating the CNS irritability described. It especially dramatized the impaired ability of post-narcotic babies to adequately organize their responses to environment. They showed lessened capacity to attend and react to noxious stimuli, to habituate disturbing events. They reacted, oriented and habituated better to sound than to visual stimuli, with optimal soothing response to human voice.

The detailed analysis of Brazelton data will follow this preliminary discussion in a later paper.

Psychological Findings The distribution of obtained scores on the Bayley Mental Scale is presented in Figure 1. The infants tested during their first five months of age display a wide range in functional level on the Mental Scale, from a high of 144 to a borderline score of 84. Examination of individual records

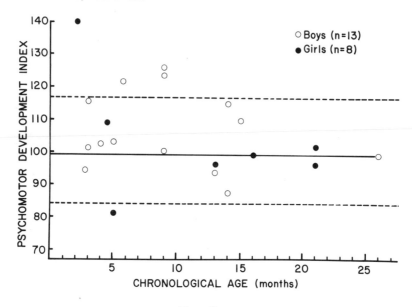

Figure 2

shows those at the higher levels to be more socially responsive, more able to reach, grasp, or to manipulate objects, and to vocalize, whereas infants with the lowest functional levels tended to be limited.

The children evaluated during the last quarter of their first year (8 to 12 months) generally fell within the normal range. Past 15 months, the trend was toward borderline or a definite lag in mental development. This appears to be related primarily to poor verbal ability. When performance reflecting the receptive understanding or the expressive use of language is considered, these children are estimated at two to four months below the expected.

Figure 2 presents the distribution of scores obtained on the Motor Scale. Although there is a wide dispersion in overall functional level at the youngest ages (from a low of 81 to a high of 140), it may be noted that motor performance of a significantly large proportion of infants falls above the mean of 100. Of the twelve children evaluated between 2 and 8 months of age, ten achieved motor scores above the mean and two below (p. 0.038). Of these, five exhibited accelerated motor development (scored past 116), and only one child exhibited signs of significant lag (motor scores of 81). Evaluation of motor function during this period of development is based largely on behaviors reflecting postural adjustments, balance, muscular strength and tonus and midline arm and hand coordinations. From examination of individual protocols, no particular type of motor skill appeared to contribute to the observed trends. Good motor performance was exhibited by the children evaluated during the second year of life with scores distributed within the normal range.

DISCUSSION

According to our observations based upon a body of neurological semeiological data, nearly every post-narcotic newborn presents, usually within four days and not later than seven, a constellation of subtle but significant behavior changes which merit designation as "minor" withdrawal, in distinction to the more dramatic "major" withdrawal.

In too many of these cases, nursery staff and physicians may diagnose "no symptoms of withdrawal," and this has thwarted treatment and misled to theories of feto-placental drug-metabolic idiosyncrasies.

Thus, we suggest the concept of "late," "subacute," or "rebound" withdrawal to be largely the result of semeiological oversight: rather these often represent preventable exacerbations of manifest "minor" or remited major withdrawal, for which special nursing and maternal handling could have been therapeutic or prophylactic.

This has important social implications. If medication is not required, the child can be released home and estrangement avoided, with obvious benefit to the mother-child relationship. The economies thus realized can more than defray the often critically essential homemaker-nurse assistance.

Cooperative mothers are easily trained by an enlightened staff and motivated to handle the specific behavior of these infants. The concept of the baby's hyperexcitability and his lowered threshold to external and internal stimuli is readily grasped, and the mothers then respond better to their irritable, seemingly inconsolable charges. This is doubly valuable because of the fragile self-confidence of these mothers.

The increased oral drive sucking can be handled with pacifier, and by prone posture or swaddling in fetal position to give finger pacification to the neonate. Hyperirritability and tremors yield to swaddling, coddling, and soothing; for the last the soft voice is very effective. Distressing hyperkinesis and coarse tremors are attenuated by prone positioning and swaddling.

The mother needs reassurance about the temporary nature of the insufficient and restless sleep which may endure for weeks. Preliminary EEG studies in newborns suggest that physiological alterations of drug-abstinent states include rebound REM increases with disorganization of cyclic phenomena (Schulman, 1969).

It is interesting to note that turning over, postural reflexes, and sequencing of primitive automatisms are advanced by weeks or months; this may not previously have been reported. Furthermore, these subjects are often hyper-alert with wide-open eyes. However, a higher cortical basis is not suggested by the neurological findings: most of this is of sub-cortical mediation, and the advance is not sustained when processes known to be expressive of higher cortical function supervene.

The clinical findings in neonatal withdrawal, the hypertonicity and particularly, the ophisthotonus, the diarrhea, myclonic jerks (and, rarely, seizures), sleep disturbance, and the hyper-alert state are reminiscent of hyperserotoninemia syndromes in the newborn. This would be consistent with well-known findings of rebound REM sleep associated with rebound increased brain serotonin in the adult withdrawing from narcotics (Kay et al, 1969; Hartman, 1967; Oswald et al; and Way et al, 1968). It does raise questions as to the role of serotonin and other neurotransmitters in withdrawal phenomena.

Although no conclusions may yet be drawn from the present psychometric data, the trend toward acceleration of motor behavior appears limited to the early developmental period, most notably the first eight months, with average performance between one and two years. No deleterious effects on development are indicated. However, tendencies for black infants to be more advanced in early motor performance have been reported (Bayley, 1965), with the difference disappearing after age twelve months. Others have reported similar findings which may be related to environmental conditions, socio-economic status, and related childrearing practices. (Knoblock and Pasamanick, 1954; Pasamanick, 1946; Williams and Scott, 1953).

Comparisons of developmental trends exhibited by methadone infants with those of carefully selected control subjects are being undertaken by our group at this time. The aforementioned deviant characteristics observed during the immediate postnatal period will be related to subsequent patterns of social interaction and development.

RELATED QUESTIONS AND FORMULATIONS

It appears that the motor, sensory, and cognitive behaviors observed during the early weeks and months of life are temporary and exclusively drug-induced. Nevertheless, an enduring effect on the child's subsequent development cannot yet be excluded.

Opiates may induce chemical and structural changes in the brain and other organs of the chronically exposed fetus, particularly in the synthesis, turnover, or disposition of catecholamines, serotonin, or dopamine (Kay et al, 1969; Hartman, 1967; Oswald et al; Way et al, 1968; Bowers et al, 1971; and Wyatt et al, 1970). What are these changes, specifically, and to what extent are they and their consequences reversible after exposure?

As to these behaviors and their underlying lesions, we should strive to elucidate their incidence, longitudinal evolution, neurophysiological correlates (auditory and visual evoked responses), and correlation with later outcome. All these require carefully designed prospective studies monitored from as early prenatally as possible, to include comparison with carefully selected control subjects not exposed to addictive drugs.

SUMMARY

The semeiology and significance of neonatal "minor withdrawal" are developed. Its treatment and the consequent prevention of rebound, late, or classical withdrawal are proposed. Basic research implications are formulated.

Acknowledgments

We wish to thank Dr. William Washington, Director of the Narcotics Treatment Administration, Department of Human Resources, District of Columbia, for his support of this work, and Ms. Margery Carr, R.N., Treatment Coordinator, and the staff of the Perinatal Treatment Program, NTA, for their contributions.

Part of this work was done with support of NIH Grant # DA00398-01.

References

Barnet, A.B., and Lodge, Ann, Click evoked EEG responses in normal and developmentally retarded infants. *Nature*, 214 (5085), 252-255, 1967.

Barnet, A.B., Ohlrich, E.S., and Shanks, Betty. EEG evoked responses to repetitive auditory stimulation in normal and Down's syndrome infants. *Develop. Med. Child Neurol.*, 13: 321-329, 1971.

Barnet, A.B., and Goodwin, A.M. Average evoked eletroencephalographic responses to clicks in the human newborn. *Electoenceph. and Clin. Neurophysiol.* 18: 441-450, 1965.

Barnet, A.B. EEG audiometry in children under three years of age. *Aeta-Oto-Laryngol.*, 72, 1-13, 1971.

Bayley, N. *Bayley Scales of Infant Development.* Psychological Corp., New York, 1969.

Birch, H., and Gussow, J.D. *Low Birth Weight and Handicap: Disadvantaged Children.* New York and London: Grune and Stratton, Inc., 46-80, 1970.

Blatman, S. Personal communications, 1972, 1973.

Blinick, G., Wallach, R., and Jerez, E. Pregnancy in methadone detoxification programs. *Am. J. of Ob-gyn.*, 105: 997, 1969.

Bowers, Kleber, and Davis. Acid monoamine metabolites in cerebrospinal fluid during methadone maintenance. *Nature*, 1971 (August), 232 (5312), 581-582.

Bowes, W., Brackbill, Y., Conway, E., and Steinschneider, A. *Effects of Obstetrical Medication on the Infant's Sensory Motor Behavior.* Monographs in Social Research and Child Development No. 137, 34, June, 1970.

Brazleton, B. Effects of maternal medication: psychophysiological reactions in neonates. *J. of Pediatrics*, 58: 5133, 1961.

Brazleton, B. Effects of drugs in the neonate. *Am. J. of Psychiatry*, 126: 9, 1970.

Brazelton, B. Neonatal Behavioral Assessment Scale. *Clinics in Developmental Medicine*, No. 50, Spastics International Medical Publications, 1973.

Chappel, J.N., and Davis, R.C. *A Comparison of Management Methods for Pregnant Narcotic Addicts.* State of Illinois Drug Abuse Rehabilitation Program Preliminary Report, January, 1972.

Cobrinick, R.W., Hood, R.T., Jr., and Chusid, E. The effect of maternal narcotic addiction on the newborn infant. *Pediatrics*, 35(2): 288, 1959.

Davis, M.M., Brown, B.S., and Glendinning, S.T. Neonatal effects of heroin addiction and methadone treated pregnancies. *Proceedings, Fifth National Conference on Methadone*, Washington, D.C., February, 1973.

Davis, M.M. Impact of technology on human development: the offspring of methadone-treated heroin-addicted mothers. Paper presented at the American Academy of Sciences, San Francisco, February 22, 1974.

Desmond, M.M., Rudolph, A., Hill, R., Claghorn, J., and Dreesen, P. Behavioral alterations in infants born to mothers on psychoactive medication during pregnancy. *Sumposium on Mental Retardation*, Texas Institute of Mental Sciences. Austin, Texas: University of Texas Press, p. 235, 1969.

Drillien, C.M. The small-for-dates infants: etiology and prognosis. *Ped. Clin. of N. Amer.*, 17: 9, 1970.

Dustman, R.E., and Beck, E.C. The effects of maturation and aging on the wave form of visually evoked potentials. *J. of Electroenceph. and Clin. Neurophysiol.* 26: 2, 1969.

Ellingson, R.J. *Developmental Neurophysiology: Drugs and Poisons in Relation to the Developing Nervous System.* P.H.S. Publication # 1791, 1967.

Engel, R., and Butler, B.V. Appraisal of conceptual age of newborn infants by EEG methods. *J. of Pediatrics*, 63: 386-393, 1963.

Engel, R. Maturational changes and abnormalities in the newborn EEG. *Dev. Medicine Child Neurol.*, 498-506, 1965.

Ertl, J.P., Schafer, E.P. Brain response correlates of psychometric intelligence. *Nature*, 223: 421-422, 1969.

Feinberg, I., Braun, M., and Schulman, E. EEG sleep patterns in mental retardation. *J. of Electroenceph. and Clin. Neurophysiol.*, 27: 128-141, 1969.

Harper, R.G., Solish, G.I., Purow, H.M., Sang, E., and Panepinto, W.C. The effect of methadone treatment programs upon pregnant heroin addicts and their newborn infants. *Pediatrics*, 54(3): 300, 1974.

Hartman, E.L. Effect of L-tryptophan on the sleep dream cycle in man. *Psychon. Sci.*, 8: 295-296, 1967.

Hill, R.M., and Desmond, M.M. Management of the narcotic withdrawal syndrome in the neonate. *Ped. Clin. of N. Amer.*, 10: 67, 1963.

Kay, D.C., Eisenstein, R.B., and Jasinski, D.R. Morphine effects on human sleep REM state, waking state and NREM sleep. *Psychopharmacologia* (Berl) 14: 404-416, 1969.

Khazan, N., Weeks, J.R., and Shroeder, L.A. EEG, Emg, and behavioral correlates during a cycle of self-maintained morphine addiction in the rat. *J. of Pharmacol., Exp, Ther.*, 155: 521-531, 1967.

Kron, R. Newborn sucking behavior affected by obstetrical sedation. *Pediatrics*, 37: 1012, 1966.

Kron, R.E., Litt, M., and Finnegan, L.P. Behavior of infants born to narcotic addicted mothers. *Proceedings of the Committee on Problems of Drug Dependence*, National Research Council, 1973.

Kron, R.E., Stein, M., and Goddard, K.E. Newborn sucking behavior affected by obstetric sedation. *J. of Pediatrics*, 37(6): 1012, 1966.

Lewis, S.A., Oswald, I., Evans, J.I., Akindele, M.O., and Tompsett, S.L. Heroin and human sleep. *J. of Electroenceph. and Clin. Neurophysiol.*, 28: 374-381, 1970.

Maternal Nutrition and the Course of Pregnancy. National Research Council Report, National Academy of Science, 1970.

Ohlrich, E.S., and Barnet, A.B. Auditory evoked responses during the first year of life. *J. of Electroenceph. and Clin. Neurophysiol.*, 32: 161-169, 1972.

Oswald, I., Evans, J.I., and Lewis, S.A. Addictive drugs cause suppression of paradoxical sleep with withdrawal rebound, in H. Steinberg (ed.), *Scientific Basis of Drug Dependence*. London: Churchill, 243-257.

Paine, R. and Donovan, D. Prognostic implications of neurologic abnormalities in the neonatal period. *Neurol.*, 12: 910, 1962.

Prechtl, M., and Beintema, D. The neurological examination of the full-term, normal infant. *Little Club Clinics in Developmental Medicine*, No. 12, London: Heineman, 1964.

Rosenthal, T., Patrick, S.W., and Krug, D.C. Congenital neonatal narcotic addiction: a natural history. *Am. J. of Public Health*, 58(8): 1252, 1964.

Rosenwaike, I. *Influence of Socioeconomic Status on Incidence of Low Birth Weight*. H.S.M.H.A. Health Reports, 86: 641, 1971.

Schutt, J. *Social Adaptation of the Pregnant Addict*. 4th National Conference on Methadone Treatment, San Francisco, January 9, 1972.

Shulman, C.A. Alterations of the sleep cycle in heroin addicted and "suspect" newborn. *Neuropadiatrie*, 1: 89-100, 1969.

Soule, A.B., Standley, K., Copans, S.A., and Davis, M.M. Clinical uses of the Brazelton Neonatal Scale. Paper presented at Society for Research in Child Development, Philadelphia, March, 1973. Also, *Pediatrics*, in press.

Statzer, D.E., and Wardell, J.N. Heroin addiction in pregnancy. *Am. J. of Ob-gyn.*, 113(2): 273, 1972.

Way, E.L., Low, H.H., and Shen, F.H. Morphine tolerance and synthesis of brain 5-HT. *Science*, 162: 1290-1292, 1968.

Winick, M. Cellular growth in intrauterine malnutrition. *Ped. Clin. of N. Amer.*, 17: 9, p. 69, 1970.

Wyatt, R.J., et al. Effects of 5-HTP on the sleep of normal human subjects. *J. of Electroenceph. and Clin. Neurophysiol.*, 1971 (June), 30(6): 505-509.

Zelson, C., Rubio, E., and Wasserman, E. Neonatal narcotic addiction: a 10 year observation. *Pediatrics*, 48: 178, 1971.

Zelson, C. Personal communication, August, 1972.

DISCUSSION

Q. *Dr. Statzer*: I would like to add only a couple of comments. I am now a full-time clinical obstetrician, no longer involved in this type of program, and am now in the research area. For many years, obstetricians have been handing pediatricians babies in various states of health. I think that as obstetricians, our feelings relating to this are sometimes very complex. We have a mother who has some type of either physical, social, or psychic trauma, not necessarily in the area of drugs, but in other areas as well. The problem for us as obstetricians is to handle that mother through her prenatal course, and give to the pediatrician the best possible baby. With the methadone program and the drug addiction program, this is even more of a problem. In our early studies in Detroit, for instance, we knew very well that we were addicting babies. However, with the very high means of psychosocial treatment available to us in our maternal-infant care project, we were able to proceed with a very good program, and end up with very good results. Basically, we realize that we were handing the pediatrician babies who were addicted at that point, but if we did not do this, we were not handing him a baby at all. So I think that the whole thing has to be put into perspective. Your points relating to the development of this and relating to the babies afterwards are everyone's concerns, and these are very well taken. As a clinician, I want to reiterate the fact that to assess properly it has to be a team effort to put the whole thing in the perspective and get the best possible baby.

Q. *Dr. Statzer*: I think in the early phases of treating addicted mothers we did not understand or were not concerned enough with the total picture. I think this has changed. We used low-dosage methadone from the beginning in Detroit, purely because we wanted to use the very minimal dose that would keep the patients in the program, keep them symptom-free, with the idea that we were very much concerned about what it would do to the baby. I support this whole-heartedly and I am a firm believer in the low-dosage area, which is, I think, being supported by the meeting. But what I meant to say was that we handed you the best possible baby, addicted or not, that we could, and I think that it is very important to study this very well, and to find out whether or not this is truly the best baby we can give you.

Q. *Dr. Krasnegor:* I have a general comment which applies to the general field of neonatal research and has to do with informed consent with respect to human subjects. I wonder how the various people who do research with neonates inform the mothers about what is being done with their children, and if there is a specific kind of informed consent that is used?

A. *Dr. Lodge: It is required that we use informed consent and, as you know, we actually try very much to involve the mothers. They hold the infants, they observe the testing, and we use the testing as a feedback kind of educational procedure. We have found that actually subjects in this general category of addiction are usually much more receptive and responsive to going ahead with this kind of testing, especially in the early stages. As a result, we have the advantage (in a cold research sense) of their feelings about the situation at the time, but we try and deal with this in a positive way. Our EEG lab is painted up and has posters, music, and this kind of thing. We try not to make it a frightening procedure despite all the tape recorders, and actually have had much more difficulty getting consent from mothers who were unaware or denied a problem in their infants, or from normal parents and babies, than from this particular group. It is an important issue certainly.*

Q. *Dr. Krasnegor:* In the experimental design, do you match these patients for dosages of methadone?

A. *Dr. Lodge: It is more after the fact. We take every one we can get and then we specify the group afterwards, because there are such variations in the dosage level.*

Q. *Dr. Krasnegor:* So you choose those patients which you will use, for example, for these numbers that you showed us?

A. *Dr. Lodge: Well, there is a wide range of dosage in all of the groups and I suspect that the findings that might appear to be heroin-related could, of course, be dosage-related, because these are quite possibly the ones that are getting the least amount of any kind of drug. The methadone-heroin group is probably a phenomenon that is not related to the characteristics of either drug. This is a problem with this kind of grouping. I do not know how to deal with it at this time.*

Q. *Dr. Connaughton:* I just want to know if you think that when you test these babies with the mothers there you can be completely objective, knowing, I assume, when you are talking to them that they are methadone patients or methadone-heroin patients before you start testing? Does this not influence how you interpret the results of the test?

A. *Dr. Lodge: It certainly could and it would be preferable to have a double-blind. I am a firm believer in the double-blind. If I had a large staff, I would do this much more. I do with the addicted infants; I know which infants are normal and which are not in the addicted group because I really have to dig them out of the nursery. With the others, I characteristically do not know which drug group they are in because by the time I get them, it all happens so fast. Afterwards, I find out which ones are addicted.*

Q. *Dr. Ostrea:* I would like to ask a question of Dr. Davis and Dr. Lodge regarding the reference you made to the Farston and Strauss paper and our studies in Detroit. We have come to the same findings as you, as far as the response of the addicted newborn to stimuli—like sound and light. There is, however, something that has bothered us. We were studying the effects of environment and grouping withdrawal into different grades of severity. The data we presented yesterday, as far as the methadone dose is concerned, show that there seems to be a higher dose for the mother, either initial, final, or average, if the baby is having severe withdrawal. The P-value here was less than .025 and these were babies in a controlled environment, that is, they were in a regular nursery. In another situation, babies whom we had in the dark nursery room where we controlled everything, developed moderate to severe withdrawal, and there was no correlation at all between the dose of the mother's intake to the severity of the withdrawal. In other words, is there a minimal form of environmental stimulus that would soothe the baby? There have been studies in the past where the rhythmic heartbeat sound of a mother would soothe a baby. If we remove this completely, are we going to produce more irritability rather than soothing the baby?

A. *Dr. Lodge: I wonder if I can quote from your study another thing that I think is related to this, that I thought was beautifully stated in the report? The study says "it appears that the basic cognitive structures of the addicted infants are not organically impaired, for when in an alert state they perform as well as their nonaddicted counterparts on the first day of life. As narcotic withdrawal proceeds, however, the level at which the addicted infants are able to explore their environment becomes less mature. This performance decrement is evident even during those rare periods of alertness experienced by the addicted neonates. Although the addicted neonates become less able to orient to auditory stimuli while alert, they do show normal ability to habituate to most stimuli while asleep; and show less than normal ability to habituate to visual stimulation." They did report that there was some ability of the infants to have a self-quieting behavior, that is, with the hand-to-mouth facility, and also, I think that the* *point that Dr. Davis made is that these babies are very responsive to holding, and cuddling, and to voice stimulation, which might not be as available even in a controlled dim light.*

Dr. Davis:

There is no question that affected infants have a lowered excitability threshold whether stimuli will be irritating or soothing depends not only upon its intensity but also upon its quality. Our preliminary clinical and Brazelton tests observations suggest that soft voice or similar tones, the human face, coddling and moderate light are soothing stimuli to affected babies.

In summary, expansion of the concept of the symptomalogy to include "minor" withdrawal, incidence of morbidity can be more validly determined and infants more effectively treated.

Addictive Diseases: an International Journal 2 (2): 227-234 (1975)
© 1975 by Spectrum Publications, Inc.

Neonatal Addiction: A Two-Year Study

PART I

Clinical and Developmental Characteristics of Infants of Mothers on Methadone Maintenance

CYRIL M. RAMER
ANN LODGE
*Children's Hospital,
San Francisco, Calif.*

Insufficient clinical experience exists regarding the management of the pregnant heroin addict who enters a methadone-maintenance treatment program or the female who conceives and delivers while consuming methadone. Comprehensive long-term studies of the outcome and course of the infants born to these mothers are also inadequate and sometimes contradictory.

This study presents a review of the neonatal course and a report of the early growth and development of thirty-five infants born to addicted mothers over a two-year time period.

STUDY

Between April, 1972 and September, 1974, 35 infants were born to 32 mothers registered in the San Francisco city-operated Methadone Maintenance Treatment Program. One mother delivered twins and two mothers each delivered two infants during the course of study. All the mothers in the program received methadone and comprehensive rehabilitative services from the Center for Special Problems, a division of the San Francisco Health Department. (Ramer, 1973). Their medical and obstetrical services were provided by the High Risk Pregnancy Clinic, Children's Hospital, San Francisco. The infants were examined and treated in the Intensive Care Nursery at Children's Hospital. Hospital pediatric care and outpatient follow-up on all 35 infants were provided by the same pediatrician, the co-author. The infants were assessed daily during their hospitalization for presence and severity of withdrawal signs and symptoms. Daily urines were collected for presence of narcotic metabolites; serum bilirubin, glucose, calcium, CBC, VDRL, SGOT were obtained as well.

In June 1972, the Infant Development Research Laboratory at Children's Hospital began a longitudinal study of the development of these infants.

RESULTS

Obstetrical Complications Of the 35 infants, 34 were born at or near term and one at 36 weeks' gestation—this infant was delivered prematurely by Caesarian section for abruptio placenta. The mother had a history of significant uterine bleeding for 2 months prior to delivery of the infant.

One infant expired at 12 hours of age from severe bilateral aspiration pneumonia, despite extensive resuscitative measures. The mother was admitted to the hospital shortly before the delivery was completed by emergency Caesarian section. For 12 hours prior to hospital admission, the mother was passing meconium-stained fluid. The fetal monitor on admission revealed a heart rate of less than 40, Apgar scores were 1 and 2, and the infant had severe meconium stain. The mother had been stabilized on 5 mgms of methadone for several months. An extensive autopsy revealed no congenital abnormalities. Two other infants were born following Caesarian section.

Sex There were 26 females and 9 males, a ratio of 2.9:1.

Congenital Abnormalities There were no congenital abnormalities noted in any infant except for bilateral rudimentary extra digits on one infant.

Apgar scores Apgar scores were at least 8 and 9 except for one transiently depressed infant and for the one severely depressed infant who expired.

Birth Weight The average birth weight for all single births was 3015 gms. However, when the infants were divided into two groups; those whose mothers were heroin addicts at the time of conception and later entered the methadone-maintenance pregnant addicts program (16 infants), versus those infants whose mothers were enrolled and stabilized on methadone maintenance when conceived (17 infants), a significant weight difference is demonstrated ($t = 3.447$; $p > .01$, 2-tailed test).

The average birth weight of infants conceived while mothers were using heroin was 2775 gms; the average birth weight of infants conceived while mothers were taking methadone was 3240 gms, a difference of 465 gms.

In addition, the mother of the largest infant of the heroin conceived group (3320 gms) entered the methadone program in her first trimester and received methadone for eight months of her pregnancy.

Laboratory Results Serum bilirubin levels were obtained on all infants on the

2nd and 3rd day of life. One infant developed an ABO incompatibility confirmed by the presence of a positive Coombs test. Another infant developed an elevated bilirubin level (14 mgs %) on the 3rd day of life. Both infants responded well to phototherapy. The bilirubin levels of all other infants (32) were below 7 mgms %.

CBC, serum calcium, glucose, and SGOT were all normal. VDRL results were positive in 4 infants whose mothers also demonstrated falsely positive VDRL's. FTA results on all four were negative.

Daily urine specimens were obtained on 31 of the infants (91%) and tested for narcotic metabolites. Twenty infants (65%) demonstrated urines positive for methadone at least once. Fifteen infants had methadone present in urine specimens for two days; seven for three days, and three infants for four days. In addition to methadone, six infants also demonstrated morphine (a breakdown product of heroin) in their urines.

Withdrawal Of the 34 surviving infants, eleven (32%) showed no symptoms of withdrawal during the entire hospital course. Nine infants (27%) showed mild symptoms of withdrawal, including minimal irritability, being tremulous only when stimulated, minimal regurgitation, and being comfortable when swaddled. Ten infants (29%) showed moderate signs of withdrawal, including irritability, being tremulous without stimulation, accompanied by a high pitched cry for periods of several hours, easy regurgitation unless gavage fed and usually requiring medication for comfort. Only four infants (12%) showed severe symptoms of withdrawal, including high irritability, tremulousness, constant crying, inconsolability, regurgitation of most feedings and the need for sedative medication several times each day. In addition, three of these infants developed transient seizures.

Of the 11 infants discharged as asymptomatic during hospitalization, three subsequently developed mild but definite symptoms of withdrawal, primarily irritability and tremulousness at 7 to 10 days of age. If the frequency of withdrawal symptoms is considered for the entire neonatal period, 8 remain asymptomatic (24%), 12 showed mild symptoms (35%), 10 moderate (29%), and 4 severe (12%).

Treatment Treatment was individualized and aimed at making each infant comfortable. Valium, 1 mgm, IM every 6 to 8 hours as needed, was used successfully in most moderate and severe cases. Two infants with the most severe symptoms required paregoric as well. Some moderate infants responded favorably to Donnatal, 1cc by mouth every 6 to 8 hours. 14 infants (41%) required medication during their hospitalization, six (18%) more were started on Donnatal after discharge, and 14 (41%) required no medication at all.

Length of Hospitalization The length of hospitalization ranged from 3 to 26 days with the average being 6 days.

Follow-Up Care 88% of the infants were available for follow-up care and study. Many infants failed to gain weight during the first and second weeks of life,

TABLE I
Mean Bayley Infant Scale Mental and Motor Indices of Infants Born to
Mothers on Methadone Maintenance

Monthly Age Interval		Mental (MDI)		Motor (PDI)
1 month	$\bar{x}$	89.80*	$\bar{x}$	121.00*
(1-30 days)	S.D.	10.94	S.D.	18.72
n=20	R	73-111	R	81-145
2-3 months	$\bar{x}$	117.30	$\bar{x}$	136.40
(31-90 days)	S.D.	16.56	S.D.	18.67
n=10	R	87-140	R	117-177
4-6 months	$\bar{x}$	116.43	$\bar{x}$	116.29
(91-150 days)	S.D.	17.91	S.D.	19.20
n=7	R	92-144	R	92-147
7-9 months	$\bar{x}$	110.40	$\bar{x}$	110.40
(151-240 days)	S.D.	31.41	S.D.	30.26
n=5	R	57-136	R	65-140
10-15 months	$\bar{x}$	113.57	$\bar{x}$	105.71
(241-420 days)	S.D.	13.25	S.D.	14.65
n=7	R	93-128	R	90-120
16-24 months	$\bar{x}$	99.25	$\bar{x}$	107.25
(421-690 days)	S.D.	16.76	S.D.	18.70
n=4	R	82-116	R	89-133

*Scores for the one-month age group are derived according to the method described by Bayley (1969, p. 22) using the NIH norms based on the 1958-60 version of the scales.

despite more than adequate caloric intake (150 to 250 cal/K). These infants seemed exceptionally hungry and required frequent feedings to remain comfortable. During the 3rd week of life, there was some weight gain, and in the 4th week they seemed to gain at an accelerated rate.

Thirteen infants (38%) continued to have mild irritability, excessive crying, and some tremulousness until 2-5 weeks of age. All were symptom-free by 6 weeks of age with no relapses.

Growth and development have continued normally in all infants but the one with abruptio placenta who has mild cerebral palsy. The general health of all infants has remained good.

There has been one case of child battering. This mother had terminated the methadone program and had returned to the use of heroin. She has since reentered the methadone program, has regained custody of her child and has delivered her second child, while on methadone. Both children appear to be normal and developing well.

Developmental Test Results During the neonatal period, the infants were examined using the Brazelton Neonatal Behavioral Assessment Scale. The Bayley Scales of Infant Mental and Motor Development are given at three-month intervals during the first year, and at six-month intervals during the second and third years. Auditory and visual evoked EEG potentials are also being investigated at these same test intervals.

Table I presents a summary of developmental test results thus far obtained with infants born to mothers in the methadone-maintenance program. Since only 11 infants have as yet been tested between the ages of one and two years, the trends suggested by these scores are necessarily preliminary and inconclusive. During the neonatal period the babies born to mothers who received methadone during pregnancy received a mean Mental Developmental Index (MDI) on the Bayley of 89.80, or low average, while their mean Psychomotor Development Index (PDI) was 121, or above average. The somewhat lowered scores of the neonatal methadone group on the "mental" portion of the Bayley Scale seemed largely based on poor attentiveness to visual stimuli and lack of sustained visual following. On the Brazelton, methadone infants were rated as showing less alertness than normals, and significantly depressed visual orientation and following responses. However, the methadone babies proved highly responsive to auditory stimuli and oriented well to sound. The neonatal behavioral and electrophysiological findings are presented in detail in Part II of this study.

The overall motor development of the methadone infants appears to progress rapidly during the second and third month and tends to remain above average during the first six to nine months. By one year of age, there appears to be some leveling off of this rapid rate of sensorimotor development. The Bayley Mental Scale results also appear generally indicative of rapid developmental gains during the second and third months, after initial withdrawal symptoms have subsided, with a mean MDI of 117.30 (above average) during this period. In our group, the average MDI has remained in the high average range during the first year, then has approached closer to average ($\overline{X}=99.25$) by year two.

SUMMARY

Thirty-five infants born over a two-year period to mothers participating in a methadone-maintenance treatment program were studied. The average birthweight was normal (3240 gms) for infants born to mothers who conceived while taking methadone, and 465 gms less (2775 gms) for infants conceived while their mothers were taking heroin (p<.01).

Sixty percent of the infants demonstrated mild or no symptoms and 40% developed moderate or severe symptoms. The infants whose symptoms were most severe were born to mothers who had documented histories of polydrug abuse. Many infants were slow to gain weight in the neonatal period. Thereafter growth and development have remained generally within the normal range.

References

Nathenson, G., et al., 1971: Diazepam in the management of the neonatal narcotic withdrawal syndrome: *J. Pediat.* 48:523-526

Ramer, B., et al., 1973: Experiences with the pregnant addict: *Proceedings, Fifth National Methadone Conference*, Washington D.C.

Reddy, A.M.: 1971: Observations on Heroin and Methadone withdrawal in the newborn: *J. Pediat.* 48:353-358.

Zelson, C., et al., 1971: Neonatal Narcotic Addiction: Ten Year Observation: *J. Pediat.* 48:178-189

DISCUSSION

Previous studies of infants of heroin-addicted mothers (Zelson *et al*, 1971) report a high incidence of smallness for gestational age, low birthweight infants with increased incidence of prematurity as well. An important finding in our study is that infants who were conceived while their mothers were receiving methadone demonstrated normal birthweights (3240 gms). Since these infants were significantly larger (465 gms) than those infants whose mothers conceived while taking heroin (and later entered the methadone-maintenance program), we speculate that the variation may represent a substantial difference in the lifestyles of the two groups. Heroin addicts during the early stages of pregnancy, before entering the program, often suffer from poor nutrition, and this may well account for the lower birthweights. However, even the infants who were conceived while their mothers were on heroin were larger than the infants of heroin addicts reported in other studies throughout the country. (Reddy, 1971; Zelson, *et al*, 1971) This may be explained by the improved nutritional state during the latter stages of pregnancy when these patients were actively treated and stabilized on the methadone program.

Jaundice has been described as an uncommon finding in congenital narcotic addiction. (Zelson *et al*, 1971). It appears that the imposed early metabolization of narcotics in utero stimulates the liver microsomal enzyme system to mature earlier. Physiologic clinical jaundice (bilirubin over 8 mgms %) occurs in approximately 40% to 50% of normal newborn infants. Only one infant in our study (except for one with documented hemolytic ABO incompatability) developed an elevated bilirubin level (14 mgms %), and all others were below 7 mgms %.

The sex ratio of 2.9 female to 1 male is certainly an interesting finding, but its significance is unknown.

An attempt to correlate severity of withdrawal symptoms of infants with mothers' methadone dose and history of polydrug abuse was made. Pregnant addicts were usually stabilized on 30 to 40 mgms methadone per day after entering the program. In the last trimester this dose is gradually tapered as long as the mother remains comfortable. However, if the mother has a history of documented chronic polydrug abuse (primarily heroin, barbiturates, or alchol) she is maintained at 40 to 60 mgms methadone in an attempt to blockade her use of illicit drugs.

Three of the four infants with the most severe withdrawal signs and symptoms were born to mothers who had documented records of sustained and chronic polydrug abuse. Four of the mothers of the ten infants who demonstrated moderate symptomatology also had histories of polydrug abuse, although less frequently than those mothers whose infants suffered severe symptoms.

All infants whose mothers were on less than 20 mgms of methadone demonstrated mild or no symptoms, while those on 20 to 40 mgms daily had moderate, mild, or no symptoms.

Six infants with the most severe symptoms showed morphine (a heroin metabolite) as well as methadone in their urine.

The severity of withdrawal symptoms appeared to be primarily related to the degree of polydrug abuse of the mothers enrolled in the program and secondarily related to the mothers' dose of methadone.

Valium has been reported (Nathenson *et al*, 1971) as a useful treatment for congenital narcotic addiction. It was used successfully in our study and in some cases not only resolved all the symptoms, but also seemed to shorten the duration of the withdrawal syndrome. Valium was unsuccessful in our two most severe cases, and paregoric was substituted with excellent results.

Several infants, during their hospitalization and later at home, demonstrated milder symptoms of discomfort, primarily increased irritability and excessive crying. Donnatal elixir completely reversed these symptoms in all cases.

While the developmental test data are not yet sufficient to permit generalization, they do suggest that infants born to mothers who received methadone during pregnancy may possess a unique pattern and rate of development in various areas. Most of our older infants have shown age-appropriate development in the area of vocalization and language. Their performance on perceptual motor tasks has proven somewhat less adequate. However, it has not yet been possible to assess the relative impact of genetic, prenatal and subsequent environmental factors upon the overall developmental picture. It should also be remembered that developmental quotients during these early years, while useful in identifying areas of strength and weakness, are not predictive of subsequent intelligence quotients. In any case, the present results lend encouragement to the possibility that the provision of a modified methadone maintenance program which includes good prenatal care and nutrition, neonatal care, and continued support and encouragement to the mother after the birth of the child may offset the detrimental effects of the neonatal withdrawal experience for the infant and foster an environment which may facilitate development within the normal range.

Addictive Diseases: an International Journal 2 (2): 235-255 (1975)
© 1975 by Spectrum Publications, Inc.

PART II

Behavioral and Electrophysiological Characteristics of the Addicted Neonate*

ANN LODGE,
MARILYN M. MARCUS,
and CYRIL M. RAMER

The focus of this report will be upon the comparison of some of the neonatal characteristics of 29 infants whose heroin-addicted mothers received varying degrees of methadone treatment during pregnancy with those of a control group of 10 normal infants. The relationship of auditory and visual evoked response characteristics to the clinical symptom picture as well as to behavioral response patterns will be examined. This report will update neonatal findings presented in two earlier papers (Lodge and Marcus, 1973; Ramer and Lodge, 1974). A subsequent report will deal with longitudinal follow-up data which are not yet complete. The Infant Development Research Laboratory at Children's Hospital

* This investigation was conducted as a collaborative effort between Children's Hospital of San Francisco, the Brain-Behavior Research Center of Langley Porter Neuropsychiatric Institute, University of California, and the Center for Special Problems, a division of the San Francisco Department of Public Health. This research was also supported in part by contracts awarded to Dr. Marilyn M. Marcus from the Department of Maternal and Child Health, California State Department of Health. The technical assistance of Fred New, Mitzi Speer, Paula Kleinfeld, Karen Lou, Sue Nelson, Mercedes Cameron, Douglas Murray and Noellene Sommer in carrying out this study is gratefully acknowledged. The cooperation of Dr. June Brady, Dr. Toshiko Hirata, and the staff of the Newborn Nursery and the Newborn Intensive Care Unit of Children's Hospital of San Francisco is also deeply appreciated.

235

of San Francisco began the study of addicted infants in June, 1972, as part of a more general research effort directed towards the exploration of interrelationships between behavioral and electrophysiological development of infants at risk for central nervous system damage during the critical first three years of life. The long-range aim of this research has been to provide a comprehensive diagnostic profile of the infant from birth as a basis for possible intervention during the formative stages ofhbrain development before potential learning, perceptual and behavioral problems gain an irreversible foothold.

The symptoms of neonatal withdrawal to both heroin and methadone have been extensively described and are currently the subject of much controversial attention (Cobrinik et al., 1959; Hill and Desmond, 1963; Liu-Fu, 1967; Stone et al., 1971; Zelson et al., 1971). Nevertheless, information concerning electrophysiological and behavioral status during the perinatal period is scarce, and there have been few systematic longitudinal studies to clarify important questions concerning the long-range developmental picture of these children. In both the neonatal and follow-up studies, there has been difficulty in differentiating the effect of such significant prenatal factors as prenatal care and nutritional status and subsequent environmental conditions which may affect the child's development from developmental consequences directly attributable to action of the drug and the experience of withdrawal at birth upon the infant's developing nervous system.

Although placental drug transfer mechanisms are not well understood, there is evidence that both heroin and methadone may cross the placental barrier (Davis et al., 1952; Fabro, S., 1973). While several of the effects of methadone upon the adult human brain have been described, possible effects upon the developing central nervous system of the human fetus are unknown, although cns and autonomic involvement is clearly indicated by the symptoms of the neonatal withdrawal syndrome. Such symptoms typically include hypertonicity, tremulousness, jitteriness and, sometimes, seizures. Yawning, sneezing, vomiting, diarrhea and constant gastrointestinal distress are also common. While these babies often make persistent attempts at sucking on their hands and fingers, their capacity for sustained efficient sucking has been reported to be poor, and adequate food intake and retention is frequently a problem (Kron et al., 1973). Swaddling appears to have a quieting effect and medical treatment has included barbiturates, paregoric, Donnatal, chlorpromazine, Valium, and even methadone.

SUBJECTS

One approach to isolating the possible drug effects is to attempt to optimize environmental factors which favor good development. The subjects of our study were largely drawn from the Pregnant Addict Program, a methadone

treatment program of the San Francisco Department of Public Health in operation for the past two years. In addition to rehabilitation counseling and other
therapeutic services, this program provides comprehensive medical treatment,
including prenatal counseling, delivery services and pediatric care at Children's
Hospital under the direction of Dr. Cyril Ramer.

With subjects drawn from this population we have not generally seen the
low birthweights, high incidence of prematurity and subsequent poor development to the extent which has been reported in some other studies (e.g., Stone et
al., 1971; Wilson et al., 1973; Zelson et al., 1971; Zelson and Lee, 1973). Thus
far the longitudinal study of 29 infants was begun during the neonatal period.
Because of the small number of subjects, it has been necessary in much of our
analysis to treat the addicted infants as a homogeneous group; however, because
important differences may exist between the effects of heroin, methadone, or a
combination of the two resulting in much higher dosage, the overall group has
been further divided into the three following subgroups:

1. Methadone (n = 13); regular use of methadone during pregnancy with no
   "cheating" on heroin.
2. Heroin (n = 9); received little or no methadone during pregnancy or
   began methadone during last month of pregnancy.
3. Methadone-heroin (n = 7); regular and simultaneous use of heroin as
   well as methadone during pregnancy.

The characteristics of these subject groups are summarized in Table I.

The overall group of 29 addicted neonates consists of 19 females and 10
males with an average birthweight of 2895 gms. Average Apgar ratings for 1
and 5 minutes were 7.93 and 8.90, respectively. Fourteen of the babies are white,
9 are black, and 6 are of mixed black/white parentage. Average age of the
mothers was 24.52, and average birth order 2.79. Age of testing ranged from 1
to 25 days of age; however, babies tested at the older ages were generally from
the 9 of the total group who were judged 2-4 weeks premature. The variables of
birthweight, Apgar rating, maternal age and racial composition did not differ
significantly between the heroin, methadone and methadone-heroin subgroups.
However, there were some indications of a possible trend for the one-minute
Apgar of the methadone-heroin subgroup ($\overline{X} = 6.86$) to be lower than that of either the methadone subgroup ($\overline{X} = 8.08$) of the heroin subgroup ($\overline{X} = 8.56$). Nine
babies whose birthweights were less than 2500 grams were distributed in roughly
similar proportions between the methadone subgroup (38%) and heroin subgroup (33%), but only one of the 7, or 14%, of the babies in the methadone-
heroin subgroup fell into the low birthweight category. It should be noted that
100% of mothers in both the methadone and methadone-heroin subgroups received consistent prenatal care averaging about six visits, while only 67% of
mothers in the heroin subgroup received such care.

Birth order tended to be somewhat higher for the methadone subgroup,
with a mean of 3.31, as compared with 2.71 for the methadone-heroin subgroup

TABLE I
Characteristics of Subject Groups

Subject Group		Birth-weight (gms)	Apgar 1'	Apgar 5'	Baby's Age (days)	Mother's Age (yrs)	Parity	Symptom Severity*
NORMAL n=10	X̄	3354	8.50	9.30	2.80	27.00	2.50	0
	S.D.	223.55	0.85	0.48	0.63	3.89	1.35	0
	R	2715-4780	7-10	9-10	2-4	18-32	1-5	0
OVERALL ADDICTED n=29	X̄	2895	7.93	8.90	6.76	24.52	2.79	1.34
	S.D.	472.94	1.58	1.29	5.73	3.20	1.78	0.86
	R	1910-3720	2-9	3-10	1-25	20-33	1-7	0-3
ADDICTED SUBGROUPS Methadone n=13	X̄	2885	8.08	9.00	7.73	24.77	3.31	0.92
	S.D.	533.43	0.95	0.58	6.55	2.28	1.60	0.86
	R	1910-3720	6-9	8-10	2-25	22-29	1-6	0-3
Methadone-Heroin n=7	X̄	3037	6.86	7.86	5.07	25.57	2.71	2.29
	S.D.	519.70	2.73	2.19	3.86	4.24	2.21	0.49
	R	2370-3710	2-9	3-9	2-13	21-33	1-7	2-3
Heroin n=9	X̄	2800	8.56	9.56	6.67	23.33	2.11	1.22
	S.D.	354.12	0.53	0.53	5.96	3.46	1.62	0.44
	R	2225-3250	8-9	9-10	1-17	20-31	1-6	1-2

*Rated according to scale: none=0, mild=1, moderate=2, severe=3.
**Race: W=White; B=Black; M=Mixed White/Black.

DISTRIBUTION BY PER CENT

Subject Group	Female	Race** W	B	M	Prenatal Care	Medication for Withdrawal Symptoms
NORMAL	50	60	40	0	100	0
OVERALL ADDICTED	66	48	31	21	90	52
Methadone	77	46	54	0	100	54
Methadone-Heroin	43	43	28	28	100	71
Heroin	67	56	0	44	67	33

and 2.11 for the heroin subgroup. Severity of withdrawal symptoms was rated according to the following scale: none = 0, mild = 1, moderate = 2, severe = 3. Infants in the methadone subgroup received a mean rating of .92, or mild, while the heroin subgroup received a mean rating of 1.22, or within the mild to moderate range according to these criteria, and the infants in the methadone-heroin subgroup received a mean symptom-severity rating of 2.29, or between moderate and severe. The findings of greater severity of withdrawal symptoms according to these ratings in the methadone-heroin subgroup as compared with either the methadone or the heroin subgroups was significant at less than the .01 level of probability according to the results of two-tailed t-tests. Seventy-one percent of the babies in the methadone-heroin subgroup were deemed in need of medication for alleviation of withdrawal symptoms, as compared with 54% of the babies in the methadone subgroup, while only 33% of infants in the heroin subgroup received such medication. While the infant's comfort and safety is the guiding concern, in general a fairly conservative policy as regards medication has been followed at Children's Hospital. Infants in distress are swaddled and receive extra holding and comforting when possible. Donnatal is usually given to relieve significant gastrointestinal distress, with phenobarbital and Valium used to alleviate more severe symptoms.

The control group consisted of 6 white and 4 black babies (5 boys, 5 girls), who were tested between the ages of 1 and 3 days. Mean birthweight was 3354 grams, mean Apgar ratings for 1 and 5 minutes were 8.50 and 9.30, respectively, and all infants were judged to be in good birth condition. Mean maternal age was 27.00 years, and mean birth order was 2.50. Thus, while control group mothers were a little older on the average than the mothers of the addicted infants, the normal and addicted infant groups were fairly well matched in terms of Apgar scores and parity. The difference in birthweights, however, between the normal and addicted infant groups was significant ($t = 2.93$; p<.01; two-tailed test), as was the greater mean age of testing ($\bar{X} = 6.76$ days) of addicted infants in comparison with the younger controls ($\bar{X} = 2.80$ days; $t = 2.16$, .05 p<.02, two-tailed test).

All babies in both the addicted and normal infant groups were delivered under local or no anesthesia, with the exception of four babies in the addicted group who were delivered by Caesarian section.

METHOD

The clinical symptom picture of the addicted infants was evaluated by Dr. Ramer and the staff of the Newborn Intensive Care Unit, where the babies were kept for observation and treatment. Behavioral assessment was carried out by Dr. Lodge and assistants either in the infant research laboratory or in a quiet corner of the nursery, utilizing the Brazelton Neonatal Behavioral Assessment Scale (1973) and the Bayley Infant Scales of Mental and Motor Development

(1969). For the electrophysiological studies the baby was brought to the laboratory from the nursery, and Beckman miniature silver-silver chloride electrodes were taped to the vertex (Cz) and occipital (Oz) areas as well as to the right shoulder in the area of the trapezius muscle. The right ear lobe was used as a reference for monopolar EEG recordings. The baby was then held in a seated or propped-up position in the lap of his mother or one of the examiners in a dental chair located inside a small, darkened, electrically shielded room.

Evoked potentials to auditory and visual stimulation were obtained using the average of 50 presentations for each condition. Two sets of 50 stimuli were presented when feasible in order to examine habituation. The test stimuli included an 80 decibel click, an unpatterned white light flash and a black and white checkerboard pattern of intermediate complexity. Control recordings which average ongoing EEG and muscle activity in the absence of stimulation were also carried out. An attempt was made to randomize the order of stimulus presentation, although this decision was determined to some extent by the infant's state. Each stimulus was triggered manually at a rate which varied between 2 and 8 seconds and had a pulse duration of 10 milliseconds. The auditory stimulus was delivered through an amplifier to an 8-inch speaker located in the center of the booth about 60 centimeters above the infant's head. The visual stimuli consisted of 8" x 10" rectangles mounted in Plexiglass and horizontally oriented on a sliding frame located 30 centimeters directly in front of the infant's eyes. A rectangular opening at the back of the booth covered with translucent white plastic made it possible to illuminate and diffuse the light produced by the Grass PS II photostimulator set at intensity 8 and mounted behind the visual stimulus.

The electrical output from the subject was amplified by means of a Bastin amplifier (which has a gain of 100) located within the electrically shielded stimulation chamber. The amplified signal was simultaneously monitored on a Tektronix oscilloscope, recorded from 1-100 hertz on an Ampex FM tape recorder and fed into a Krohn-Hite Variable Filter with a band pass of 3 to 20 hertz with a 24 db roll-off for visual responses and 3 to 30 hertz for auditory responses. From the filter the signal is fed into a CAT 1000 with a sample rate of 2 milliseconds, and the results of averaging of responses recorded during the first 500 ms. following stimulation written out on a Hewlett-Packard X-Y plotter.

The baby's apparent behavioral state during the stimulation was recorded descriptively and rated on a scale from 1 to 6 according to Brazelton's (1973) adaptation of the method developed by Prechtl and Beintema (1964). For most of the analyses of EEG data to be considered here, responses recorded during drowsiness and active or quiet sleep stages (states 1-3) were combined and treated separately from responses obtained during awake, alert or active states (states 4-5) which were similarly combined. Most of the click data was collected during sleep when these responses tend to be enhanced, while most of the visual data was collected during an awake state.

TABLE II
Bayley Infant Scale Mental (DIQ) and Motor (DMQ) Developmental
Quotients for Normal and Addicted Infant Groups*

Subject Group		Mental (DIQ)	Motor (DMQ)
NORMAL	x	96.60	126.60
(n=10)	S.D.	10.11	14.14
	R	80-111	105-145
TOTAL ADDICTED	x	90.41	121.30
(n=27)	S.D.	13.06	18.89
	R	73-125	81-145
ADDICTED SUBGROUPS			
Methadone	x	90.67	121.67
(n=12)	S.D.	9.95	19.43
	R	76-104	81 145
Methadone-Heroin	x	83.33	118.33
(n=6)	S.D.	9.21	20.66
	R	73-94	89-137
Heroin	x	94.78	122.78
(n=9)	S.D.	17.51	19.09
	R	73-125	97-153

*Scored according to the method described by Bayley (p.22, 1969)
using the NIH norms obtained with one-month-old infants on the
1958-60 version of the scales.

RESULTS

Behavioral findings

Behavioral test results with the neonatal subject groups are summarized in Tables II and III. On the Bayley Scales, the addicted infants as a group attained a mean Mental Development Quotient of 90.4 and a mean Motor Development Quotient of 121.3, as compared with a mean MDQ of 96.6 and PDQ of 126.6 for the normal babies. Thus, while the addicted babies were somewhat lower in their overall mental score than the control group, due largely to poor visual attention and orientation which constitute a substantial portion of the test at this age, the scores of both were within the average range. Both groups were somewhat above the norm in their overall motor development. Despite the high activity levels, hypertonicity, exaggerated reflexes and indications of motor precocity in such areas as head control and hand-mouth facility seen in many addicted infants, individual item analysis indicated that the addicted heroin and methadone-heroin infant subgroups (but not the methadone subgroup) differed significantly from the control group on only one item from the motor portion of the test, i.e., their hands were more tightly fisted (p<.05, according to Fisher's exact probability test).*

* Two-tailed tests of significance are used throughout in reporting results.

(Final)

TABLE III
Per Cent of Infants in Each Subject Group
Passing Bayley Mental Scale Items

Item No.	Age Place- ment (Months)	Item	Normal n=10	Total Addicted n=27	Methadone n=12	Methadone- Heroin n=6	Heroin n=9
1	0.1	Responds to sound of bell	100	100	100	100	100
2	0.1	Quiets when picked up	100	100	100	100	100
3	0.1	Responds to sound of rattle	100	96	92	100	100
4	0.1	Responds to click	100	92	92	100	89
5	0.1	Momentary regard of red ring	100	77	83	50	89
6	0.2	Regards person momentarily	100	92	100	67	100
7	0.4	Prolonged regard of red ring	90	66	75	50	67
8	0.5	Horizontal eye coordination: red ring	90	59	58	50	67
9	0.7	Horizontal eye coordination: light	60	18	8	0	44
10	0.7	Eyes follow moving person	40	18	8	33	22
11	0.7	Responds to voice	100	92	92	100	89
12	0.8	Vertical eye coordination: light	40	7	0	0	22
13	0.9	Vocalizes once or twice	20	33	33	17	44
14	1.0	Vertical eye coordination: red ring	70	15	8	0	33
15	1.2	Circular eye coordination: light	0	0	0	0	0
16	1.2	Circular eye coordination: red ring	10	7	0	0	22
17	1.3	Free inspection of surroundings	30	7	8	0	11
18	1.5	Social smile: E talks and smiles	0	0	0	0	0
19	1.6	Turns eyes to red ring	0	3	0	0	11
20	1.6	Turns eyes to light	0	0	0	0	0
21	1.6	Vocalizes at least 4 times	0	11	25	0	0
22	1.7	Anticipatory excitement	0	0	0	0	0
23	1.7	Reacts to paper on face	100	81	75	100	77
28	2.2	Searches with eyes for sound (bell or / rattle)/	20	51	58	33	55
29	2.3	Eyes follow pencil	0	3	0	0	11
33	2.6	Manipulates red ring	0	22	33	0	22
36	2.8	Simple play with rattle	0	3	0	0	11
39	3.2	Fingers hand in play	0	18	17	0	33
44	3.8	Carries ring to mouth	10	25	42	0	22

On the Mental Scale, addicted infants displayed a somewhat different pattern of performance from controls in certain areas of behavior. While these trends did not always reach statistical significance, this performance pattern appeared to be generally characterized by a pronounced degree of auditory responsiveness and orientation, below average visual following and exploration, more vocalization, and a greater degree of manipulation and mouthing of objects and fingering hands together, as compared with controls (Table IV). Individual item analysis (using the Fisher exact probability test) revealed that infants in the methadone subgroup displayed significantly less horizontal eye coordination in response to a light stimulus (p=.05); and that infants in both the methadone (p=.02) and methadone-heroin (p=.05) subgroups displayed significantly less vertical eye coordination than did non-addicted controls in response to the red ring, while the heroin subgroup did not differ significantly from controls on these items.

The Brazelton Scale ratings for normal and addicted infant subgroups based on a 9-point scale are summarized in Table V and presented graphically for several areas of behavior in Figures 1 and 2. Pooled results obtained for auditory orientation items (#6 and #8) and for visual orientation items (#5 and

TABLE IV
Summary of Brazelton Scale Scores for Subject Groups

Item	Normal n=10 $\bar{x}$	S.D.	Total Addicted n=27 $\bar{x}$	S.D.	Methadone n=12 $\bar{x}$	S.D.	Methadone-Heroin n=6 $\bar{x}$	S.D.	Heroin n=9 $\bar{x}$	S.D.
1. Response decrement to light	5.90	2.96	4.78	2.21	4.40	2.12	6.33	1.86	4.00	2.24
2. Response decrement to rattle	6.20	2.70	6.52	2.27	6.80	1.23	7.00	1.79	5.71	3.59
3. Response decrement to bell	5.80	2.44	5.88	2.77	6.60	1.96	6.33	2.66	4.62	3.54
4. Response decrement to pinprick	3.10	1.91	4.12	1.98	3.70	1.49	4.67	2.25	4.25	2.43
5. Orientation inanimate visual	5.30	1.34	3.68*	2.14	3.64	1.69	2.67	1.86	4.50	2.73
6. Orientation inanimate auditory	4.50	1.58	4.60	1.71	4.91	1.81	4.00	1.67	4.62	1.68
7. Orientation animate visual	5.30	1.34	3.92*	1.55	4.09	1.04	2.67	1.63	4.62	1.68
8. Orientation animate auditory	5.90	1.37	5.72	1.62	5.82	1.40	6.00	1.90	5.38	1.85
9. Orientation animate visual & auditory	5.70	1.25	4.29*	1.55	4.00	1.41	3.50	1.22	5.25	1.58
10. Alertness	5.40	1.84	3.84**	1.70	3.73	1.62	3.50	1.76	4.25	1.91
11. General tonus	5.10	0.88	6.80**	1.35	6.54	0.82	7.50	1.87	6.62	1.51
12. Motor maturity	4.30	1.25	4.76	1.48	5.09	1.45	4.33	1.97	4.62	1.19
13. Pull-to-sit	4.90	1.73	5.84	1.95	6.00	2.10	5.50	1.64	5.88	2.17
14. Cuddliness	5.20	1.14	5.20	1.19	5.36	1.43	4.83	0.98	5.25	1.04
15. Defensive movements	5.90	1.85	5.79	2.00	5.90	2.08	5.33	1.86	6.00	2.20
16. Consolability	6.30	1.34	5.44	1.66	5.36	1.80	5.33	1.75	5.62	1.60
17. Peak to excitement	4.60	1.58	6.04*	1.57	6.00	1.34	6.50	1.38	5.75	2.05
18. Rapidity of buildup	4.90	2.02	4.08	1.47	5.20	1.75	5.83	0.41	6.50	1.41
19. Irritability	3.80	1.14	5.54*	2.02	5.50	1.84	5.83	1.94	5.38	2.50
20. Activity	4.80	1.23	5.80*	1.35	5.36	1.12	7.00	0.00	5.12	1.64
21. Tremulousness	5.00	1.70	5.88	2.33	6.00	1.79	5.50	3.62	6.00	2.14
22. Startle	3.60	1.35	3.72	1.88	3.27	1.95	4.17	1.94	4.00	1.85
23. Lability of skin color	3.80	1.99	4.60	1.96	4.45	2.02	4.67	1.63	4.75	2.31
24. Lability of states	3.90	1.20	5.32**	1.31	5.18	1.25	6.00	1.41	5.00	1.31
25. Self-quieting activity	5.20	1.55	5.68	1.91	5.36	1.80	5.33	1.75	6.38	2.20
26. Hand-mouth facility	5.30	2.31	7.28*	1.86	6.91	2.30	7.33	1.86	7.75	1.16
27. Smiles	1.00	1.41	1.12	1.92	1.45	2.38	1.33	2.16	0.50	0.76
Combined Scores:										
Auditory response decrement (2 + 3)	6.00	2.51	6.19	2.53	6.70	1.59	6.67	2.19	5.13	3.48
Visual orientation (5 + 7)	5.30	1.30	3.80**	1.85	3.86	1.39	2.67	1.67	4.56	2.19
Auditory orientation (6 + 8)	5.20	1.61	5.16	1.74	5.36	1.65	5.00	2.00	5.00	1.75

Note: Starred items indicate significance levels (*p <.05; **p <.01) for comparison of normal and total addicted group means according to results of two-tailed t tests.

7), which combined findings with human as well as inanimate stimulation, are seen on the left-hand side and center of Figure 1, while the right-hand side of the figure presents responses to the human face and voice combined (item # 9). While the groups did not differ with respect to auditory orientation, the overall addicted infant group showed significantly depressed visual orientation and following responses when compared with non-addicted controls ($t = 3.304; p<.01$), due predominantly to the poor performance of infants in the methadone and methadone-heroin subgroups. A similar pattern is seen in the lowered responsiveness of the methadone ($t = 2.847; p<.02$) and methadone-heroin ($t = 3.430; p<.01$) infant subgroups to the combined stimulation of both face and voice (item # 9) as compared with non-addicted controls. No significant differences were found in the comparison of scores of the addicted infant subject groups

COMPARISON OF NORMAL AND ADDICTED NEONATES
ON VISUAL AND AUDITORY ORIENTATION

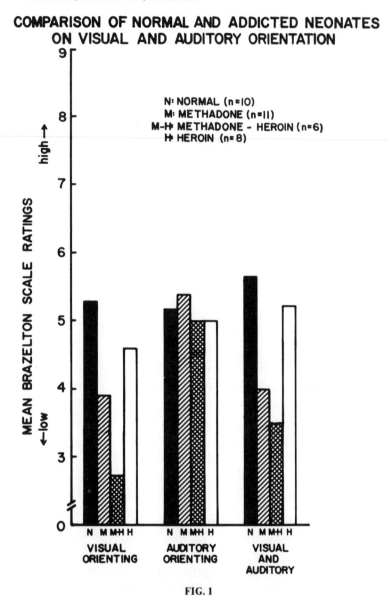

FIG. 1

with those of the normal control group on behavioral response decrement or habituation to either repeated visual (item # 1) or auditory (items # 2 and # 3) stimulation or to pinprick (item # 4). However, it is of interest that the heroin infants are found to show less visual response decrement than normals, while infants in the methadone-heroin subgroup displayed a greater degree of visual response decrement than was found with the normal group. The significance of

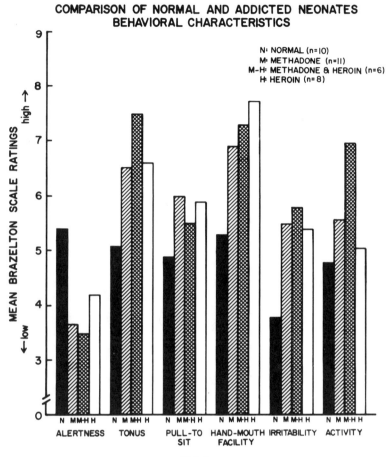

FIG. 2

the difference between the heroin subgroup mean rating of 4.00 and the methadone-heroin subgroup mean rating of 6.33 fell between the .05 and .10 level, suggesting that this relationship may reflect a possible trend. Soule et al., 1973, and
Lessen-Firestone et al., 1974, both report that methadone-addicted neonates
displayed less response decrement to light than non-addicted neonates. The capacity for rapid habituation is generally viewed as representing a greater degree
of adequacy or higher maturational level in the development of perceptuocogni-
tive capacities.

The addicted neonates as a group were found to display significantly less
alertness (item #10) than normal infants ($t = 2.398$; $p < .05$); however, the difference between the normal and heroin subgroups was not significant with respect to this variable (Figure 2). The addicted infant group was rated significantly
higher than the non-addicted group in general tonus (item #11: $t = 3.658$,

p<.001); peak of excitement, or intensity and duration of greatest arousal in response to test stimuli (item # 17: $t=2.451$, p<.05); irritability (item # 19: $t=2.545$, p<.02); lability of states (item # 24: $t=2.958$, p<.01); hand-mouth facility (item # 26: $t=2.654$, p<.02); and activity level (item # 20: $t=2.023$, p>.05) (Figure 2). However, ratings for infants in the heroin subgroup with respect to lability of states, peak of excitement, irritability and activity did not differ significantly from non-addicted controls. Of the addicted infant subgroups, heroin babies were rated most similar to normals in amount of activity; methadone infants tended to be somewhat more active, while infants in the methadone-heroin subgroup displayed a significantly greater amount of both spontaneous and elicited activity when compared with either the normal group ($t=4.322$, p<.001) or with the heroin subgroup ($t=2.768$, p<.02).

It is worthy of note that despite their difficulties, particularly in the regulation of arousal states, the addicted neonates are found to possess many adaptive behavioral capacities that would appear to have significance for their handling, for example, their ability to respond with orienting and quieting to the human voice and their hand-mouth facility which provides some source of gratification of their frantic sucking needs. Our results also indicate several areas where normal or near-normal behavioral responsiveness was found, including reactions to being held, rocked and cuddled, some aspects of self-quieting activity, consolability and overall motor maturity. In addition to the well-known calming effect of swaddling, it is suggested that the use of behavioral soothing techniques such as Davis has emphasized (1974) should be more widely recognized and utilized by both the mother and the nursing staff as an integral part of the treatment program.

Several of the present findings appear consistent with those reported by Soule et al. (1973), who reported lower visual as compared with auditory orientation, and by Lessen-Firestone et al. (1974). The latter study concluded that methadone-addicted infants showed some ability to control their high levels of arousal but manifested disturbances in alertness and were less successful in responding appropriately to environmental stimulation.

The present analysis has attempted to examine the possible relative impact of methadone and heroin addiction in the neonate, although these findings can only be regarded as tentative in view of the small number of subjects and the difficulty in assessing the quality and dosages of drugs involved. Nevertheless, the results obtained with these subjects suggest that there are differences in behavior patterns during withdrawal among the addiction categories examined here, with infants in the methadone-heroin subgroup displaying a behavior pattern which deviates most from that obtained with normal controls, while the pattern of performance of infants in the heroin subgroup generally appeared more similar to that obtained with the normal infants. It appears likely that infants in the methadone-heroin subgroup were exposed to a higher overall dosage level of narcotics prenatally, while infants in the heroin subgroup were probably exposed to considerably less narcotics due to impurities in their sources of supply. Nevertheless, when the neonatal behavior patterns of a group of four infants whose mothers' methadone dosage at delivery were between 40-60 mg ($x = 46.25$) was compared with those of six infants whose mothers were receiving 5-20 mg of methadone ($x = 15$), no significant differences between the groups could be demonstrated. It appears that more definitive evaluation of the selective impact of these drugs is a highly complex issue involving considerable individual variability and must await the availability of more refined biochemical assessment techniques.

EVOKED RESPONSE FINDINGS

Both visual and auditory evoked electroencephalographic (EEG) potentials recorded from newborn addicted infants proved in general to be more irregular and unreliable than those of the control group. Even when the addicted infant appeared relatively quiet and asleep, identification of significant evoked response components was often complicated by the presence of dysynchronized high frequency activity distributed throughout the record. Both visual and auditory records of addicted infants were characterized frequently by the appearance of sharp high amplitude components which were particularly prominent during the first 100 ms. following stimulation. Figure 3 compares both the unstimulated averaged EEG and the auditory evoked vertex (C_z) response of an addicted and a normal newborn female infant.* The normal record shown on the right-hand side of the figure is better integrated than that of the methadone-heroin infant, and the most prominent component is the positive-negative deflection (P_2N_2) which begins around 200 ms. In the record of the addicted infant, early sharp waves are also prominent and the P_2N_2 component tends to be obscured by dysynchronous high frequency activity. High amplitude response components in this early latency range of simultaneously acquired electromyographic (EMG) recordings from both addicted and normal infants did not appear to be clearly synchronized with the averaged EEG response components, as is illustrated in a record of a heroin addicted infant in Figure 4. While the origin both of the high frequency activity and early peaks in the evoked response records has not yet been determined, it appears likely that they may represent characteristics of CNS irritability, although the possibility of neuromuscular contamination must be considered (Bickford et al., 1964; Weitzman et al., 1965). The appearance of these high frequency components is particularly noteworthy in view of the narrow bandpass used in this study (3-30 hz). Sleep stage may also play an important role in vertex derived recordings particularly, especially in view of Schulman's report (1969) of disturbed sleep patterns in heroin-addicted infants which include a predominance of disorganized REM periods and ab-

---

* Positive is up in all figures which present electrophysiological data.

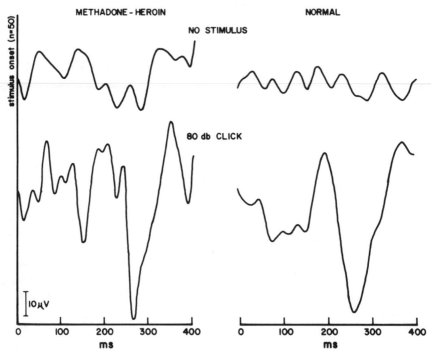

AUDITORY EVOKED VERTEX RESPONSES IN ADDICTED AND NORMAL NEWBORN FEMALE INFANTS

FIG. 3

sence of normal periods of quiet sleep. Weitzman and Graziani (1968) have reported finding a very early evoked response component (= 15 ms) which they interpret to be of probable muscle origin and which they report displays higher amplitude during active as compared with quiet sleep.

In general, the evoked response records of the heroin subgroup appeared to contain less of this high-frequency activity than did babies in the methadone-heroin subgroup, an observation of interest in view of the heroin babies' significantly lower activity ratings in comparison to that of the methadone-heroin babies. Nevertheless, many of the behaviorally quieter heroin babies also displayed short latency evoked response components of relatively high amplitude. Figure 5 presents both auditory (left-hand tracing) and visual (right-hand tracing) evoked responses obtained with a one-day-old heroin-addicted infant on no medication with mild withdrawal symptoms. A subsequent recording obtained from this subject at 7 days is shown in the lower tracing; by this time withdrawal symptoms had subsided and he was about to be discharged from the hospital. The click response which had been characterized by a prominent P_{100} component and lower amplitude P_{300} component at one day of age is now characterized by a lower amplitude early positive component and a higher amplitude later

SIMULTANEOUSLY RECORDED VERTEX AND SHOULDER MUSCLE
ACTIVITY FOLLOWING AUDITORY STIMULATION (80 db CLICK) IN
II DAY OLD HEROIN-ADDICTED MALE INFANT

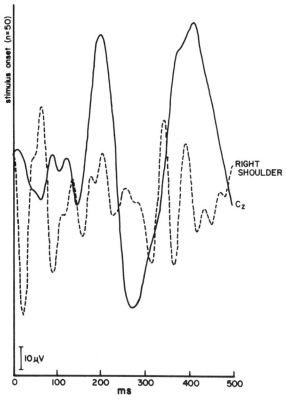

FIG. 4

positive component more similar to that found with the normal neonate in quiet
sleep. Occipital flash responses for this baby are poorly differentiated and obscured by high-frequency activity at both 1 and 7 days of age. In general, the occipital visual evoked responses of the addicted infants were difficult to evaluate
because, again in contrast to the normal control infants, they were rarely in the
quiet alert state optimal for recording such responses, and responses obtained
even in an apparently quiet watchful state frequently contained a great deal of
high-frequency activity. However, in the small percentage of infants for whom
satisfactory waking records were obtained, a positive component in the normal
latency range of 190 ms. could frequently be detected (Ellingson, 1964). Differential responding to flash and patterned input has been reported (Harter and
Suitt, 1970; Marcus, 1970), and though this differential in the form of amplitude
modulation of the P_2 component was found with most of the normal babies, this
did not appear to be true with the addicted infants.

TABLE V
Differences in Hertz of Visual Evoked Responses and Auditory Evoked Responses Between Addicted and Non-Addicted Infants

Flash (C_z-A_2)	Flash (O_z-A_2)	Click (C_z-A_2)	Non-Addicted n	Non-Addicted $\bar{x}$ %	Addicted n	Addicted $\bar{x}$ %	t (pooled variance)*
26–50			9	31.0	11	30.9	0.03
	26–50		9	32.0	13	31.6	0.11
		26–50	9	27.6	14	30.6	-1.08
18–25			9	28.4	11	26.1	2.56**
	18–25		9	27.3	13	27.6	0.18
		18–25	9	25.1	14	23.9	0.70
13–17			9	12.7	11	13.9	-1.08
	13–17		9	12.8	13	13.9	-0.99
		13–17	9	13.6	14	12.6	0.82
8–12			9	9.3	11	10.5	-0.62
	8–12		9	9.3	13	9.1	0.13
		8–12	9	11.1	14	9.4	1.12

* No significant differences between groups; pooled variances used.

** p=.02

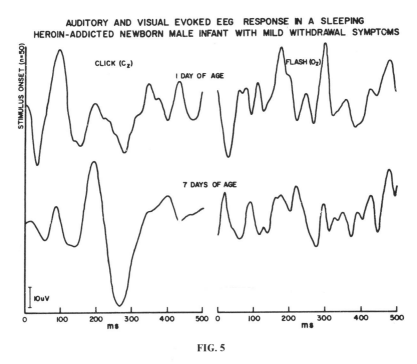

AUDITORY AND VISUAL EVOKED EEG RESPONSE IN A SLEEPING
HEROIN-ADDICTED NEWBORN MALE INFANT WITH MILD WITHDRAWAL SYMPTOMS

FIG. 5

Ellingson et al., (1974) conclude that the auditory evoked response matures earlier than the visual evoked response according to several criteria and that 7 components are present in the full-term newborn, although $N_1P_2N_2$ which are most prominent during quiet sleep (P_2 in particular) have been the ones most consistently detected and reported on in previous studies. Earlier components ($P_0M_0P_1$) are reported more variable and generally absent during quiet sleep, although they were present in one of their 6 subjects (Ellingson et al., 1974). Weitzman and Graziani (1968) report the emergence of a 90 ms. low amplitutde vertex positive component in the auditory evoked response by 37-38 weeks gestational age. Ohlrich and Barnet (1972) identify a component with a mean latency of 63 ms. for neonates. Amplitude was reported to increase with age, but latency remained relatively constant for this component, in contrast to the decreasing latency found with P_2 during the first year (Ohlrich and Barnet, 1972). They found, however, that this early component was clearly defined in only 33% of their normal neonatal sample during Stage 2 sleep.

A preliminary analysis of latency, amplitude and frequency characteristics of evoked responses has been carried out on a sample of 15 addicted neonates (5 in each addiction subgroup), and the results compared with those obtained with our normal sample (n = 10). All of the normal infants displayed a positive component in the 50-100 ms. range with a mean latency of 69 ms. in auditory evoked response recordings obtained predominantly during quiet sleep. Mean latency for the P_2 component in the normal group was 211 ms. Latencies for the most prominent early component in the records of the addicted infants showed considerably greater variability than was found with normal infants, making comparisons difficult. However, all but one of the addicted infants was found to have an identifiable P_2 component in response to click stimulation with a mean latency of 202 ms. for the group. P_2 latency was shortest for the heroin subgroup (n = 5, $\overline{X}$ = 18₂ ms.) and longest for the methadone subgroup (n = 5, $\overline{X}$ = 215 ms.), with the methadone-heroin subgroup intermediate between the two in P_2 latency (n = 5, $\overline{X}$ = 205 ms.). Mean latencies for those auditory response components which permitted comparison (N_0, P_2, N_2) were not found to differ significantly between the normal and addicted subject samples. Response amplitudes showed a great deal of intraindividual variability (as recently described by Ellingson et al., 1974) and were not found to differentiate between groups or to be correlated with behavioral ratings for tonus, activity level or auditory response decrement. Latency of the P_2 component, however, was found to have a significant negative correlation with behavioral auditory orientation ratings for both normal and addicted subjects ($r = -0.549$, $p = .018$; shorter P_2 latency associated with more adequate auditory orientation).

In order to further evaluate the characteristics of evoked responses of normal and addicted infants, the frequency distribution for all stimulus conditions was analyzed using a time interval histogram program on a Lab 8/E computer. Four frequency ranges were examined: 8-13 Hz.; 14-17 Hz.; 18-25 Hz.; and 26-50 Hz. The results of this analysis are summarized in Table V. A comparison of the normal and addicted infant groups for each of these frequency ranges for click from the vertex (C_z) and flash from the vertex (C_z) and occipital (O_z) regions show only one significant difference ($t = 2.56$, $p = .02$) and that is in the vertex response to flash stimulation in the 18-25 Hz. range. The distribution of frequencies in this 18-25 Hz. range showed the highest intra- and inter-reliability within groups. The finding of a significantly lowered vertex arousal response to visual stimulation corresponds to the diminished visual attention noted behaviorally for addicted babies. Furthermore, the absence of significant difference between groups on the flash occipital response suggests that it is the arousal feature of visual input rather than sensory processing which differentiates both behaviorally and electophysiologically between our normal and addicted babies (Watanabe et al., 1973). The lack of a significant difference between the groups for the vertex click response, on the other hand, appears congruent with the more adequate auditory behavioral responses of addicted infants.

SUMMARY

The neonatal withdrawal period was characterized by heightened auditory responsiveness and orientation, lowered overall alertness and poor attentiveness to and following of visual stimuli. Electroencephalographic recordings revealed high-frequency dysynchronous activity suggestive of cns irritability. Analysis of evoked response data further corroborated the behavioral findings with evidence for low arousal value of visual stimulation in the vertex frequency characteristics and poorly defined occipital responses. Auditory evoked responses appeared better integrated, and a significant correlation was found between auditory orienting ability and latency of the P_2 component. The long-range developmental significance of these neonatal characteristics awaits further follow-up investigation.

References

Bayley, N. *Bayley Scales of Infant Development: Birth to Two Years*, New York: Psychological Corp., 1969.

Bickford, R.G., Jacobson, J.L., and Cody, D.T.R., Nature of average evoked potentials to sound and other stimuli in man. *Ann. N.Y. Acad. Sci. 112*: 204-218, 1964.

Brazelton, T.B. *Neonatal Behavioral Assessment Scale*, London: William Heinemann Medical Books, 1973.

Breakey, A. Ocular problems in kernicterus. In *Kernicterus in Cerebral Palsy*. Conference presented by the American Academy for Cerebral Palsy. Springfield, Ill.: Charles C. Thomas, 1961.

Cobrinik, R.W., Hood, R.T., and Chusid, E. The effect of maternal narcotic addiction in the newborn infant. Review of the literature and report of 22 cases. *Pediatrics, 24*: 288-304, 1959.

Davis, M. Neurological and behavioral characteristics of the infant and the addicted mother. Paper presented at NIDA/Vanderbilt Perinatal Addiction Research Conference, Nashville, Tenn., September 1974.

Davis, M.E., Andros, G.J., and King, A.G. Use of methadone-scopolamine in obstetric analgesia. *J.A.M.A., 148*: 1193-1198, 1952.

Ellingson, R.J. Cerebral electrical responses to auditory and visual stimuli in the infant (human and subhuman studies). In Kellaway, P., and Petersen, I. (Eds.), *Neurological and Correlative Studies in Infancy*, New York: Grune and Stratton, 1964.

Ellingson, R.J., Danahy, T., Bessmarh, N, and Lathrop, G.L. Variability of auditory evoked potentials in human newborns. *EEG Clin. Neurophysiol., 36*: 155-162, 1974.

Fabro, S. Passage of drugs and other chemicals into the uterine fluids and preimplantation blastocyst. In *Fetal Pharmacology*, Boreus, L (Ed.), New York: Raven Press, 1973.

Hagne, I. Development of the waking EEG in normal infants during the first year of life: A longitudinal study including automatic frequency analysis. In Kellaway, P., and Petersen, I. (Eds.), *Clinical Electroencephalography of Children*. New York: Grune and Stratton, 1968.

Harter, M.R., and Suitt, C.D. Visually-evoked cortical responses and pattern vision in the infant: A longitudinal study. *Psychon. Sci. 18*: 235-237, 1970.

Hill, R.M., and Desmond, M.M. Management of the narcotic withdrawal syndrome in the neonate. *Pediatric Clinics of North America, 10*: 67-87, 1963.

Kron, R.E., Litt, M., and Finnegan, L.P. Behavior of infants born to narcotic-addicted mothers. *Pediatric Res. 7*: 292/64, 1973.

Lessen-Firestone, J.K., Strauss, M.E., Starr, R.H. Jr., and Ostrea, E.M. Behavioral characteristics of methadone addicted neonates. Technical Report No. 02-74. Spencer Foundation. Wayne State University, Detroit, 1974.

Liu-Fu, J.S. *Neonatal Narcotic Addiction*. U.S. Dept of Health Education & Welfare Administration, Children's Bureau, U.S. Government Printing Office, 1967.

Lodge, A., and Marcus, M.M. Evoked EEG response characteristics of infants born to methadone-treated mothers. Paper presented at the Third Annual Meeting of the Society for Neuroscience, San Diego, Calif., November, 1973.

Marcus, M.M. Developmental change and age related waveforms in the visual evoked response. *Psychophysiology. 8*: 271, 1971.

Marcus, M.M. VEPs to flash and pattern in normal and high risk infants. In Desmedt, J.E. (Ed.) *Evoked Potentials in Man.* In press.

Ohlrich, E.S., and Barnet, A.B. Auditory evoked responses during the first year of life. *EEG Clin. Neurophysiol. 32*: 161-169, 1972.

Pert, C., and Snyder, S.H. Opiate receptor: Demonstration in nervous tissue. *Science. 179*: 1011-1014, 1973.

Prechtl, H., and Beintema, O. *The Neurological Examination of the Full-Term Newborn Infant.* London: William Heinemann Medical Books, 1964.

Ramer, C.M., and Lodge, A. Neonatal addiction: A two year study. Paper presented at the National Drug Abuse Conference, Chicago, Ill., March 1974.

Schulman, C.A. Alterations of the sleep cycle in heroin-addicted and "suspect" newborns. *Neuropadiatrie 1*: 89-100, 1969.

Sigman, M., Kopp, C.B., Parmelee, A.H., and Jeffrey, W. Visual attention and neurological organization in neonates. *Child Development, 44*: 461-466, 1973.

Slotkin, T. Sympatho-adrenal development in perinatally addicted rats. Paper presented at NIDA/Vanderbilt Perinatal Addiction Research Conference, Nashville, Tenn., September 1974.

Soule, B., Standley, K., Copans, S., and Davis, M. Clinical implications of the Brazelton Scale. Paper presented at the annual meeting of the Society for Research in Child Development, Philadelphia, 1973.

Stechler, G. Newborn attention as affected by medication during labor. *Science, 144*: 315-317, 1964.

Stone, M.L., Salerno, L.J., Green, M., and Zelson, C. Narcotic addiction in pregnancy. *Am. J. Obstet. Gyn. 109*: 716-723, 1971.

Watanabe, K., Iwase, K., and Hara, K. Visual evoked responses during sleep and wakefulness in preterm infants. *EEG Clin. Neurophysiol., 34*: 571-577, 1973.

Weitzman, E.D., Fishbein, W., and Graziani, L. Auditory evoked responses obtained from the scalp electroencephalograms of full-term human neonate during sleep. *Pediatrics, 35*: 458-462, 1965.

Weitzman, E.D., and Graziani, L.J. Maturation and topography of the auditory evoked response of the prematurely born infant. *Developmental Psychobiology, 1*: 79-89, 1968.

Weisel, T.N., and Hubel, D.H. Single-cell responses in striate cortex of kittens deprived of vision in one eye. *J. Neurophysiol., 26*: 1003-1017, 1963.

Wilson, G.S., Desmond, M.M., and Verniaud, W.M. Early development of infants of heroin-addicted mothers. *Am. J. Dis. Child 126*: 457-462, 1973.

Zelson, C., and Lee, S.J. Neonatal narcotic addiction: Exposure to heroin and methadone. *Pediatric Res. 7*: 289/61, 1973.

Zelson, C., Rubio, E., and Wasserman, E. Neonatal narcotic addiction: Ten year observation. *Pediatrics 48*: 178-189, 1971.

DISCUSSION

Identification of correlative electrophysiological and behavioral response systems may help to clarify the processes underlying unique developmental aspects of addiction and the withdrawal experience in infancy. The results of this study indicate some aspects of these relationships for two sensory modalities. In the relatively mature auditory system, behavioral adequacy in orientation and heightened responsiveness is found with addicted infants. This appears to be reflected at an electrophysiological level in auditory evoked responses which correspond essentially in their latency, amplitude and frequency characteristics to those of normal infants despite their poorer integration, variable early components, and dysynchronous high-frequency activity. The correlation of P_2 latency with adequacy of auditory orientation is found with both the addicted and non-addicted subject group. Possible hypersensitivity to auditory stimulation may indicate a need for protection from overstimulation in this area. A recent study with morphine-sensitized baby mice indicated that even brief early exposure to a loud stimulus such as a doorbell predisposed them to subsequent audiogenic seizures (Slotkin, 1974).

In the relatively less mature visual modality which undergoes a significant degree of postnatal development, there is evidence for a diminished vertex arousal response as indicated by EEG frequency characteristics associated with behavioral deficits in visual attentiveness and following in addicted infants during the neonatal period. Even if this is a temporary deficit associated with withdrawal, the work of Wiesel and Hubel (1963) indicates that adequate early visual input, especially with regard to pattern stimulation, may be essential to the normal development of the visual system. Neonatal visual deficits in the realm of attention, following and pattern perception appear to be intimately associated with disturbance in overall neurological organization, and have been implicated as a predominant symptom in infants at risk for central nervous system damage due to such factors as prematurity, low birthweight, hyperbilirubinemia, respiratory distress and drug toxicity (e.g., Marcus, in press; Sigman et al., 1973; Stechler, 1964). Damage to the basal ganglia resulting from kernicterus has been associated with disturbance of upward gaze (Breakey, 1961); however, it should be noted that addicted infants have been reported to manifest a low incidence of neonatal jaundice (Zelson et al., 1971). Nevertheless, opiate receptor binding has recently been demonstrated to be greatest in the corpus striatum in the rat brain when compared with a number of other areas including cerebral cortex, midbrain, brainstem and cerebellum (Pert and Snyder, 1973). One might speculate as to a possible relationship between the apparent involvement of the visual system in neonatal withdrawal symptoms and the anatomical proximity of a brain area demonstrated to be significantly involved in opiate receptor binding with an area which has been associated with regulation of vertical eye movements.

The possible long-range significance of these neonatal findings in addicted infants must await further longitudinal follow-up. Clarification of nutritonal and dosage factors as well as further specification of both facilitating and detrimental environmental influences appear to be essential in evaluating reported differences between methadone and heroin addiction in neonates. Further research into the role of state variables and neuromuscular organization also appears to be a prerequisite for more definitive interpretation of the electrophysiological and behavioral characteristics of the addicted neonate.

Addictive Diseases: an International Journal 2 (2): 257-275 (1975)
© 1975 by Spectrum Publications, Inc.

The Assessment of Behavioral Change in Infants Undergoing Narcotic Withdrawal: Comparative Data from Clinical and Objective Methods

REUBEN E. KRON
Department of Psychiatry
University of Pennsylvania
School of Medicine; and Eastern
Pennsylvania Psychiatric Institute
Philadelphia, Pa.

LORETTA P. FINNEGAN
Department of Pediatrics
University of Pennsylvania
School of Medicine;
Philadelphia General Hospital
Philadelphia, Pa.

STUART L. KAPLAN
Department of Psychiatry
University of Pennsylvania
School of Medicine
Philadelphia, Pa.,

MITCHELL LITT
Department of Chemical and
Biochemical Engineering
University of Pennsylvania
Philadelphia, Pa.

MARIANNE D. PHOENIX
Department of Psychiatry
University of Pennsylvania School of Medicine
Philadelphia, Pa.

The neonatal narcotic abstinence syndrome is an important health hazard for the newborn infant and may have significant consequences for subsequent physical growth and psychological development. Burgeoning usage of illicit drugs by inner-city populations, during the past decade, has increased to near epidemic proportions the numbers of infants delivered at city hospitals who must undergo the rigors of narcotic withdrawal within the very first days of life.

257

In Philadelphia, it is estimated that 1% of the population are narcotic addicts and that in some neighborhoods over half of the residents are on drugs. Included among the 20,000 Philadelphia narcotic addicts are 4,000 women, the majority of child-bearing age. Philadelphia has a number of out-patient treatment centers for addicts, and the methadone clinics associated with the Philadelphia General Hospital (PGH) care for about 400 addicted adults, of whom approximately 100 are women. At any given time, 10 to 20 of these women are pregnant. Almost all attend the prenatal clinic for addicts, and eventually deliver their infants at PGH, where special nursery facilities are available for the treatment and study of the neonatal narcotic abstinence syndrome. During the past 4 years more than 200 infants residing in the newborn nurseries at PGH have been diagnosed and treated for narcotic withdrawal syndrome. About 1 in 3 of these infants was born to a street addict, the others to clients of the methadone clinics. Not all passively addicted infants develop a clinically significant abstinence syndrome, but about 4 out of 5 babies do require pharmacologic treatment for withdrawal symptoms. Occasionally the maternal addict takes a very large dose of narcotic immediately prior to presenting herself for delivery, in which case her infant may be born in respiratory distress as reflected in a low Apgar score. However, in our experience at PGH, most of the infants born to addicts appear physically normal at the time of delivery, but the majority develop signs of narcotic withdrawal between 6 and 24 hours of postnatal life.

Narcotic withdrawal is manifested by a wide variety of non-specific symptoms. Most frequent are those of central nervous system (CNS) irritability, i.e. restlessness, incessant shrill crying, inability to sleep, increased muscle tone, hyperactive reflexes, tremors, and, in severe cases, generalized convulsions. Gastrointestinal symptoms are frequent. The infants may frantically mouth their hands as if in extreme hunger, yet feedings are taken poorly, and vomiting, diarrhea, and progressive weight loss are common. Other symptoms include yawning, sneezing, stretching, sweating, nasal stuffiness, and skin pallor. Poor temperature regulation and fever tend to signify severe withdrawal syndromes. In some infants constant squirming causes excoriation of the skin on knees, toes, and face.

Despite this large catalog of withdrawal symptoms, there are difficulties in diagnosing the narcotic withdrawal syndrome in the absence of prior knowledge of maternal addiction. The problem of missing the diagnosis is greatest among infants born to street addicts on heroin, who usually attempt to escape detection, whereas clients of the methadone clinics generally acknowledge their drug dependence. Because of the wide variety of non-specific signs, narcotic withdrawal in the newborn can be readily misdiagnosed as meningitis, gastroenteritis, or brain injury. Furthermore, routine laboratory studies of blood or urine may fail to detect evidence of narcotic addiction. However, in recent years highly specific techniques have been developed to isolate and measure the minute quantities of drug metabolites present in the maternal and infant blood and urine. Such techniques are now routinely used to monitor "cheating" in methadone clinics; however, false "positives" and "negatives" may account for a high percentage of the test findings, so that at present there is no absolute laboratory method for detecting the abstinence syndrome in the infant born to a mother who does not present obvious stigmata (such as needle tracks), and does not otherwise admit to her addiction.

It is difficult to separate the medical complications caused by long-term *in utero* narcotic exposure of the infant from those generated by the multiple health problems of the addicted mother. The free-living heroin addict receives little, if any, prenatal care, and most street addicts do not seek medical attention until they enter labor. Since many female addicts support their habit by prostitution, there is a high incidence of venereal disease. There tends to be an increased frequency of obstetrical complications. Toxemia of pregnancy, premature labor, and breech presentation are common. Additional complications are related to low birthweight (almost half are under 2,500 grams), because such infants are highly susceptible to infection resulting from general debilitation, skin excoriation, and exposure to maternal venereal diseases. In most cases the mother is unmarried and the pregnancy is unplanned. In the past many of the infants of street addicts were deserted or given up for adoption, and thereby became part of the placement pool of infant care agencies. (Most mothers who attend methadone clinics keep their infants.) The low standard of maternal self-care is reflected in malnutrition and infectious disorders. Serum hepatitis, thrombophlebitis, and abscesses are common among "mainliners."

Unless the heroin-addict mother is able to obtain the drug while in the obstetrical ward, she begins to experience withdrawal symptoms within 6 to 24 hours postpartum and usually will sign out, against medical advice, to obtain drugs. Our initial interest in the neonatal abstinence syndrome was spurred by an experience with two newborn infants who were delivered at PGH within a short period some 5 years ago. Each baby weighed under 2500 grams but was otherwise normal at the time of delivery. However, each infant developed unusual progressive signs of CNS hyperirritability by the second day of life. Extensive neurological workups, including EEG and spinal taps, were unrevealing, and the diagnosis of narcotic abstinence syndrome was not made until one mother signed out of the hospital to obtain a fix.

In contrast to free-living heroin addicts who have a greater than 50% incidence of prematurity among their babies, the mothers who attend the methadone clinic enjoy the advantages afforded by an excellent prenatal-care program. The methadone mothers do not differ significantly in prematurity rate from non-addict mothers at PGH—about 1 in 5 infants under 2500 grams.

Unless the newborn infant of the addict is managed properly, it may suffer formidable morbidity. Failure to make a timely diagnosis of the withdrawal syndrome may jeopardize the life of the infant. If the infant is misdiagnosed or incorrectly managed, progressive dehydration, electrolyte imbalance, inanition,

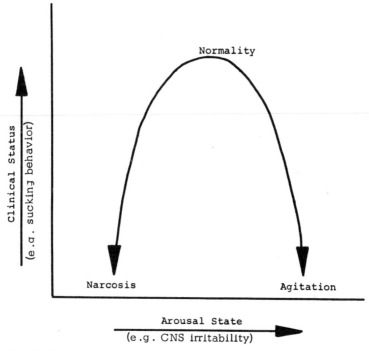

FIG. 1.   Model of relation between clinical status and state of arousal in the neonatal narcotic withdrawal syndrome

coma, and shock may result from inadequate food intake and diarrhea. Even among infants who are treated, there is a significant mortality rate, and many infants are poorly controlled. The number of treatment methods described in the literature, and the variability in response to these recommended therapies, indicate the importance of evaluating the effectiveness of available modalities (Hill and Desmond, 1963; Cobrinik et al., 1959; Stern, 1966; Goodfriend et al., 1956; Krause et al., 1958; Vincow and Hackel, 1963; Rosenthal et al., 1964; Slobody and Cobrinik, 1959). However, up to this time there have been no objective methods for comparing the usefulness of various therapies.

The definitive medical management of the neonatal narcotic withdrawal syndrome has yet to be described. Supportive therapy and close observation in a special nursery are indicated. If there is significant dehydration and electrolyte imbalance, parenteral fluids are administered; in the presence of incessant motor activity, frequent feedings and increased caloric intake are required. A number of pharmacologic agents are being used with varying degrees of success. These include paregoric, methadone, barbiturates, Demerol, Valium, and chlor-promazine. It is usually recommended that treatment be instituted with the onset of clinically significant withdrawal symptoms, and that dosage be modified depending upon the response. Treatment is generally continued for a few days to a few weeks. Severe cases may require medication for 6 weeks to 2 months. It is suggested that the dosage be "individualized" for each infant so that neither agitation nor narcosis occurs. However, routine clinical evaluation tends to be insensitive to nuances in the newborn infant's state of arousal (level of CNS excitation or depression), and therefore it has been difficult to accurately titrate the level of drug therapy to match the needs of the infant. Our experience at PGH indicates that fine-grained clinical approaches and objective methods for monitoring treatment can be important adjuncts to standard clinical procedures. Figure 1 illustrates the concept of the optimal behavioral and neurological state in which the infant undergoing narcotic withdrawal should be maintained. In actual practice the withdrawal symptoms tend to be inadequately regulated. Using standard clinical approaches for prescribing dosage levels many infants are still quite agitated days after treatment is instituted, while others are oversedated by amounts of medication being administered. Further, it has not been possible to objectively compare the effectiveness of different treatment modalities in the absence of clear-cut criteria for application and dosage.

It has long been recognized that the characteristics of behavior reflect the activity of the CNS. In order to use the characteristics of infant behavior in the assessment of CNS functioning, it is necessary to have reliable methods for measuring behavior; however, there are few precise clinical methods applicable to the newborn. During the past decade a number of fine-grained behavioral approaches [such as the clinically based neonatal neurobehavioral assessment scale devised by Brazelton (1972) and the abstinence scoring system of Finnegan (1974), and the objective method for recording nutritive sucking behavior invented by Kron (1966)] have been reported as useful in detecting and measuring changes in CNS functioning due to drug effects. It has been our goal to refine these techniques in order to provide a practical, valid, and reliable method for measuring drug effects in the nursery, and to develop means to better monitor the narcotic abstinence syndrome and its therapy.

PROCEDURES

The Neonatal Assessment Scale

Brazelton (1972) has developed a neonatal behavioral scale which includes a wide range of behaviors that are thought to reflect the status of the infant's CNS. The Brazelton contains a short neurological evaluation, but the core of the exam consists of the assessment of 26 behavioral items scored on a scale of 1 through 9 (Table I). The infant's responses to a variety of graded perturbations and interventions are rated. For example, in one test the crying infant's reaction to being cuddled and consoled by the examiner is evaluated; and in another the baby is subjected to a variety of stimuli such as the sounding of a bell, the shin-

TABLE I

Brazelton Findings in the Neonatal Abstinence Syndrome

Brazelton Behavioral Items	Significant Differences: Experimental Group (n-16) Compared to Control Group (n 10)	Significant Correlations: Brazelton Item Versus Sucking Rate (Experimental Group n=16)
1 Response Decrement: Light		
2 Response Decrement: Rattle		
3 Response Decrement: Bell		
4 Response Decrement: Pin		
5 Response to Bell (Inan Vis)		
6 Response to Rattle (Inan Aud)		X
7 Response to Face (An Vis)		
8 Response to Voice (An Aud)		X
9 Response to Face and Voice		
10 Alertness		X
11 Tonus		
12 Motor Maturity	X	X
13 Pull to Sit		X
14 Cuddliness		
15 Defensive Movements		
16 Consolability	X	
17 Peak of Excitement	X	
18 Rapidity of Buildup	X	
19 Irritability	X	
20 Activity	X	X
21 Tremulousness		
22 Startles		
23 Color Lability		
24 State Lability		
25 Self-Quieting		
26 Hand to Mouth Activity		

ing of a light, and the removal of bedclothes, etc. Soule (1973) applied the Brazelton scale to the study of infants undergoing narcotic withdrawal and reported significant differences between the scores of such infants and a normal control group; also, that certain subsets of behavioral items within the Brazelton were significantly better discriminators of drug effects than were others. Our own work with similar research populations has confirmed both of these findings (Kaplan et al., 1974). Hopefully, a shortened and refined version of the Brazelton may provide a standardized, reliable clinical method for assessing drug effects on the newborn, and also prove useful for validating more objective techniques for measuring drug effects.

Objective Measures of Sucking Behavior

Measures of newborn sucking and other adaptive behaviors may provide objective tools for evaluating the influence of sedative, narcotic, and stimulant

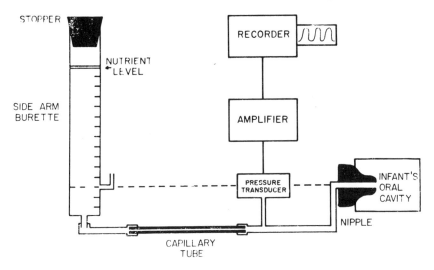

FIG. 2.   Diagram of instrument to measure newborn sucking behavior

drugs. Prior studies (Kron et al., 1966, 1968) have revealed that nutritive sucking in the newborn is significantly modified by drug effects, which are reflected
in altered sucking rates, pressures, and amounts of nutrient consumed per unit
time. Figures 2, 3, and 4 show the sucking instrument being used in the newborn
nursery and the type of sucking records generated. This method has been applied to study a variety of perinatal factors. For example, we have shown that
routine doses of obstetric sedation (i.e., secobarbital) given to the mother during
labor have a prolonged depressant effect upon spontaneous nutritive sucking
throughout the first week of life (Figure 5). These effects are generally not detected by standard clinical methods, such as Apgar scores, or by routine neurological evaluation. Also, when measures of sucking are used to study infants undergoing narcotic withdrawal, there are significant differences found between
the sucking behavior of such infants and normal controls, and between infants
being treated with different pharmacologic agents, e.g., Valium and phenobarbital depressed sucking much more than did paregoric (Kron et al., 1973, 1974).

The Clinical Scoring System

In order to further refine the clinical assessment of the infant undergoing
narcotic withdrawal, Finnegan et al. (1974) devised a scoring system for rating
the severity of narcotic withdrawal and regulating drug-dosage levels during
therapy. The ratings are performed periodically throughout the infant's stay in
the newborn nursery. The scoring system consists of 32 items ranging in severity
from minor symptoms, such as "yawning" and "sneezing," which are given a
score value of 1 point, through "continuous high-pitched crying," which is rated
at 3 points, to "generalized convulsions," which earn 5 points. The total score
earned by the infant determines the medication-dosage level. An infant who

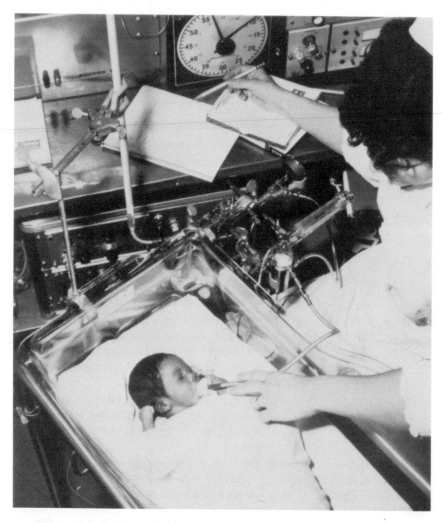

FIG. 3.   Infant being tested with sucking instrument

scores less than 8 points will receive no medication, while an infant having 8 points or more will receive proportionately greater dosages. The goal is to maintain the infant at a minimal level of symptomatology using the least amount of medication. (A detailed description of this method and its application are to be found in the paper by Finnegan et al. in this journal.)

The three above-described approaches were applied concurrently to study the behavior of passively addicted infants in comparison to various control groups. The infants born to addicts entered these studies on a "as you come" basis as they were admitted to the PGH high risk nursery. The majority of the

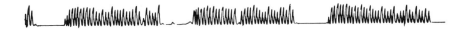

FIG. 4A.   Infant A—Two minute sample of high-rate, rhythmic sucking recorded from a clinically healthy newborn

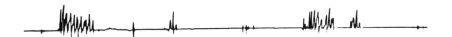

FIG. 4B.   Infant B—Two-minute sample of slow rate, dysrhythmic sucking as may be found in infants whose narcotic abstinence syndrome is poorly regulated, i.e., either suffering from CNS depression or hyperirritability

addict mothers had been attending the methadone-maintenance clinics associated with PGH; a smaller number of mothers were street addicts on heroin. However, in the studies reported herein, except where noted, only infants born to mothers attending the methadone clinic were included in the experimental group in order to minimize confounding with the unknown drug effects prevalent among free-living addicts. Control groups consisted of populations drawn from the same high risk nursery at PGH as the experimental group in order to provide a similar extrauterine environment for both the experimental and control groups, and also to provide control infants from the same social and racial background as the experimental group. The control infants were also selected on an "as you come" basis, excluding only those infants born to narcotic addicts, and those considered by the pediatric staff to be "too ill" to participate in the study.

PART I:
DRUG EFFECTS, THE CLINICAL SCORING SYSTEM
AND SUCKING

Studies were performed to compare the sucking behavior of two groups of infants undergoing narcotic withdrawal whose treatment was prescribed and monitored either by the application of the clinical scoring system (Finnegan et al., 1974) or by routine clinical methods. In the PGH newborn nursery, infants undergoing narcotic withdrawal are treated with phenobarbital or with paregoric. There was an improvement in the sucking behavior of barbiturate-treated infants whose dosage was prescribed under the abstinence scoring system (*vis a vis* standard clinical approaches), probably because of the greater precision in dosage afforded by this method. However, under either method, infants treated with paregoric evidenced better sucking performance than those treated with barbiturates (Table II). The data indicate that opiates have less of a depressant

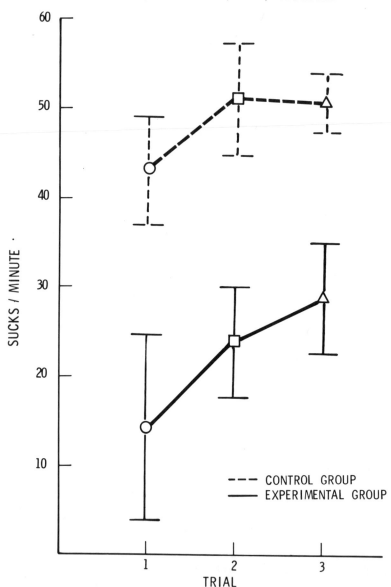

FIG. 5. Effects of obstetric sedation. Differences in sucking behavior between matched groups of newborn infants within the first week of life. The infants were studied at 24, 48, and 72 hours of age (Trials 1, 2 and 3). The data illustrate that the rate of nutritive sucking is significantly affected by drugs administered to the mother during labor and delivery. The experimental group was born of mothers who received a single dose of sedation during labor (200 mg secobarbital), while the control group was delivered of mothers who received no sedation. Although clinical methods including the Apgar score were insensitive to the drug effect, the infants' responsivity during objective measures of nutritive sucking was significantly depressed.

TABLE II

Dose Prescribed by:	Treatment Drug for Neonatal Abstinence Syndrome		
	Paregoric	Phenobarbital	None Prescribed
Standard Clinical Method	30. 5 ± 3. 0* (n = 5)	19. 4 ± 2. 3 (n =28)	23. 2 ± 4. 3 (n = 8)
Abstinence Scoring System	29. 0 ± 2. 5 (n = 12)	24. 1 ± 2. 5 (n = 13)	24. 5 ± 2. 5 (n = 13)

*Sucking Rate ± SD in sucks/min during test feeding.

effect upon infant-sucking behavior than do barbiturates, and these results are in keeping with the pharmacologic nature of the drugs: both barbiturates and opiates relieve CNS irritability associated with narcotic abstinence; however, barbiturates accomplish this through CNS depressant effects, whereas opiates alleviate the underlying narcotic abstinence syndrome. Imprecision in prescribing dosage levels, as is likely to occur when standard clinical approaches are used, tends to be more troublesome with barbiturates, since overdosage will depress adaptive behaviors much more than will excess opiate dosage. The paregoric-treated infants sucked at near normal rates, and were even higher than those infants who were not deemed to require any pharmacologic treatment for their abstinence symptoms (Table II). Another important finding among the experimental group was that the sucking performance of the infants was inversely correlated with the length of time that the mothers had been attending the methadone clinic and with the maternal methadone dosage (Table III). Infants born to addicts who entered the methadone program shortly before delivery had significantly higher sucking rates than infants of those who were on methadone for a long period of time. This finding is supported by similar differences in sucking behavior between infants born to street addicts and those attending methadone clinics, i.e., the sucking rates of babies born to methadone mothers are more depressed during the first week of life (Kron et al., 1973, 1974).

CONCLUSIONS

Our findings using the sucking instrument support the usefulness of the abstinence scoring system for monitoring drug therapy of the neonatal abstinence syndrome. The sucking data reveal important differences between infants born to street addicts and infants born to mothers attending the methadone clinic, and also differential effects caused by the pharmacologic agent used in the treatment of the neonatal abstinence syndrome.

TABLE III
Sucking Rates Arranged by Duration
of Maternal Methadone Treatment and Average Dose

Treatment Duration	N	Rate, sucks/min.	Average Daily Methadone Dose (mg)
Group 1 (< 2 weeks)	6	32. 6	<15*
Group 2 (1-4 months)	15	24. 3	28
Group 3 (> 9 months)	12	21. 6	52

*Four received no methadone, and two received
only a few small doses prior to delivery

PART II:
THE NEONATAL ASSESSMENT SCALE AND SUCKING

The experimental and control infants were administered the Brazelton assessment between the 3rd and 7th days of life. Using the standard operating procedure as described in prior publications (Kron et al., 1963, 1968, 1971), sucking behavior was measured on three consecutive days, on one of which the Brazelton was also given. The infant's sucking performance on the third day was used for comparison with the Brazelton. (The first two days were considered practice sessions.) For the purposes of this report, only the results with sucking rate will be discussed, since they are representative of the findings with the other sucking measures.

The Brazelton evaluations were performed by two examiners (Kaplan and Phoenix) trained by Brazelton, who have achieved interrater reliabilities of .85 or higher on repeated testing. The Brazelton was performed with both examiners present, each recording his ratings independently. Therefore, each Brazelton examination also served as a retest for interrater reliability. The examiners were not blind to whether the infant belonged to the experimental or control group; however, they were not aware of the infant's performance on the sucking instrument.

The Brazelton and sucking data were statistically analyzed to test for significant differences between the experimental (methadone) and control groups; also the Brazelton and sucking data were tested for significant correlations. On the Brazelton, each of five items that measured *irritability* (consolability, peak of excitement, rapidity of build-up, irritability, and tremulousness) revealed significant differences between the experimental and control groups (Table IV). When the five items were combined into an irritability factor, the significance of differences between groups achieved a p .001 level. In regard to two *motor* items (motor maturity, activity), infants of addicts were different from the controls. When these items were combined to generate a single factor, the difference

TABLE IV
Summary of Brazelton Results

Brazelton Factor	Experimental Group (n=16) Compared to Control Group (n=10) p <	Brazelton versus Sucking (Experimental Group n=16) r
Irritability	0.001	n. s.
Motor	0.05	0.50
Alertness	n. s.	0.57

between experimental and control groups was significant at the p .05 level. *Alertness* items did not distinguish infants born to addicts from controls.

Three *motor* items (motor maturity, pull to sit, activity) and three *alertness* items (response to rattle, response to voice, and alertness) showed significant correlations between sucking measures and Brazelton findings (Table IV). When the *alertness* and *motor* items were combined, the correlation between Brazelton and sucking was very high (r = .673, p .005).

CONCLUSIONS

These findings are of great clinical importance, since the behavioral items of the Brazelton represent a much more fine-grained and reproducible method for clinical evaluation of the behavioral manifestations of narcotic withdrawal than is usually applied in the nursery.

The above findings also indicate that certain Brazelton items are highly correlated with sucking, and that almost half of the variability of the *motor* and *alertness* behaviors measured by the Brazelton can be expressed in terms of a single sucking measure.

DISCUSSION OF BRAZELTON RESULTS

Irritability items of the Brazelton significantly distinguish between experimental and control infant populations. Measures of irritability have a high degree of face validity in regard to the expected clinical findings of the neonatal narcotic withdrawal syndrome, which includes many signs of CNS excitation. Thus it can be predicted *a priori* that infants undergoing withdrawal will score differently on an irritability scale than would a normal control population. Our findings confirm that the *irritability* items of the Brazelton are a valid measure of neonatal narcotic withdrawal. In a comparable study by Soule et al. (1973), who administered the Brazelton to infants born to addict mothers on methadone, they found increased irritability in the experimental population *vis a vis* normal controls. However, *irritability* items did not show a linear correlation with sucking measures in our studies. This is because sucking performance is related to CNS arousal as a "U" shaped function (Figure 1) in which either high or low levels of CNS arousal would be expected to result in decreased sucking performance. For example, in prior studies (Kron, 1966, 1968) it was found that infants born to mothers who receive obstetric sedation suck poorly, and the sucking performance of these infants falls in the lower left side of the "U" curve in Figure 1. Infants with a high degree of CNS arousal (irritability) fall on the right side of the curve, and here also sucking is poor. Infants who are not receiving enough medication for the narcotic abstinence syndrome usually demonstrate a high level of CNS irritability, while those getting excessive pharmacologic treatment tend to be behaviorally depressed. The *irritability* items of the Brazelton directly monitor the level of CNS excitation and therefore, as can be seen in Figure 4B, infants with either high *or* low irritability scores may show similar sucking performance. The linear correlation between Brazelton *irritability* items and sucking is quite low, since sucking performance reflects the magnitude but *not* the polarity of CNS irritability. Brazelton *motor* items correlate highly with sucking measures and also distinguish between experimental and control groups. A possible explanation of the former finding is the close relationship that exists between measures of motor ability on the Brazelton and measures of sucking behavior—i.e., sucking is a motor ability. In addition, *motor* items distinguish infants of addicts from controls because narcotic withdrawal and its treatment directly influence the quantity and quality of motor performance. For example, infants undergoing withdrawal are more active than control infants. Therefore, a linear (monotonic) model for the relationship between sucking and *motor* items is suggested by our findings.

Alertness items do not distinguish between addicts and controls; however, they correlate highly with sucking measures. A possible explanation for the correlation between alertness and sucking is that the Brazelton *alertness* items measure both the infant's initial orienting response to a stimulus, and also the infant's ability to sustain attention to the stimulus. For example, the infant is presented with a ball to test whether he alerts and then follows with his eyes and head. The following of the ball is a measure of the infant's capacity to maintain visual contact. The ability to maintain contact with a stimulus may also be revealed in the infant's rate of sucking, which is a measure of the amount of time spent actively attending to the nipple. Thus the infant's ability to remain attached to a stimulus may account for the linear correlation between alertness and sucking.

In regard to the specific Brazelton findings, the experimental group (born to methadone addicts) was more excited, more rapidly excited, more irritable, more tremulous, less easily consoled, less motorically mature, and more active than were controls.

CONCLUSIONS

The definitive medical management of the neonatal narcotic withdrawal syndrome has yet to be described. Standard clinical methods for evaluating the infant undergoing withdrawal tend to be insensitive to nuances in neonatal behavior that reflect important changes in CNS functioning. Fine-grained clinical and objective methods of assessing the adaptive behavior of the infant, such as the Brazelton neonatal scales, the abstinence scoring system, and objective measures of sucking behavior, may help to better define the optimal pharmacologic treatment and dosage schedules for the abstinence syndrome.

SUMMARY

Studies comparing objective measures of sucking with data from fine-grained clinical assessments of the neonate have shown significant correlations between painstaking and time-consuming clinical methods which may only be reliably applied by highly trained clinician-investigators, and the data generated by a simple technique which can be rapidly and precisely administered in the nursery by nurses or technicians. Within a few minutes the sucking instrument can generate data that explain 50% or more of the variance in certain relevant factors of the Brazelton neonatal neurobehavioral assessment scale, which in our hands requires the participation of two trained clinician-investigators for a period of almost one hour for each test and recording session. There are certain limitations to the information directly available from the sucking measures. Clinical observations must be made in order to correctly interpret some of the findings such as the biphasic relationship between irritability and sucking. For example, an infant may not suck at all because it is obtunded, or it may not suck because it is overexcited. In the case of *irritability,* sucking performance provides a measure of the magnitude, but not of the polarity of the CNS arousal state. In the case of monotonic factors, such as *motor* activity and *alertness,* sucking correlates directly and gives a good estimate of both polarity as well as amount of these behaviors. Objective measures of sucking behavior are a convenient and reliable means for measuring drug effects in the nursery and may be useful in regulating therapy of the newborn.

Acknowledgement

The studies described here were performed within the Newborn Nurseries of the Philadelphia General Hospital, laboratories of the Departments of Psychiatry and Pediatrics of the University of Pennsylvania School of Medicine and the Department of Chemical and Biochemical Engineering of the University of Pennsylvania. We are grateful to the Departments of Obstetrics and Gynecology, and Pediatrics, of the Philadelphia General Hospital for their support, and especially to Dr. John P. Emich, Director of the Department of Obstetrics, and the Staff of the Newborn Nurseries of the Philadelphia General Hospital for their cooperation. Also, we extend our thanks to Mr. Don Newman for help in data reduction.

Supported in part by Research Grant HD-06009 from the NICHD, Research Grant DA-00325 from the NIDA, and small Grant MH-19052 from the NIMH, also a Research Contract from the Commonwealth of Pennsylvania Governor's Council on Drug and Alcohol Abuse, and the Department of Public Welfare through the Eastern Pennsylvania Psychiatric Institute.

Requests for reprints should be addressed to Reuben E. Kron, M.D. Piersol Bldg., Rm. 202, Hospital of Univer. of Penna., Philadelphia, Pa. 19174.

References

Brazelton, T. B., et al., Neonatal behavioral assessment scale. Unpublished manual, Harvard University, 1972.

Cobrinik, R. W., Hood, R. T., and Chusid, E., The effect of maternal addiction in newborn infants, *Pediat.* 24:288, 1959.

Finnegan, L. P., Kron, R., Connaughton, J. F., and Emich, J. P., A scoring system for evaluation and treatment of the neonatal abstinence syndrome: a new clinical and research tool, *Proceedings of the International Symposium on Perinatal Pharmacology, Milan, Italy* (in press) 1974.

Goodfriend, M. J., Shey, I. A., and Klein, M. D., The effects of maternal narcotic addiction on the newborn, *Amer. J. Obstet. Gyn.* 71:29, 1956.

Hill, R. M., and Desmond, M. M., Management of the narcotic withdrawal syndrome in the neonate, *Pediat. Clinics N.A.* 10:67, 1963.

Kaplan, S. L., Kron, R. E., Litt, M., Finnegan, L. P. and Phoenix, M. D., Correlations between scores on the Brazelton neonatal assessment scale, measures of newborn sucking behavior, and birthweight in infants born to narcotic addict mothers, Abstract in *Pediat. Res.* (1974).

Krause, S. O., Murray, P. M., Holmes, J. B., and Burch, R. E., Heroin addiction among pregnant women and their newborn babies, *Amer. J. Obstet. Gyn.* 75:754, 1958.

Kron, R. E., Litt, M., and Finnegan, L. P., Behavior of infants born to narcotic addicted mothers, abstract in *Pediat. Res.* (1973).

Kron, R. E., Litt, M. and Finnegan, L. P., Effect of maternal narcotic addiction on sucking behavior of neonates, abstract in *Pediat. Res.* (1974)

Kron, R. K., Stein, M., and Goddard, K. E., Newborn sucking behavior affected by obstetric sedation, *Pediat.* 37:1012, 1966.

Kron, R. E., Ipsen, J. and Goddard, K. E., Consistent individual differences in the nutritive sucking behavior of the human newborn, *Psychosomat. Med.* 30:151, 1968.

Kron, R. E., Stein, M., and Goddard, K. E., A method of measuring sucking behavior of newborn infants, *Psychosomat. Med.* 25:181, 1963.

Kron, R. E., and Litt, M., Fluid mechanics of nutritive sucking behavior: the sucking infant's oral apparatus anlayzed as a hydraulic pump, *Med. Biol. Eng.* 9:45, 1971.

Rosenthal, T., Patrick, S. W., and Krug, D.C., Congenital neonatal narcotic addiction: a natural history, *Amer. J. Pub. Health* 54:1252, 1964.

Slobody, L., and Cobrinik, R., Neonatal narcotic addiction, *Quart. Rev. Pediat.* 14:169, 1959.

Soule, B., et al., Clinical implications of Brazelton assessment, presented at the Biennial Meeting of the Society for Research in Child Development, Philadelphia, Pa., 1973.

Stern, R., The pregnant addict: a study of 66 case histories 1950-1959, *Amer. J. Obstet. Gyn.* 94:253, 1966.

Vincow, A., and Hackel, A., Neonatal narcotic addiction," *Gen. Pract.* 22:90, 1963.

DISCUSSION

Q. *Dr. Garrettson:* My first question is: I am unclear about the response in sucking to the treatment with opium; does it increase sucking rate, or just not change it? Or does phenobarbital decrease sucking rate? And the second question is a simple technical question: do you use a different size capillary depending upon the size of the baby?

A. Dr. Kron: *The second question is the easier one to answer. The size of the capillary does not change. It has been chosen to provide an amount of nutrient which would provide the same amount of nutrient as the babies would normally get in their routine feedings. We have chosen a capillary of a given diameter and a given length which will provide, at 100 mm Hg of constant pressure over a 1-minute time, 10 milliliters of the given nutrient. Different nutrients have different viscosities; therefore, if you are feeding water you have to use a different capillary tube than if you are feeding a full-strength formula. And that has to be different from the one you would use for a half-strength formula. One has to calibrate the instrument for the nutrients, not for the baby. Now, as to the first question, as to what is the effect of phenobarbital upon sucking, I showed a slide (Figure 5) which demonstrates the effects of barbiturates. Barbiturates do depress the sucking response and a variety of other adaptive behaviors over a prolonged period of time. Our data indicate that, throughout the first week of life, the babies' sucking responses are considerably depressed; but we have not followed these babies long enough to see the timing-out of that depression. As far as the opiates are concerned, the opiates do, indeed, improve sucking response. They bring it up very close to normal levels. These babies are lively and good suckers and their sucking is well organized. Apparently, because of the great latitude that one has in using the opiates, it is possible to get equally good effects, at least according to our data, using clinical (standard) approaches, or using very refined behavioral approaches, such as we have at Philadelphia General Hospital. This is not possible with phenobarbital; even the most careful attempts to modulate the dosage of phenobarbital result in a depression of adaptive behavior.*

Q. Dr. Shuster: Could I, perhaps, rephrase that first question in a different way? What would happen to a normal baby if you gave him paregoric? Would there be any change in the sucking behavior?

A. Dr. Kron: *That is a good question. We have not tested that.*

Q. Dr. Nuite: Another area which might shed some light on Dr. Shuster's question is, have you observed a difference in the dose of paregoric that you have to titrate a methadone baby as compared to a heroin baby? They do not exhibit the same syndrome, or have the same qualitative syndrome.

A. Dr. Kron: *I am sorry I cannot answer that; it is a very worthwhile question. Actually, we have the data, but I do not know whether they have been analyzed as yet. Maybe we could do that and send you the information.*

Q. Dr. Nuite: But you do appear to have more trouble with a mother who has been on methadone for a longer period of time and who is on a higher dosage. If you are lucky and get the correlation well, you would assume you have to give a lot more paregoric to control the syndrome quantitatively.

Q. Dr. Finnegan: The amount of heroin that people on the streets of Philadelphia are getting is very minimal, so that when we compare the low dosage of heroin to a very good dosage of either 10 or 20 mg of methadone that is taken every day, obviously the baby is going to have higher amounts of drug or more.

A. Dr. Nuite: You could say that the only effect of paregoric is to suppress the abstinence, which is what your sucking behavior measures, rather than to have any effect of its own.

A. Dr. Kron: *Right, as best we can tell.*

A. Dr. Davis: In a clinical situation, there is not a linear correlation between a dosage of methadone the mother has been receiving and the symptoms of the baby. We all know that there are patients who have been receiving large dosages, and the babies barely have any symptoms, and vice versa. So that we cannot make a prediction of the amount of drug the baby is going to need versus the amount the mother has received.

A. Dr. Kron: *That is not the intention of the data.*

Q. Dr. Nuite: I realize that there are a lot of other factors that enter into how much the mother is consuming, how much she reverts to other drugs, and all the other factors. That is why I said if you are lucky, you will get the correlation which you would theoretically assume.

A. Dr. Kron: *It is actually the data that we are not presenting which are more pertinent in terms of answering some of Dr. Davis' questions, because the correlations that are important are those within the individual infant. I have just shown you group data. The individual correlations occur when one measures what is happening, with fine-grained measures of behavior like the Brazelton and sucking, within the same infant. In that case, you find a really extraordinary correlation. You can predict what takes place. In our laboratory, we have two experienced Brazelton examiners, who have been trained by Berry Brazelton in Boston, and they do the exams simultaneously on the same infant. They come up with .85 and higher inter-rate reliabilities consistently. It takes them one hour each to do the exam and the scoring. The sucking method I showed you here, once you have the setup, takes only 10 minutes to do the procedures and you get data which explain about 50% of the variance in certain subsets of items on the Brazelton. Now that, in terms of practicality, in terms of being able to work in the nursery and get data quickly, data which may have clinical application, is something we are trying to develop at Philadelphia General Hospital.*

Q. Dr. Kahn: Have you observed any depression of the respiratory center when you use paregoric, instead of methadone, in the methadone-addicted infant? One would expect this to happen because there is very little depression, if any, with methadone. Also, I wonder why, in methadone-addicted babies, you do not use methadone for the control of symptoms.

A. Dr. Kron: *I Think Dr. Finnegan can best answer that.*

A. Dr. Finnegan: In general, we have not observed respiratory depression with the use of paregoric because, if you noted from the dosages that we are using, they are very minimal and it is amazing that we do not have to use the higher doses on the scale in order to alleviate the symptoms. Now, as far as the nursing staff is concerned, if you ask them which drug is better in our nurseries, they will say phenobarbital, because the babies are all sleeping, as Dr. Zelson said, from feeding to feeding, and the nurses do not have to be concerned. The paregoric babies are always a little up, they are not having such severe tremulousness or gastrointestinal disturbances that they need any further treatment. As far as the other question about the use of methadone—we have not used methadone yet. We have looked at the effects of paregoric and phenobarbital, and we will be looking at methadone next.

Addictive Diseases: an International Journal 2 (2): 277-292 (1975)

Perinatal Narcotic Addiction in Mice: Sensitization to Morphine Stimulation

L. SHUSTER
G.W. WEBSTER
G. YU
Department of Biochemistry and Pharmacology
Tufts University School of Medicine
Boston, Massachusetts

INTRODUCTION

Several hypotheses that have been invoked to explain the phenomena of narcotic tolerance and physical dependence postulate the induced synthesis of proteins in the central nervous system. It has been suggested that repeated administration of narcotic drugs may lead to an increased synthesis of either neurohormone-synthesizing enzymes (Shuster, 1961; Goldstein and Goldstein, 1961), or neurohormone receptors (Collier, 1965) in the brain. Experimental evidence for these hypotheses is still meager. There are reports that narcotic tolerance and physical dependence can be prevented by treatment with cyclohex-imide, an inhibitor of protein synthesis (Loh et al., 1969). There is also evidence that treatment with narcotic drugs may increase the turnover of several neuro-hormones in the central nervous system (Way et al., 1973; Clouet and Ratner, 1970; Domino and Wilson, 1973).

We have observed that the addition of morphine to cells cultured from the brains of chick embryos increased the amount of two enzymes involved in ace-tylcholine metabolism—choline acetyltransferase and acetylcholinesterase (Peterson et al., 1974). Similar results were obtained when morphine was injected into the yolk sacs of embryonated chick eggs. When mice bearing a neuroblas-toma tumor were implanted with a subcutaneous pellet of morphine base there was an increase in the acetylcholinesterase activity of the tumor, but not in the brains of the mice (Shuster, 1974). These findings led us to suspect that we might be dealing with an effect of morphine upon growing or developing nervous tissue. For this reason we began to treat baby mice with morphine.

Our objectives in this work were: 1) to demonstrate that pretreatment of baby mice would alter their subsequent response to narcotic drugs, and 2) to look for biochemical changes that may be responsible for the altered response. We have achieved the first objective and are now approaching the second.

The data to be presented here indicate that pretreatment of baby mice with morphine increases their responsiveness to the stimulant effects of narcotic drugs. For such treatment to be effective it should be administered after the animals are 14 days old. Pretreatment of adult mice also sensitizes the animals to morphine. Adult mice have been used to define some of the characteristics of this response.

METHODS

The mice used in these experiments were B6AF₁/J hybrids produced by crossing an A/J male with a C57Bl/6J female. They were housed in plastic cages lined with chipped hardwood bedding, and fed Purina chow. The animal room was maintained at 22° with a lighting cycle of 12 hours light and 12 hours darkness.

Baby mice were left with their mothers until they were between 3 and 4 weeks old. After this time they were weaned and the two sexes were kept in separate cages. It was often necessary to combine two litters born within 1 or 2 days of each other in order to have 6 males and 6 females for a given experiment. When litters were combined, the babies were randomized and 3 mice of each sex were placed with each mother. One of the resulting litters was injected with morphine and the other was injected with saline.

The method of Dews (1953) was used to measure motor activity. Food and water were removed just before testing. Mice were usually tested individually in clear plastic cages, 28 cm x 16 cm x 13 cm deep, containing about 1 cm of bedding chips. In some cases 3 mice were run in 1 cage. Each cage was placed lengthwise between the light source and photocell of an Autotron Model SIAC photoelectric counter (Autotron, Inc., Danville, Ill.) Spontaneous activity was determined for the first four 15-minute periods after the mouse was put in the cage. The mice were then injected intraperitoneally with morphine sulfate, and activity was recorded every 15 minutes for the next 2 hours. The running response was the number of light beam interruptions during the first 90 minutes after the injection of morphine.

The tail flick method of D'Amour and Smith (1941) was used to determine analgesic response to morphine. The latency to response of uninjected mice was

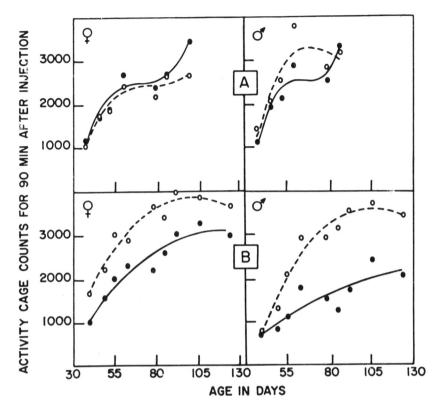

FIG. 1. Running response of adult mice that had been pretreated with morphine as babies. Group A was injected from 10 through 14 days of age; group B, from 13 through 17 days. Treated mice in each group were injected subcutaneously with 10 mg per kg morphine sulfate twice on the first day of injection, and with 25 mg per kg twice on each of the following four days. Control mice were injected with 0.15 M NaCl. Each point represents the number of light beam interruptions by a group of 3 mice during the first 90 minutes after an intraperitoneal injection of 25 mg per kg morphine sulfate. Open circles indicate morphine-pretreated mice. Solid circles indicate saline-pretreated controls. This figure is taken from Shuster et al. (1974) by permission of the *Journal of Pharmacology and Experimental Therapeutics.*

about 2 seconds, and the lamp was switched off automatically at the end of 8 seconds, so that the maximal possible increase in latency was 6 seconds.

Morphine sulfate (Merck), cocaine hydrochloride (Merck), and d-amphetamine HCl (Amend) were purchased from Gilman Bros., Boston. Naloxone hydrochloride was donated by Endo Laboratories, Garden City, N.Y. Levorphanol bitartrate and dextrorphan bitartrate were donated by Hoffman-Laroche, Inc., Nutley, N.J. Cycloheximide was purchased from Nutritional Biochemicals, Cleveland, Ohio.

Statistical significance of the difference between means was determined by the Mann-Whitney U-test (Goldstein, 1971).

TABLE I

Effect of Morphine Pretreatment on Running Response to Morphine

Mice were injected subcutaneously with morphine sulfate twice daily and tested for running response as indicated under Methods. Except where indicated values are for 3 mice per cage. Controls were injected with 0.15 M NaCl.

Experiment	Sex	Pretreatment Days	Age at Testing	Running response to morphine sulfate, 25 mg/kg	
				Counts per 90 min	
				Control	Treated
2[a]	F	10–14	32	932	461
24	M	10–14	39	1210	1616
25A	F	10–14	46	830	1295
25B	F	10–14	46	1400	1480
3	F	10–15	29	263	822
13	M	12–16	35	645	1068
15[b]	F	20–24	52	540	1031
	M	20–24	52	418	816
16A	F	16–20	45	635	1108
16B	F	19–23	45	635	1249
17A	M	16–20	56	1010	2695
17B	M	19–23	56	1010	2759
22	F	45–49	68	615	2216

Footnotes

a : 4 mice per cage

b : 2 mice per cage

RESULTS

Pretreatment of baby mice. Mice were injected subcutaneously with morphine sulfate twice daily for 5 days. The dose of morphine was 10 mg per kg for each injection on the first day, and 25 mg per kg on the next 4 days. The same animals were tested tepeatedly with 25 mg per kg morphine sulfate, starting at about 5 weeks of age. At least 10 such experiments were carried out. Representative results from 2 of them are illustrated in Figure 1. There was no consistent sex difference. The following additional conclusions can be derived from these data:

(1) The running response to morphine was always quite low at the time of the first test. This response increased two- to three-fold during the succeeding tests.

(2) Mice that had been pretreated with morphine when they were older than 15 days consistently showed a higher running response to morphine than controls that had been pretreated with saline. Figure 1B, for example, shows the response of mice that had been treated between 13 and 17 days of age.

(3) Mice that had been pretreated with morphine when they were less than 15 days old showed an increased running response in some experiments, but no increase in other experiments. Thus, Figure 1A shows that pretreatment on days 10-14 had no effect.

Data from additional experiments presented in Table I suggests that for pretreatment to be effective the mice should be at least 15 days old, and that they can be sensitized even when they are fully mature.

Running response to morphine in mice of different ages. As shown in Figure 1, the running response of saline-pretreated mice increased when they were tested repeatedly after 35 days of age. One possible explanation for this finding was that responsiveness to the stimulant effects of morphine might increase with age. Saunders et al. (1973) have described an age-related increase in the responsiveness of rats to several drugs that act on the central nervous system. We therefore examined the running response of 8 groups of untreated mice ranging in age from 35 to 115 days. The results of 2 separate experiments are shown in Figure 2. There was no correlation between the age of the mice and their running response to 25 mg per kg morphine sulfate. Running activity ranged from 300 to 650 counts per 90 minutes. Similar variability was encountered between different shipments of mice of the same age. It is clear that the increased responsiveness shown in Figure 1 cannot be attributed to aging.

Effects of weekly injections. The possibility remained that the increased responsiveness of control mice may have resulted from the weekly morphine injections that were used for testing. We soon found that the injection of 25 mg per kg morphine sulfate once a week for 2 or 3 weeks produced a three-fold increase in the running response of adult mice. The characteristics of morphine sensitization in adult mice are reported in detail elsewhere (Shuster et al., 1974). The salient features, together with some more recent results, can be summarized as follows:

(1) Morphine sensitization is a specific response to pretreatment with narcotic drugs. The running response of mice that were pretreated with different doses of morphine sulfate was proportional to the dose over the range 10-50 mg

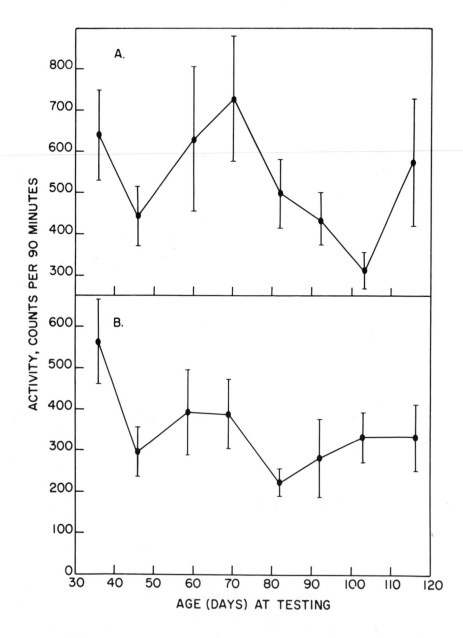

FIG. 2. Running response of mice of different ages to morphine sulfate. Each point is the mean value + S.E. obtained by testing individually a different group of 8 mice. The mice were injected intraperitoneally with morphine sulfate, either 25 mg per kg (experiment A) or 12.5 mg per kg (experiment B).

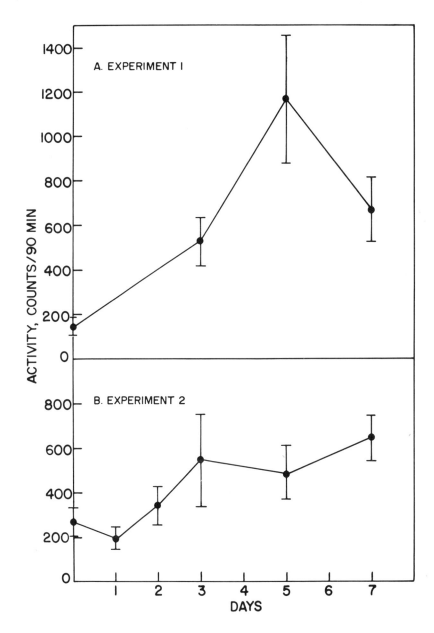

FIG. 3. Effect of a single injection of morphine on the running response. Adult mice were injected with 50 mg per kg morphine sulfate. At the times indicated, different groups of mice were tested for their running response to morphine, 25 mg per kg. Each point represents the mean activity + S.E. for 5 mice (experiment 1) or 10 mice (experiment 2).

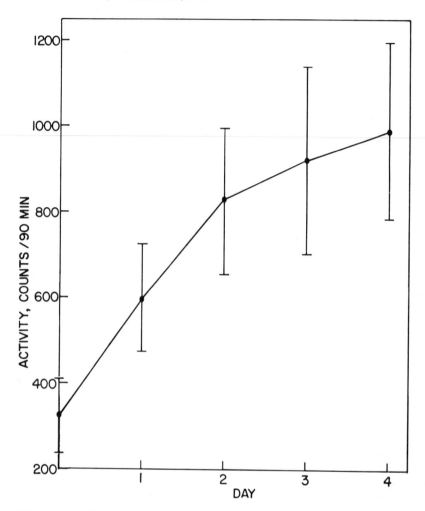

FIG. 4.   Sensitization to daily injections of 25 mg per kg morphine sulfate. Each point is the mean value for 10 mice + S.E.

per kg. Pretreatment with levorphanol increased the running response to both levorphanol and morphine. Pretreatment with dextrorphan or naloxone did not alter the response to morphine. Sensitization by 25 mg per kg morphine could be blocked completely by the simultaneous administration of naloxone, 10 mg per kg.

(2) There are marked differences among different strains of mice. There was little sensitization of adult mice from either of the two parental strains of the hybrids used in these experiments. We also found little sensitization in 5 different experiments when C57Bl/6J baby mice were pretreated with morphine.

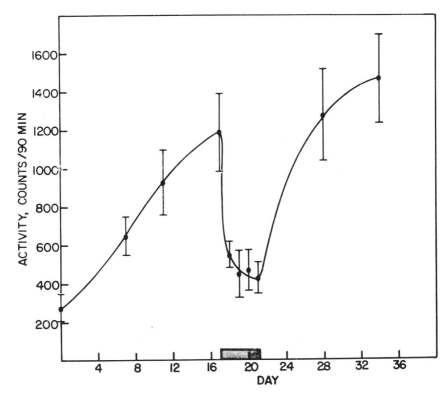

FIG. 5. Development of tolerance to morphine running in sensitized mice. During the period indicated by the shaded bar the mice received 2 injections of 25 mg per kg morphine sulfate every day. Each point is the mean response + S.E. of 10 mice to a test dose of 25 mg per kg morphine sulfate.

(3) Sensitization can be produced by a single injection of morphine sulfate. In two experiments a large number of mice were injected with 50 mg per kg morphine sulfate. At various times different groups were tested with 25 mg per kg morphine sulfate. As shown in Figure 3, sensitization appears within 3 to 5 days after a single injection.

(4) Two or three daily treatments with 25 mg per kg morphine sulfate are as effective as the same number of treatments given one week apart (Figure 4).

(5) Sensitization is fairly long-lasting. The sensitization after 4 weekly treatments with morphine lasts at least one month after the last pretreatment, but has worn off by 2 months. In the case of baby mice we have also found that sensitization lasts for at least one month.

(6) Tolerance to morphine running can be induced in sensitized mice by increasing the frequency of morphine injections to twice daily. Figure 5 shows that after only one additional injection within the first 24 hours there was a two- to

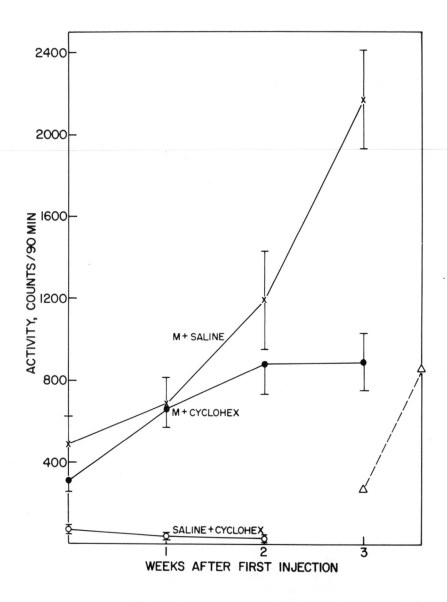

FIG. Blockade of morphine sensitization by treatment with cycloheximide. Mice were inject-ed i.p. with 25 mg per kg morphine and .15M NaCl (M + saline) or cycloheximide, 20 mg per kg. Controls received saline and cycloheximide. Each point is the mean running activity + S.E. for 10 mice. At 3 weeks after the first injection, the mice that had been receiving saline plus cycloheximide were injected with morphine sulfate, 25 mg per kg, to determine whether prior treatment with cycloheximide had impaired their ability either to respond acutely to morphine or become sensitized (open triangles).

TABLE II

Comparison of Sensitization to Audiogenic Seizures and Sensitization to
Morphine Running

	Induced audiogenic seizures	Sensitization to morphine running
Threshold age for induction	15 days	about 15 days
Induction period after stimulus	about 5 days	about 5 days
Duration of sensitization	up to 40 days	about 1 month
Genetic predisposition	yes	yes
Induction in adults	by increased stimulus	yes
Initial response	partial deafness	tolerance (?)
Denervation hypersensitivity	demonstrated	postulated

three-fold decrease in the running response. When the injections were stopped, tolerance wore off, but sensitization remained.

(7) Sensitization does not appear to result from the differential development of tolerance to the depressant effects of morphine. The analgesic response is one measure of depression of the central nervous system by morphine. Control and sensitized mice displayed the same analgesic response to 2.5 mg per kg morphine sulfate, as determined by the tail-flick assay. The injection of morphine into withdrawn rats and human narcotic addicts produces electroencephalographic tracings that indicate central nervous system stimulation rather than the depression observed in naive subjects. Such tracings have been obtained long after analgesic tolerance has worn off (Khazan and Colasanti, 1971; Kay et al., 1969).

(8) Pretreatment of adult mice with cocaine or amphetamine does not sensitize them to morphine. Adult mice that were pretreated with morphine showed a slight increase (30%) in their running response to amphetamine, 5 mg/kg, and a two-fold increase in response to cocaine, 10 mg/kg.

(9) Sensitization to morphine was not accompanied by an increase in the number of opiate receptors as determined by the naloxone-binding assay of Pert and Snyder (1973). The binding of naloxone to extracts of brains from 5 control mice, expressed as counts + S.E. stereospecifically bound per mg protein, was 97 + 18. The corresponding figure for a group of morphine sensitized mice was 898 + 33. This finding is not unexpected, because genetic studies in our laboratory have indicated that there may be some relationship between the number of opiate receptors and the analgesic response, but not the running response.

(10) Sensitization to morphine running can be blocked by treatment with cycloheximide, an inhibitor of protein synthesis (Figure 6). There have also been reports that the development of analgesic tolerance is blocked by cycloheximide (Loh, Shen, and Way, 1969). The simultaneous injection of cycloheximide, 20 mg per kg, prevented the development of sensitization to 25 mg per kg morphine sulfate.

DISCUSSION

The results presented here indicate that treatment of baby mice with morphine and other narcotics produces long-lasting sensitization to the stimulant effects of morphine. There are interesting similarities between morphine sensitization and the sensitization of baby mice to audiogenic seizures. If baby mice of the right strain are briefly exposed to a loud noise they will convulse when exposed to a similar noise several days or even weeks later. The similarities between morphine sensitization and induced audiogenic seizures are listed in Table II.

Careful investigation of induced audiogenic seizures has led to the conclusion that the initial exposure to loud noise produces partial deafness, and that subsequent sensitization probably results from denervation hypersensitivity (Henry, 1973; Gates and Chen, 1973). Initial tolerance to the running response in mice that were acutely treated with morphine (Shuster et al., 1963; Goldstein and Sheehan, 1969) might be considered analogous to the partial deafness produced by initial exposure to loud noise. Sensitization to morphine running might be attributed to a "pharmacological denervation" (Emmelin, 1961). Collier (1965) has suggested that the expansion of receptor sites resulting from denervation hypersensitivity may explain narcotic tolerance and physical dependence.

The comparison presented in Table II leads to several interesting predictions. Gates and Chen (1973) found that audiogenic seizures could be induced in adult mice if the intensity of the priming stimulus was greater than that used for baby mice. We are looking into the possibility that the amount of morphine needed to sensitive baby mice to morphine running may be considerably less than what we have been using for adult mice. The development of hypersensitivity after surgical denervation is accompanied by an increased rate of protein synthesis, and can be inhibited by treatment with cycloheximide (Kimura and Kimura, 1973). We have found that the development of morphine sensitization can be blocked by treatment with cycloheximide. Does morphine sensitization involve induced protein synthesis? Could cycloheximide block the induction of audiogenic seizures? These are some of the intriguing questions arising out of the comparison in Table II.

The observations reported here may have some relevance to certain aspects of narcotic addiction in humans. The long-term effects of perinatal addiction in infants born to addicted mothers have not been explored. In the case of adult patients it has been shown that ex-addicts experience considerably more euphoria in response to narcotic drugs than do subjects who have never been addicted (Lasagna et al. 1955).

Little is known about the nature of the central nervous stimulation produced by narcotic drugs. The running response to morphine in mice has been attributed to the release of catecholamines (Rethy et al., 1971), or to the action of both catecholamines and serotonin (Carrol and Sharp, 1972). We are presently examining neurohormone metabolism in the brains of pretreated mice, and attempting to alter the sensitization process with drugs that can change the concentration and turnover of neurohormones in the brain.

SUMMARY

The injection of morphine sulfate into baby mice twice daily for 5 days increased their running response to morphine when they were tested as adults. If treatment was completed before the mice were 15 days old there was no effect. Sensitization to morphine running was longer-lasting than either analgesic tolerance or tolerance to morphine running. Sensitization was blocked by concurrent administration of either naloxone or cycloheximide. It is suggested that sensitization to morphine running may be a form of denervation hypersensitivity that has several features in common with noise-induced sensitization to audiogenic seizures.

Note

This work was supported by grants Nos. DA00022 and DA00323 from the National Institutes of Health of the U.S. Public Health Service. We wish to thank Gary Kalan for excellent technical assistance in some of the experiments described here.

References

Carol, B. J., and Sharp, P. T. Monoamine mediation of the morphine induced activation of mice. *Brit. J. Pharmacol.*, 1972, *46*, 124-139.

Clouet, D. H., and Ratner, M. Catecholamine biosynthesis in the brains of rats treated with morphine. *Science,* 1970, *168,* 854-855.

Collier, H. O. J. A general theory of the genesis of drug dependence by induction of receptors. *Nature,* 1965, *205,* 181-182.

D'Amour, F. F., and Smith, D. L. A method for determining loss of pain sensation. *J. Pharmacol. Exp. Ther.,* 1941, *72,* 74-79.

Dews, P. B. The measurement of the influence of drugs on voluntary activity in mice. *Brit. J. Pharmacol.* 1953, *8,* 46-48.

Domino, E. F., and Wilson, A. E. Enhanced utilization of acetylcholine during morphine withdrawal in the rat. *Nature,* 1973, *243,* 285-286.

Emmelin, N. Supersensitivity following "pharmacological" denervation. *Pharmacol. Rev.* 1961, *13,* 17-37.

Gates, G. R., and Chen, C. Priming for audiogenic seizures in adult Balb/c mice. *Exp. Neurol.*, 1973, *41*, 457-463.

Goldstein, A. *Biostatistics: An Introductory Text.* New York: Macmillan, 1964.

Goldstein, D. B., and Goldstein, A. A possible role of enzyme inhibition and repression in drug tolerance and addiction. *Biochem. Pharmacol.*, 1961, *8*, 48.

Goldstein, A., and Sheehan, P. Tolerance to opiod narcotics 1. Tolerance to the running fit caused by levorphanol in the mouse. *J. Pharmacol. Exp. Ther.*, 1969, *169*, 175-184.

Henry, K. R. Increased adult auditory responsiveness resulting from juvenile acoustic experience. *Federation Proceedings*, 1973, *32*, 2098-2100.

Kay, D. C., Eisenstein, R. B., and Jasinski, D. R. Morphine effects on human REM state, waking state and REM sleep. *Psychopharmacologia (Berl.)*, 1969, *14*, 404-416.

Khazan, N., and Colasanti, B. EEG correlates of morphine challenge in post-addict rats. *Psychopharmacologia (Berl.)*, 1971, *22*, 56-63.

Kimura, M., and Kimura, I. Increase of nascent protein synthetis in neuromuscular junction of rat diaphragm induced by denervation. *Nature New Biology*, 1973, *241*, 114-115.

Lasagna, L., von Felsinger, J. M., and Beecher, H. K. Drug-induced mood changes in man. Observations in healthy subjects, chronically ill patients, and "post-addicts". *J. Am. Med. Assoc.*, 1955, *157*, 1006-1020.

Loh, H. H., Shen, F., and Way, E. L. Inhibition of morphine tolerance and physical dependence development and brain serotonin synthesis by cycloheximide. *Biochem. Pharmacol.*, 1969, *18*, 2711-2721.

Pert, C. B., and Synder, S. H. Properties of opiate-receptor binding in rat brain. *Proc. Nat. Acad. Sci. U.S.A.*, 1973, *70*, 2243-2247.

Peterson, G. R., Webster, G. W., and Shuster, L. Effect of narcotics on enzymes of acetylcholine metabolism in cultured cells from embryonic chick brains. *Neuropharmacology*, 1974, *13*, 1-12.

Rethy, C. R., Smith, C. B., and Villareal, J. E. Effects of narcotic analgesics upon the locomotor activity and brain catecholamine content of the mouse. *J. Pharmacol. Exp. Ther.*, 1971, *176*, 472-479.

Saunders, D. R., Miya, T. S., and Paolino, R. M. Increased responsiveness of male rats to depressant and stimulant drugs as a function of age. *The Pharmacologist*, 1973, *15*, 199.

Shuster, L. Repression and de-repression of enzyme synthesis as a possible explanation of some aspects of drug action. *Nature*, 1961, *189*, 314-315.

Shuster, L. Some biochemical effects of morphine on cultured brain cells. *Intra. Science Chem. Rept.*, 1974, *8*, 149-160.

Shuster, L., Hannam, R. V., and Boyle, W. E. Jr. A simple method for producing tolerance to dihydromorphinone in mice. *J. Pharmacol. Exp. Ther.*, 1963, *140*, 149-154.

Shuster, L., Webster, G. W., and Yu, G. Increased running response to morphine in morphine-pretreated mice. *J. Pharmacol. Exp. Ther.*, 1974, *192*, 64-72.

Way, E. L., Ho, I. K., and Loh, H. H. Relations of brain serotonin to the inhibition and enhancement of morphine tolerance and physical dependence, in Mandell, A. T. (ed) *New Concepts in Neurotransmitter Regulation*, 1973, New York. Plenum Press, p. 279-295.

DISCUSSION

Q. *Dr. Braude:* Did you have a chance to observe your mice during the 90-minute period, to see if, by chance, you found seizures in these mice at these dose levels?

A. *Dr. Shuster: No. Now, this question of seizures in addicted babies really*

puzzles me, because I do not believe anyone has reported seizures as a feature of withdrawal from a narcotic drug. It is quite common after withdrawal from barbiturates, but I have not seen seizures in my studies. Actually, I have addicted my mice very strongly in the past. What I tend to find is a period of depression during withdrawal. But I have found nothing like seizures.

A. *Dr. Zemp: In the deviant 2-J strain of mice, which is genetically susceptible to audiogenic seizures without priming, cycloheximide or possible acetyl cycloheximide has been demonstrated to block the seizures. This was reported in* Science *about two years ago.*

Q. *Dr. Shuster:* That is very interesting. Did you do the work yourself?

A. *Dr. Zemp: No, we did not.*

A. *Dr. Schuster: Dr. Way, from San Francisco, blocked narcotic tolerance using cycloheximide.*

Q. *Dr. Nuite:* You say that you blocked the final sensitization effect as you measured it after three days of withdrawal with naloxone, which is demonstrative of blocking a classical narcotic effect. Have you ever treated the animals chronically with naloxone to see if you can block the development of sensitization similar to blockage of tolerance development with narcotics?

A. *Dr. Shuster: I guess I did not make myself clear—I could block the development of sensitization completely by giving the mice a mixture of morphine and naloxone.*

Q. *Dr. Nuite:* Did you give a ratio throughout the period of development of sensitization, rather than just on the final day?

A. *Dr. Shuster: Yes. Do you mean to sensitize, and then on the final day to give naloxone? That would be most amazing if naloxone did anything at that point. It might be worth a try.*

Q. *Dr. Davis:* Have you mentioned the effects on the serotonin and have you tried to block some of the effects you have spoken of with parachloraphenylalanine?

A. *Dr. Shuster: No, I have not tried parachloraphenylalanine blockade, that is one of the things we want to look at. Actually, right now, we are concentrating on catecholamines rather than serotonin, because there is good reason to believe that dopamine is the neurogenic amine that is most involved in the running behavior.*

Addictive Diseases: an International Journal 2 (2): 293-306 (1975)
© 1975 by Spectrum Publications, Inc.

Sympatho-Adrenal Development in Perinatally Addicted Rats

THEODORE A. SLOTKIN
THOMAS R. ANDERSON
Department of Physiology and Pharmacology
Duke University Medical Center
Durham, North Carolina

INTRODUCTION

The adrenal medulla is an integral part of the sympathetic nervous system and participates in the maintenance of normal autonomic functions. For practical reasons, the adrenal has often been used as a model of adrenergic neurons: both tissues arise embryonically from the neural crest and both have the ability to synthesize, store and secrete catecholamines. Both contain storage vesicles which can take up amines by a mechanism which is stimulated by ATP and Mg^{2+} (Kirshner, 1962; Carlsson et al., 1962); the vesicles contain dopamine β-hydroxylase, chromogranins and adenine nucleotides in addition to catecholamines, and it is generally accepted that the catecholamines and adenine nucleotides (primarily ATP) form a storage complex in a molar ratio of 4 to 1.

The biosynthesis of catecholamines is shown in Figure 1. Two of the enzymes involved in the synthetic pathway, tyrosine hydroxylase (TH) and dopamine β-hydroxylase (DBH), demonstrate the phenomenon termed "trans-synaptic inductions," i.e., their levels are increased by increments in the rate of neural input to the tissue. (For review, see Thoenen, 1974). These stimulation-induced changes in TH and DBH activity are of functional significance because: (1) TH is rate-limiting in synthesis and increased TH activity thus will accelerate catecholamine formation; (2) DBH is localized solely in storage vesicles (Viveros et al., 1969a) and increases in DBH activity represent an augmented storage capability of the tissue.

293

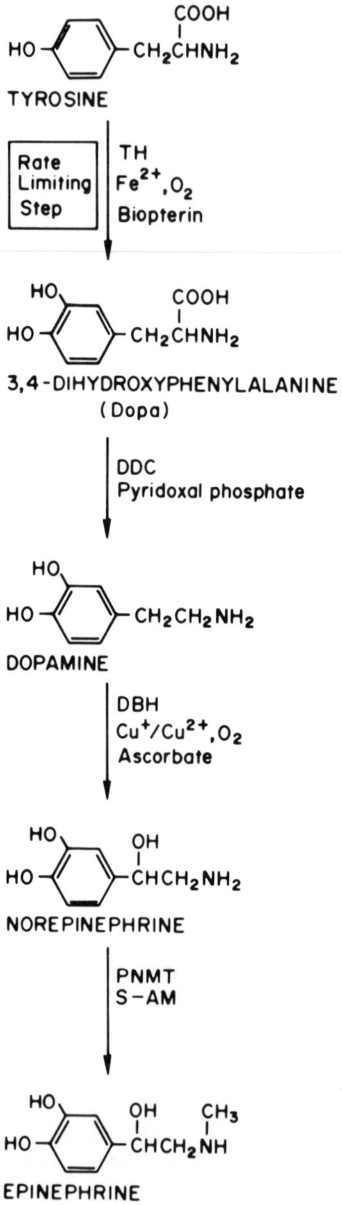

FIG. 1: Biosynthesis of catecholamines. TH, tyrosine hydroxylase; DDC, dopa decarboxylase; DBH, dopamine β-hydroxylase; PNMT, phenylethanolamine N-methyltransferase; S-AM, S-adenosylmethionine.

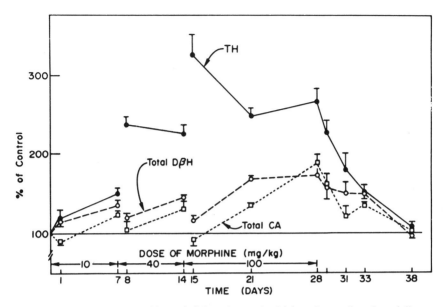

FIG. 2: Effects of morphine administration and withdrawal on adrenal medullary catecholamines (CA), tyrosine hydroxylase (TH) and dopamine β-hydroxylase (DBH). Points and bars represent means ± standard errors of 5-12 adult animals. Control values (45 animals) were: catecholamines 14.9 ± 0.4 μg/gland; tyrosine hydroxylase 2.58 + 0.2 nmol/gland/hr; dopamine β-hydroxylase 1.62 ± 0.07 nmol/gland/hr. For details, see Anderson and Slotkin, 1975.

More then sixty years ago, the morphine-induced depletion of adrenal catecholamines was first noted by Elliott (1912); subsequent investigations demonstrated that the response comprises, in part, a neurally mediated effect which can be reduced by sectioning the splanchnic nerve (Stewart and Rogoff, 1922). Recent studies from our and other laboratories have demonstrated that the maturation of the adrenal medulla is also keyed to changes in neural input (Patrick and Kirshner, 1972; Slotkin, 1973a,b), and this suggested to us that the administration of morphine in the pre-and post-natal period might produce different effects than in adults, and also that the subsequent maturation process might be altered by morphine administration. Before discussing the effects of morphine in the neonate, it is important to understand first the effects of morphine in the mature adrenal.

EFFECTS OF MORPHINE ON THE MATURE
ADRENAL MEDULLA

Adult male rats were given twice daily subcutaneous injections of morphine HCl, and doses were increased at weekly intervals. With the initiation of each dosage increment, there was a decrease in catecholamine levels resulting from neurogenic secretion (Fig. 2). As each dose was maintained, however, ca-

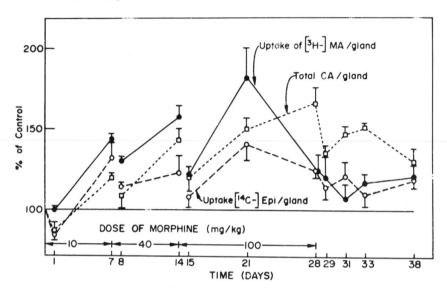

FIG. 3:   Effects of morphine administration and withdrawal on uptakes per gland of epinephrine (Epi) and metaraminol (MA). Points and bars represent means ± standard errors of 5-11 adult animals. Control values (40 animals) were: epinephrine uptake 4.07 ± 0.16 nmols/gland; metaraminol uptake 0.53 ± 0.02 nmols/gland. For details, see Anderson and Slotkin, 1975.

techolamine levels increased to supranormal levels, probably as a result of accelerated synthesis and increased storage capacity indicated by the transsynaptic induction of TH and DBH (Fig. 2). Upon cessation of morphine administration, all three parameters declined to normal in about 10 days. These data are consistent with the view that morphine increases the rate of stimulation of the adrenal medulla and further, suggest that the stimulation continues with chronic administration, i.e., that the morphine-induced stimulatory reflex does not display tolerance (Anderson and Slotkin, 1975).

We next wished to examine the effects of morphine on the properties of the adrenal storage vesicles of adult rats to determine whether the drug could alter the uptake or storage functions in any fashion. The ability of isolated vesicles to incorporate ^{14}C-epinephrine expressed in terms of nmols per gland was similar to the changes in catecholamine content (Fig. 3). This is consistent with the view that the morphine-induced stimulation of the adrenal results in changes in the number of functional storage vesicles; the initial decrease at each dosage increment represents loss of catecholamines and of intact vesicles resulting from exocytotic, quantal secretion of the vesicle contents (Viveros et al., 1969b; Slotkin and Kirshner, 1973a). The subsequent increases in uptake upon chronic treatment reflect induction of new vesicle synthesis which more than compensates for increased secretion.

Earlier studies on the mechanism of vesicle synthesis have shown that intact vesicles are formed prior to filling with soluble constituents, such as ATP

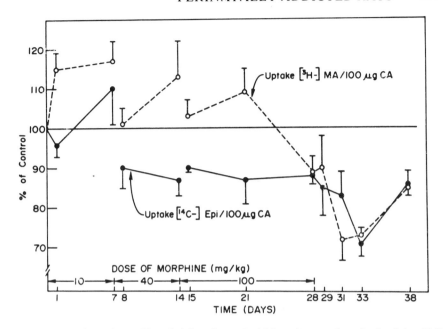

FIG. 4:   Effects of morphine administration and withdrawal on uptakes of epinephrine (Epi) and metaraminol (MA) per 100 μg endogenous catecholamines. Points and bars represent means ± standard errors of 5-11 adult animals. Control values (40 animals) were: epinephrine uptake 30.6 ± 0.7 nmols/100 μg CA; metaraminol uptake 3.97 ± 0.14 nmols/100 μg CA. For details, see Anderson and Slotkin, 1975.

and catecholamines (Viveros et al., 1971; Slotkin and Kirshner, 1973b). These partially filled, "immature" vesicles have abnormally low equilibrium densities and do not have the same capability as mature vesicles to distinguish between catecholamines and non-catecholamines, such as metaraminol (Slotkin, 1973a; Slotkin and Kirshner, 1973a,b). If morphine indeed accelerates vesicle formation, then the proportion of new, immature vesicles should increase and metaraminol uptake should show a relatively larger increase then epinephrine uptake; this hypothesis was confirmed experimentally (Fig. 3). Thus morphine administration in adult rats increased the number of vesicles but also increased the proportion of vesicles with below-normal levels of soluble consituents.

Because uptake per gland reflects to a large extent the *number* of storage vesicles present, these values do not indicate how well the individual vesicles are functioning (Slotkin and Kirshner, 1973a,b; Anderson and Slotkin, 1975). By calculating uptake per 100 μg of endogenous catecholamines, we obtain a measure of the average uptake capability of an individual vesicle relative to its endogenous content (Fig. 4). When uptake is determined in this fashion, the shift in relative uptakes of metaraminol and epinephrine is much more evident, again indicative of the presence of partially filled vesicles. However, there appears to be a defect in the ability of the vesicles to incorporate epinephrine and also, at

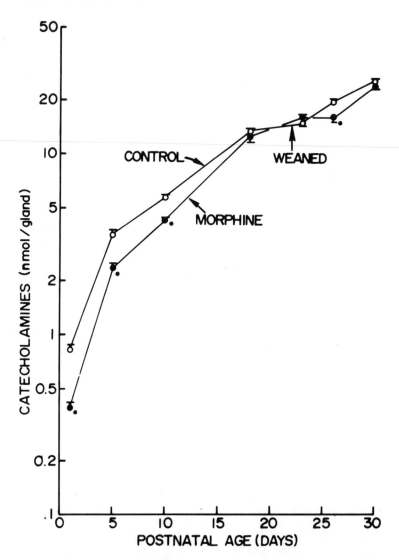

FIG. 5:   Development of adrenal catecholamines in control (o) and perinatally addicted (•) rats. Points and bars represent means ± standard errors of 5-6 determinations at each age; asterisks denote significant differences (p < 0.05 or better). Ordinate is logarithmic.

later times, metaraminol; this defect persists even after morphine is discontinued (Fig. 4). Subsequent studies have shown that vesicles from chronically morphine-treated rats have a reduced affinity constant for epinephrine (Slotkin and Anderson, 1975), suggesting a defect in the storage vesicle membrane.

The effects of morphine on the adult rat adrenal medulla can be summarized as follows: increased splanchnic stimulation leads to catecholamine secretion but also to induction of catecholamine-synthesizing enzymes and increases in the number of storage vesicles which subsequently produces above-normal catecholamine levels. A larger proportion of the vesicles are deficient in soluble constituents and display abnormal densities and an altered uptake system.

EFFECTS OF MORPHINE ON THE IMMATURE
ADRENAL MEDULLA

Studies similar to those in adult rats were carried out in developing rats. Morphine HC1 (2.5 mg/kg, s.c.) was injected twice daily to pregnant rats beginning 8 days prepartum, and the dosage was gradually increased to 40 mg/kg by day 1 postpartum and maintained at that level. The offspring thus were exposed chronically to morphine both prenatally (via the placenta) and postnatally (via the milk), and exposure was terminated at weaning. The morphine-treated animals showed a typical retardation in weight gain of about 30% through 30 days of age; however, poor nutrition per se probably had little or no effect on adrenal catecholamine biochemistry, since within age and treatment groups there was no significant correlation between body weight and any of the other parameters.

The addicted neonates exhibited a marked deficiency in catecholamines compared to controls (Fig. 5); the difference persisted through 10 days of age, but disappeared by 18 days despite the continued exposure to morphine. Four days after termination of exposure to morphine (initiated by weaning), there was again a significant, but short-lived, slowing of the maturational increase in adrenal catecholamines. These results are in marked contrast to the effects of morphine in adult rats, where acute administration produced small decreases, and chronic administration relatively large increases, in catecholamines.

Several hypotheses can be advanced to explain the morphine-induced maturational deficit in catecholamines. Morphine could inhibit catecholamine synthesis. However, measurements of the activity of TH, the rate-limiting enzyme, indicated that TH developed normally in the addicted pups (Fig. 6). On the other hand, this is once again different from the TH induction seen in mature rats given morphine.

There was a significant retardation of the age-dependent increases in DBH in morphine-addicted pups, indicating that at least part of the reduction in catecholamines resulted from the presence of fewer storage vesicles (Fig. 6). Again, this is the opposite of the DBH induction seen in adult rats. The low DBH values could not account for the entire catecholamine deficit, since the magnitudes of the morphine-induced reductions in DBH were much smaller than the reductions in catecholamines. This suggested that there might also be a reduction in the catecholamine content per vesicle, e.g., that the vesicles in morphine-treated neonates might be only partially filled. To test that hypothesis, we examined the abilities of individual vesicles to take up epinephrine and

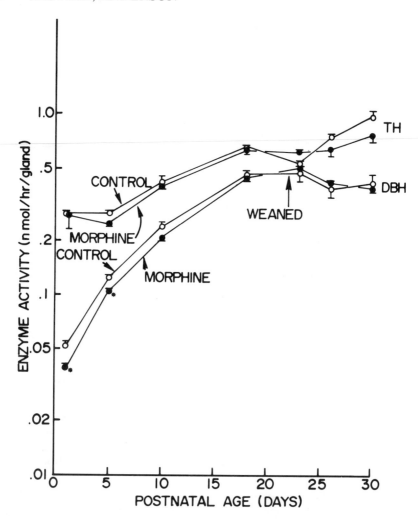

FIG. 6:   Development of adrenal tyrosine hydroxylase (TH) and dopamine β-hydroxylase (DBH) in control (o) and perinatally addicted (•) rats. Points and bars represent means ± standard errors of 5-6 determinations at each age; asterisks denote significant differences (p < 0.05 or better). Ordinate is logarithmic.

metaraminol relative to endogenous content. At 1 and 5 days of age, the perinatally addicted pups demonstrated an uptake pattern typical of partially filled vesicles, namely, an elevation in metaraminol uptake per 100μ/g of endogenous catecholamines (Fig. 7). Surprisingly, the animals failed to develop the later uptake system defect seen in adults; however, the detailed interpretation of the effects of morphine on uptake in developing rats is complicated by the fact that the uptake system itself undergoes maturational alterations (Slotkin, 1973a, 1975).

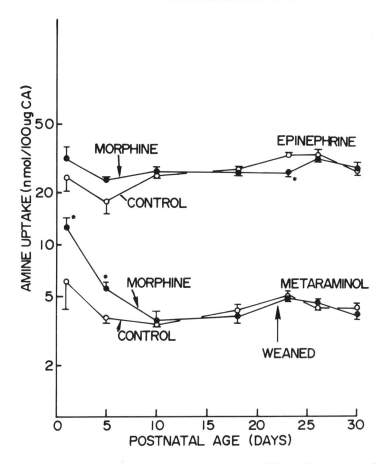

FIG. 7:   Uptake of epinephrine and metaraminol per 100 μg endogenous catecholamines in isolated adrenal vesicles from developing control (o) and perinatally addicted (•) rats. Points and bars represent means ± standard errors of 5-6 determinations at each age; asterisks denote significant differences (p < 0.05 or better). Ordinate is logarithmic.

THE ROLE OF NEURAL INPUT

Because so many of morphine's effects on the mature adrenal medulla appear to depend upon neural input to the gland, it was important to establish at what point in development the tissue became functionally innervated by the splanchnic nerve, and whether this might explain the different effects of morphine in immature rats. Measurement of catecholamines, ATP, enzyme levels and vesicle properties in untreated developing rats suggested that innervation was absent in the neonate but present by 10 days of age (Slotkin, 1973a,b). To test this hypothesis, developing rats were given injections of insulin to produce hypoglycemia, which evokes a reflex sympatho-adrenal discharge. Ca-

TABLE I
Insulin-Induced Secretion of Catecholamines from Adrenal Medullae of
Developing Rats

Age	Catecholamines (nmoles/gland)		Secretion
(days)	Control	3 hr post-insulin (20 U/kg s.c)	(%)
1	1.5 ± 0.1 (6)	1.5 ± 0.1 (6)	0 ± 4 p>0.9
10	8.4 ± 0.5 (4)	5.7 ± 0.4 (5)	32 ± 5 p<0.005
20	13.2 ± 0.5 (5)	9.8 ± 0.1 (4)	26 ± 1 p<0.001
30	29 ± 1 (5)	20 ± 1 (5)	30 ± 5 p<0.002
40	45 ± 2 (4)	29 ± 2 (4)	35 ± 5 p<0.005
50	69 ± 2 (3)	51 ± 2 (2)	26 ± 3 p<0.02

Values are given as mean ± S.E. The numbers in parentheses denote the number of determinations. Significance is determined by comparison with control values.
For details, see Slotkin, 1973b.

techolamine secretion was not observed in neonates, but 10-day old rats secreted
normally, suggesting that innervation of the adrenal was indeed nonfunctional
prepartum and at birth, but fully operational by 10 days of age (Table I).

Since trans-synaptic induction of TH and DBH requires neural input, these
data explain the inability of morphine to increase levels of those enzymes in addicted neonates. However, in the absence of functional innervation, the morphine-induced reduction in neonatal catecholamines cannot be explained by
neurogenic secretion. In this regard, Yoshizaki (1973) has demonstrated that
morphine can exert a direct catecholamine-releasing effect in chronically dener-
vated rat adrenals; and similarly, non-neurogenic secretion in response to
various other stimuli has been observed in immature adrenals of other species
(Comline and Silver, 1966). These data suggest that the catecholamine deficiency in addicted neonates might result in part from morphine-induced non-

neurogenic secretion which could not be compensated by trans-synaptic induction because of the lack of innervation. The depleting effect would be superimposed on the general slowing of adreno-medullary maturation which results from the reduced rate of development of the storage vesicles (indicated by the reduced DBH).

It is noteworthy that developing rats continuously exposed to morphine did not develop supranormal levels of TH, DBH or catecholamines even after the appearance of innervation (10 days postpartum and later); nor did they display the defect in uptake per 100 μg endogenous catecholamines seen in chronically treated adults. Further studies are required to determine whether exposure to morphine in the pre-innervation period "protects" the sympatho-adrenal system from subsequent effects or whether the regulation of catecholamine synthesis and storage has been altered.

SUMMARY

Chronic morphine administration in adult rats results in neurogenic secretion of adrenal catecholamines and compensatory increases in basal catecholamine levels, in activities of catecholamine biosynthetic enzymes and in the number of storage vesicles in the tissue. Perinatally addicted developing rats demonstrated changes completely different from those seen in adults; catecholamine levels and dopamine β-hydroxylase activity were reduced compared to controls and no induction of tyrosine hydroxylase was observed. The time course of adrenomedullary maturation was delayed through the first 10-20 days of age, with reduced numbers of storage vesicles and larger proportions of partially filled vesicles. On exposure to morphine, continued until weaning, perinatally addicted rats did not display any of the changes in catecholamine synthesis or uptake seen in adult rats. The differences between adults and developing rats can be partly explained by the absence of functional innervation of the neonatal adrenal medulla.

Notes

This research was supported by USPHS grant DA-00465 and by a Faculty Development Award from the Pharmaceutical Manufacturers Association Foundation.
Requests for reprints should be addrssed to Dr. Theodore A. Slotkin, Box 3709, Duke University Medical Center, Durham, North Carolina 27710.

References

Anderson, T.R., and Slotkin, T.A. Effects of morphine on the rat adrenal medulla. *Biochem. Pharmacol.*, 1975, in press.
Carlsson, A., Hillarp, N.-A., and Waldeck, B. A Mg^{++}=dependent storage mechanism in the amine granules of the adrenal medulla. *Med. exp.*, 1962, *6*, 47-53.
Comline, R.S., and Silver, M. The development of the adrenal medulla of the foetal and new-born calf. *J. Physiol.(London)*, 1966, *183*, 305-340.

Elliott, T.R. The Control of the suprarenal glands by the splanchnic nerves. *J. Physiol. (London)*, *44*, 374-409.

Kirshner, N. Uptake of catecholamines by a particulate fraction of the adrenal medulla. *J. Biol. Chem.*, 1962, *237*, 2311-2317.

Patrick, R.L., and Kirshner, N. Developmental changes in rat adrenal tyrosine hydroxylase, dopamine β-hydroxylase and catecholamine levels: Effect of Denervation. *Devl. Biol.*, 1972, *29*, 204-213.

Slotkin, T.A. Maturation of the adrenal medulla. I. Uptake and storage of amines in isolated storage vesicles of the rat. *Biochem. Pharmacol.*, 1973a, *22*, 2023-2032.

Slotkin, T.A. Maturation of the adrenal medulla. II. Content and properties of catecholamine storage vesicles of the rat. *Biochem. Pharmacol.*, 1973b, *22*, 2033-2044.

Slotkin, T.A. Maturation of the adrenal medulla. III. Practical and theoretical considerations of age-dependent alterations in kinetics of incorporation of catechol- and non-catecholamines. *Biochem. Pharmacol.*, 1975, *24*, 89-97.

Slotkin, T.A., and Anderson, T.R. Chronic morphine administration alters epinephrine uptake in rate adrenal storage vesicles. *Neuropharmacol.*, 1975, in press.

Slotkin, T.A., and Kirshner, N. All-or-none secretion of adrenal medullary storage vesicle contents in the rat. *Biochem. Pharmacol.*, 1973a, *22*, 205-219.

Slotkin, T.A., and Kirshner, N. Recovery of rat adrenal amine stores after insulin administration. *Mol. Pharmacol.*, 1973b, *9*, 105-116.

Stewart, G.N., and Rogoff, J.M. The action of drugs on the output of epinephrine from the adrenals. VIII. Morphine. *J. Pharmacol. Exp. Ther.*, 1922, *19*, 59-85.

Thoenen, H. Trans-synaptic enzyme induction. *Life Sci.*, 1974, *14*, 223-235.

Viveros, O.H., Arqueros, L., Connett, R.J., and Kirshner, N. Mechanism of secretion from the adrenal medulla. III. Studies of dopamine β-hydroxylase as a marker for catecholamine storage vesicle membranes in rabbit adrenal glands. *Mol. Pharmacol.*, 1969a, *5*, 60-68.

Viveros, O.H., Arqueros, L., and Kirshner, N. Quantal secretion from the adrenal medulla: All-or-none release of storage vesicle content. *Science*, 1969b, *165*, 911-913.

Viveros, O.H., Arqueros, L., and Kirshner, N. Mechanism of secretion from the adrenal medulla. VII. Effect of insulin administration on the buoyant density, dopamine β-hydroxylase, and catecholamine content of adrenal storage vesicles. *Mol. Pharmacol.*, 1971, *7*, 444-454.

Yoshizaki, T. Effect of histamine, bradykinin and morphine on adrenaline release from rat adrenal gland. *Japan J. Pharmacol.*, 1973, *23*, 695-699.

DISCUSSION

Q. *Dr. Zemp:* Let me compliment you on the elegant series of studies that you have done and ask one question. Have you done similar experiments with tissue from the central nervous system?

A. *Dr. Slotkin:* *No, we were planning to do that some time next year. There is a really big program in trying to do this in the CNS. The reason that the adrenal medulla has been used, classicially, is that it is a very clean tissue; it contains, in the rat, virtually one neuro-transmitter. The major problem we run into in the CNS is the inability to obtain purified storage vesicles with which to measure such things as uptake. The size of the vesicle in the CNS is much smaller, and is found in the microsomal fraction. It is very contaminated and we get very poor yields. But we are working on the techniques to try to do this.*

Q. *Dr. Glass:* I was not quite clear on this; what happens to norepinephrine production during acute abstinence in the neonatal animal?

A. *Dr. Shuster: I cannot really say "norepinephrine production," because we are not measuring the synthesis with a precursor. What I can say is that the tyrosine hydroxylase level, the rate-limiting enzyme, does not change in any fashion, in the neonatal animal, when you start it on withdrawal at weaning. This is in contrast to what happens in the adult animal, where morphine causes TH induction, and then on withdrawal, the tyrosine hydroxylase (TH) level just starts dropping immediately.*

Q. *Dr. Zelson:* I would like to comment on some studies we have done. We have examined the 24-hour urine specimens for catecholamines in these newborn drug-addict babies, and we have found that the levels are perfectly normal, that they relate exactly to our controls.

Q. *Dr. Slotkin:* Have you look at VMA? One of the problems is that urinary catechols (unchanged) represent only about 2 or 3 percent of the total amount of neuro-transmitter coming out in the urine.

Q. *Dr. Ostrea:* I would like to make a comment and ask a question also. I think that even in the newborn infants, there is a developmental factor in the catecholamine response to any form of stress. I say this because we know that prematures respond very poorly to cold stresses, because they cannot increase their adrenaline secretions. This is a function of time, because after 30 days they will increase. My question is, what is your explanation for that constant initial decrease in catecholamine, and dopamine beta hydroxylase levels, when you give morphine to your addicted adults?

A. *Dr. Slotkin: What you are looking at are two processes dependent on stimulation. One is the secretion process. If you do not stimulate the adrenal, it will not secrete. The other is the induction of the enzymes, and they have two time courses. Secretion is something that takes a matter of seconds, induction of an enzyme takes hours. You will see, first, a decrease in catechols, and the decrease in DBH is due to release of soluble dopamine beta hydroxylase because the mechanism of release is by exocytosis.*

Q. *Dr. Abrams:* I would not want to extrapolate from your animal experiments to the human, but as you know, the neonatal withdrawal picture is identical to hyperthyroidism. An interesting question comes up in one's mind, without any data, or anything to back it up. Is it possible that during this phase of narcotic addiction, the hypothalamus centers are suppressed, not to the extent of producing a hypothyroid situation, but suppressed enough that, on withdrawal of the drug, there is a sudden rebound release of hypothalamus-releasing factors, one of which could be TSH-releasing factor, with the concomitant, sympathetic overproduction that you would see in a neonate, adult, or child with thyrotoxicosis? I am not sure if anyone has done studies on that, and I wonder if you have any comments on that?

A. *Dr. Slotkin: My comment is an unequivocal maybe.*

Addictive Diseases: an International Journal 2 (2): 307-331 (1975)

Some Effects of Prenatal Exposure to D-Amphetamine Sulfate and Phenobarbital on Developmental Neurochemistry and on Behavior

JOHN W. ZEMP
LAWRENCE D. MIDDAUGH
*Departments of Biochemistry
and Psychiatry and Behavioral Sciences
Medical University of South Carolina
Charleston, South Carolina*

INTRODUCTION

Numerous reports and reviews (Karnofsky, 1965; Cohen, 1964) have established the teratogenic potential of psychoactive drugs administered during pregnancy. Gross anatomical deformities have been the dependent variable for most of these studies. From these studies, a number of generalizations regarding teratogenesis have been made (Wilson, 1965). Of particular interest is the finding that there are critical periods during development when the embryo is particularly vulnerable to external agents. For production of anatomical deformities, the agent must be applied at an early stage of development when areas of the embryonic disc have acquired organ-forming potential.

Dobbing (Dobbing, 1968) has extended the notion of critical periods of vulnerability well beyond the stage of organogenesis. He suggests that interference with other stages of development (e.g., during periods of rapid growth), although not capable of producing gross abnormalities of structure and function, can result in suboptimal function which might be permanent. In support of this notion, there have been a number of studies demonstrating long-term changes in behavior (Levine and Mullins, 1966; Joffe, 1969), in brain function (Dobbing,

1968; Shoemaker and Wurtman, 1971), and in endocrine function (Levine and Mullins, 1966) following *neonatal* exposure to undernutrition, irradiation, stress, and exogenously administered hormones. There is also evidence to suggest that prenatal exposure to various agents can produce long-term biochemical (Shoemaker and Wurtman, 1971; Eiduson, 1966; Sparber and Shideman, 1968; 1969 a, b; 1970), neurophysiological (Bergstrom, 1967), and behavioral (Joffe, 1969) changes.

On the basis of these studies, it appears that there are a number of developmental stages during which exposure to drugs or other agents can produce long-term changes in the behavior and physiological function of the organism.

Recently there has been increasing interest in possible subtle alterations produced by prenatal exposure to various psychoactive drugs. Behavioral studies by Werboff and co-workers (Werboff and Gottlieb, 1963; Werboff et al., 1961; Werboff and Havlena, 1962; Werboff et al., Werboff et al., 1961; Werboff and Havlena, 1962; Werboff and Kesner, 1963) and by Hoffeld et al. (Hoffeld et al., 1968; Hoffeld et al., 1965; Hoffeld et al., 1967) have established that tranquilizers given to rats during pregnancy produce long-lasting behavioral alterations in offspring. Other workers have reported long-term behavioral effects of prenatal exposure to amphetamine (Clark et al., 1970). Such changes might be the result of neurochemical alterations induced by exposure to the drug.

Research in our laboratory over the past several years has been designed to determine if maternally administered phenobarbital or dextro-amphetamine sulfate could produce neurochemical and/or behavioral changes in offspring. These drugs were chosen because:

    a. they are widely used in our culture (Kramer et al., 1967; Sadusk, 1966), including use during pregnancy (Forfar and Nelson, 1973);

    b. they have opposite effects on central nervous system activity;

    c. some of their effects on neurotransmitters (Axelrod' 1971; Brown, 1971; Lidbrink et al., 1972) and on pituitary-adrenal function (Karavolas et al., 1972) have been demonstrated; and

    d. chronic use produces brain lesions and behavioral changes in man (McColl et al., 1963; Nora et al., 1965).

Our original intent was to examine the influence of these drugs on metabolism of nucleic acids and proteins of the developing brain. The research has been extended to include an examination of the development of catecholamine systems in the brain, and possible behavioral and endocrine alterations. Emphasis was placed on the catecholamines since:

    a. their synthetic pathways and metabolic fate are to a large extent known;

    b. many important behavioral and physiological mechanisms have been postulated to be associated with these systems; and

    c. pharmacologic agents with specific effects on these systems are available.

The drugs in our studies were administered during the last third of pregnancy to reduce the probability of producing gross abnormalities and therefore to permit us to detect more subtle changes.

EXPERIMENTS WITH AMPHETAMINE

The purpose of the experiments discussed in this report was to determine if injecting pregnant mice with D-amphetamine sulfate would produce changes in the concentrations of catecholamines in the brains and in the activity of their offspring.

D-amphetamine sulfate has primary effects on catecholamine synapses, causing increased release of catecholamines into the synaptic cleft, blocked reuptake of the neurotransmitter into the terminal bouton, and possibly inhibition of monoamine oxidase (Axelrod, 1971). The catecholamine synapses, at least in the rat, are undergoing rapid development around the time of birth (Coyle and Henry, 1973). A series of studies on chicks by Sparber and Shideman (1968; 1969a, b; 1970) suggests that interference with the development of the catecholamine (CA) systems with reserpine can produce long-term alterations in CA levels and in behavior. The postulate was that pharmacologically induced changes in the level of neurotransmitters at critical stages of development could, through repression or depression, transiently or permanently alter the levels of key regulatory enzymes (Eiduson, 1966; Sparber and Shideman, 1969b, 1970). The altered level of enzymes might then produce changes in the neurotransmitter system of the brain which in turn might result in the observed behavioral changes.

Two studies using rats suggest that prenatal exposure to amphetamine produces behavioral alterations in offspring. An early study by Bell, Drucker, and Woodruff (1965) suggested that offspring of rats injected with amphetamine during the 1st or 2nd third of gestation had depressed activity at 45 days of age. More recently, Clark, Gorman, and Vernadakis (1970) reported that offspring of rats injected with amphetamine (1 mg/kg during days 12-15 of gestation) had depressed open-field activity at 21 days of age compared to offspring of rats injected with saline. Tests before and after that time revealed no difference between control and amphetamine-treated offspring. In a T-maze problem, offspring of amphetamine-treated animals ran the maze faster but did not differ from untreated animals in the number of errors made.

These two sets of experiments indicate that prenatal exposure to reserpine alters catecholamine levels and that prenatal exposure to amphetamines alters activity. Our experiments were designed to attempt to correlate the biochemical and behavioral effects of D-amphetamine sulfate.

Pregnant C57Bl/6J mice were assigned to one of three groups on the 13th day of gestation. The D-amphetamine sulfate groups (DAMS) received daily in-

TABLE I
Effects of D-Amphetamine Sulfate on Weight Gain
During Pregnancy
and on Litter Size and Pup Weight at Birth

	D[a] X+S.D.	S[b] X+S.D.	U[c] X+S.D.
Weight Gains During Last Trimester	6.2 ± 1.8g[d]	7.5 ± 1.8	8.2 ± 1.9
Litter Size At Birth	6.4 ± 1.8	6.7 ± 2.2	6.6 ± 2.1
Pup Weight At Birth	1.27 ± .09g[e]	1.27 ± .13	1.32 ± .10

[a]Drug Group animals were injected daily with D-amphetamine sulfate (5 mg/kg) during last trimester

[b]Saline Group animals were injected daily with .9% saline during last trimester

[c]Untreated Group animals were weighted only during last trimester

[d]D<U, t = 2.581, df 23, p<.025; D<S, t = 1.907, df 28, p<.1

[e]D<U, t = 2.32, df 76, p<.025; S<U, t = 1.90, df 76, p<.05

Some of the data appearing in this table was published in Devel. Psychobiol., 7(5):429-438 (1974) and is reprinted with permission of John Wiley & Sons, Inc.

jections (5 mg/kg in 0.9% saline intraperitoneally) until parturition; the saline control group (SC) received daily injections of an equivalent volume of saline; the untreated control group (UC) received no injections.

The pregnant females were selected so that the three groups would deliver on the same day. The last injection was given 12-18 hours prior to birth. On the day of birth, litters were culled to six and the pups reared by their natural

TABLE IIA
Effects of Injections of D-Amphetamine Sulfate
or Saline During Pregnancy
on Catecholamine Concentration in Brains of Offspring

	Norepinephrine ng/g brain		
	D^a	S^b	U^c
Days	$\bar{X} \pm$ S.D. (N)[d]	$\bar{X} \pm$ S.D. (N)	$\bar{X} \pm$ S.D. (N)
0	62 $\pm$ 12 (5)	115 $\pm$ 18 (8)	133 $\pm$ 15 (5)[e]
3	144 $\pm$ 46 (7)	170 $\pm$ 63 (6)	159 $\pm$ 33 (7)
7	158 $\pm$ 63 (4)	162 $\pm$ 14 (5)	175 $\pm$ 20 (6)
14	193 $\pm$ 34 (7)	175 $\pm$ 47 (4)	235 $\pm$ 27 (5)
21	294 $\pm$ 40 (6)	329 $\pm$ 17 (5)	242 $\pm$ 45 (6)[f]
30	651 $\pm$ 148 (6)	431 $\pm$ 133 (6)	325 $\pm$ 108 (12)[g]

[a]Offspring of mice injected with D-amphetamine sulfate

[b]Offspring of mice injected with saline

[c]Offspring of untreated mice

[d](N) is number of samples included in calculation of mean and standard deviation

[e]D<S, U (p<.05, Duncan's Multiple Range Test)

[f]D, S>U (p<.05, Duncan's Multiple Range Test)

[g]D>S, U (p<.05, Duncan's Multiple Range Test)

mothers until weaning at 21 days of age. Litters from each of the three groups were designated for biochemical assay or for activity measurements.

Norepinephrine and dopamine were assayed by a modification of the Anton and Sayre procedure (1962). Open-field activity was assessed by observing the mice in a 16 " x 16" box marked off into 4" squares. For mice 12-31 days old the number of squares entered/minute during a three-minute test period was recorded. For the mice tested at 75 days the number of squares entered and the number of rearing and grooming responses emitted during a three-minute period were recorded.

Table I summarizes the effect of amphetamine on weight gain during pregnancy and on litter size and pup weight at birth.

TABLE IIB
Effects of Injections of D-Amphetamine Sulfate
or Saline during Pregnancy
on Catecholamine Concentration in Brains of Offspring

	Dopamine ng/g brain		
	D	S	U
Days	$\overline{X}$ + S.D. (N)	$\overline{X}$ + S.D. (N)	$\overline{X}$ + S.D. (N)
0	224 + 110 (5)	143 + 65 (8)	163 + 71 (4)
3	103 + 73 (7)	139 + 96 (6)	155 + 49 (6)
7	198 + 89 (4)	219 + 22 (5)	257 + 46 (6)
14	445 + 59 (6)	350 + 25 (3)	480 + 87 (5)
21	727 + 198 (6)	941 + 54 (5)	634 + 87 (6)[h]
30	1550 + 153 (4)	1245 + 284 (3)	820 + 341 (8)[i]

[h]S>D, U (p<.05, Duncan's Multiple Range Test)

[i]D>U   (p<.05, Duncan's Multiple Range Test)

Animals treated with amphetamine during the last third of pregnancy gained less weight but had litter sizes comparable with control groups. Offspring of both injected groups (DAMS and SC) were slightly but significantly lighter than untreated controls at birth.

CA levels in the brains of the offspring are summarized in Tables IIA and IIB. The means given were obtained from 3 or 4 assay replications and represent brains from a minimum of 3 litters.

A 3 x 5 (Treatment x Time) analysis of variance (ANOVA) on NE concentration established a significant Treatment effect, Time effect and Treatment x Time interaction. All groups showed the expected increase in NE concentrations with increasing age, although the increase in concentration was different for the 3 groups. Subsequent data analysis within each time period established that offspring of animals prenatally exposed to amphetamine had lower NE concentrations at birth than either control group. No further significant differences were noted until day 21, at which time both the DAMS and the SC groups had higher concentrations than untreated controls. At day 30, offspring of amphetamine-treated animals had higher concentrations of NE than either control group with no significant difference between the 2 control groups.

The 3 x 5 ANOVA on DA concentrations revealed a pattern similar to that for NE with significant Treatment effects, Time effects and Treatment x Time interaction. Data analysis within each time period established no significant group differences until day 21, when saline controls had higher concentrations of DA than the other 2 groups. At day 30, offspring of the D group had higher concentrations of DA than untreated controls with no other significant group differences.

Although both injected groups (DAMS and SC) tended to have higher median open-field activity scores than the UC group on each test day, none of these differences was statistically significant. Group median scores for total activity across all test days, however, were significantly higher for both the DAMS and SC groups, compared to the UC group.

The results of this experiment established that injections of D-amphetamine sulfate during the last third of pregnancy could produce changes in CA concentration in the brains of young offspring. Activity measures, however, did not differentiate drug-treated from saline-control animals, although both of these groups were more active than untreated controls.

The purpose of the second experiment was to determine if the altered CA concentrations noted in young mice prenatally exposed to amphetamine were transient or permanent, and if the effects of amphetamine and saline on activity could be differentiated when offspring were older. In this study the analysis of activity was more comprehensive than in the previous study and the design allowed testing for possible correlation between behavioral and biochemical variables.

Three types of activity (locomotion, rearing, and grooming) were assessed when the offspring were 75 days old. Locomotion was measured by the number of squares entered. A rearing response was recorded when the animal's forepaws were removed from the floor simultaneously. No distinction was made between supported (rearing against wall) and free rearing. Grooming responses consisted of face washing with both paws. No attempt was made to record duration of the response. Scores in all 3 categories of activity were combined for each animal to provide an index of its overall activity during the 3-minute interval.

Animals were killed by decapitation between 0800 and 1200 hours 2 days after the activity test. Brains were removed, washed, and assayed for CA content, as described in the first experiment. The results of this experiment are summarized in Table III.

No significant group differences were recorded in body weight, brain weight, or CA concentrations. Treatment effects were reflected in altered activity. Most of the drug-treated animals could be readily distinguished from controls either by increased nondirected locomotion or by greatly reduced locomotion often coupled with a high frequency of grooming. These 2 measures were negatively correlated within this group.

Group means for total activity and for the 3 subcategories (locomotion, rearing, and grooming) are presented in Table III. ANOVA's revealed significant treatment effects for total activity, rearing, and grooming. The treatment

TABLE III

Effects of Intraperitoneal Injections
of D-Amphetamine Sulfate on Offspring Body
Weight, Brain Weight, Catecholamine Level, and Activity at 75 Days

	N^i	(Litter)^{ii}	Body Weight in grams $\bar{X}\pm S.D.$	Brain Weight in mg $\bar{X}\pm S.D.$	Nanograms DA per Brain $\bar{X}\pm S.D.$	Nanograms NE per Brain $\bar{X}\pm S.D.$	Total Activity^{iii} $\bar{X}\pm S.D.$	Squares Entered $\bar{X}\pm S.D.$	Rearing^{iv} $\bar{X}\pm S.D.$	Grooming*v $\bar{X}\pm S.D.$
DAMS	18	(5)	24.3±3.6	416.3±14.3	608±91	248±39	181±41	135±44	33±12	15±11
SC	8	(2)	27.3±1.8	430.1±11.2	601±55	257±16	138±34	110±27	19±7	9±6
UC	17	(4)	23.9±2.8	419.6±15.6	596±95	240±37	146±31	110±28	28±8	8±6

DAMS: amphetamine injected

SC : saline injected

UC : untreated control

i : Number of animals tested

ii : Number of litters represented

iii : DAMS >SC, (t = 2.490, p<0.025)

DAMS >UC, (t = 2.890, p<0.01)

iv : SC <UC, DAMS, (t = 2.72, 2.74, p<0.025)

v : DAMS >UC, (t = 2.26, p<0.05)

effect on the locomotion component was not significant. A comparison of group means within each category via Duncan's Multiple Range Test established heightened total activity for animals prenatally exposed to amphetamine compared to either control group. The DAMS group also had higher grooming scores compared to the UC group, but did not differ significantly from the SC group. The only other significant difference was a decreased level of rearing for the SC group, compared to the DAMS and UC groups.

The results of these experiments established that prenatal exposure to amphetamine during the last third of pregnancy produced transient changes in catecholamine levels in young mice. It appeared that some of the noted effect could be due to the stress of the intraperitoneal injection route used. Consequently studies using the subcutaneous route of administration were initiated.

Subcutaneous injections of 2.5, 5, and 10 mg/kg produced no effect on activity. Thus the effect produced is dependent on the method of administration and may be due to more rapid absorption of the drug from the peritoneal cavity, either by transport through the walls of the uterine horn directly to the fetus or, more likely, by faster absorpotion into the maternal circulation and placental transfer.

There was one remarkable effect of the subcutaneous injection. There was a drastic increase in neontal mortality with the lowest dose of amphetamine (X_2 = 21.0; p 0.001). Approximately half of the offspring in this group had died by four weeks after birth. This finding of increased neonatal mortality for lower doses of amphetamine has been reported elsewhere for rats (Seliger, 1973). We have no good explanation for this finding.

DISCUSSION

Intraperitoneal injections of amphetamine during the last third of pregnancy produced, therefore, alterations in catecholamine concentrations in the brains of offspring and changes in behavior. The alterations in catecholamines are similar to those reported following embryonic exposure to reserpine in chicks (Sparber and Shideman, 1969 a, b; 1970). Chronic exposure to either reserpine (Markiewicz, 1963) or amphetamine (Javoy et al., 1968) reduces catecholamine levels in adult animals. Our data suggest that maternally administered amphetamine also depletes CA stores in fetal brain. The time of exposure to drugs in our experiments corresponds to the time of development of the catecholamine systems in rats, and the control mechanisms for the levels of the CA neurotransmitters at this stage are similar to those in adults (Coyle and Henry, 1973). A possible mechanism therefore would be a pharmacological interference in feedback control with depletion of catecholamines in the fetal brain producing an increased concentration of norephinephrine and dopamine at 30 days. By 75 days either the synthesis has decreased to normal or the animals have compensated by increased catabolic rates. Both of these possibilities are open to investigation.

The mechanisms mediating the behavioral alterations are unknown. Alterations in activity levels have previously been associated with altered CA function (Haggendal and Lindquist, 1963). However, in the current study, activity scores and CA concentrations were not simply correlated. Further studies investigating the more dynamic aspects of CA metabolism (e.g., turnover studies) are being completed and may suggest a relationship between the neurochemical and behavioral alterations. Another possibility to be considered in accounting for the behavioral alterations is a drug-produced alteration in the mother-infant interaction. Several studies that have been reported and reviewed (Joffe, 1968) suggesting that treatment to either the mother or her offspring can alter mother-infant interactions and that this alteration can produce long-lasting changes in the behavior of the offspring. In the current study, amphetamine during the latter stages of pregnancy may have altered maternal behavior in some way. A second possibility is that the prenatal exposure to amphetamine produced subtle changes in the offspring, (e.g., lowered body weight) which in turn resulted in altered mother-infant interaction. Cross fostering and studies on maternal behavior have been initiated to investigate this possibility.

PHENOBARBITAL

Phenobarbital was chosen for study for a number of reasons. Barbiturates represent a widely used class of drugs. Phenobarbital has effects on RNA metabolism (Noach, Bunk, and Wijling, 1962) and is teratogenic in the rat in high doses (McColl, Globus, and Robinson, 1963). In man, prolonged use of this barbiturate has been reported to produce mood disorders and cerebellar damage (Reynolds, 1968). Neuropathological changes have been postulated to be the result of alterations in RNA or protein metabolism (Appel, 1966).

Phenobarbital is being ingested by an undetermined but substantial number of pregnant women. Epidemiological studies suggest that 24% to 32% of pregnant women ingest some type of sedative, frequently phenobarbital, during pregnancy (Forfar and Nelson, 1973; Hill, 1973). This occurs primarily during the last trimester (Hill, 1973). There are also a number of women with epilepsy using phenobarbital as an anticonvulsant during pregnancy (Hill, 1973; Desmond et al., 1972). In addition, phenobarbital is used by members of the "drug subculture," including pregnant females (Desmond et al., 1972). Finally, phenobarbital has been administered to gravid women shortly prior to parturition as a prophylaxis for neonatal hyperbilirubinemia (Yeung et al., 1971).

The developing brain might be particularly susceptible to interference with growth and maturation processes during periods of rapid RNA and protein synthesis, which in the mouse occurs during the perinatal period (McIlwaine, 1965). This report presents the effects of prenatal administration of phenobarbital on nucleic acid and protein levels in the brains of C57BL/6J mice and on some long-lasting behavioral deficits produced by the prenatal exposure.

Although a possible mechanism for potential long-term behavioral effects of prenatal exposure to phenobarbital has been postulated, there is currently little empirical support for the existence of behavioral abnormalities in mature organisms prenatally exposed to the drug. To help elucidate potential effects of prenatal exposure to phenobarbital, we have been conducting experiments on offspring of C57BL/6J mice injected daily with subanesthetic doses of phenobarbital for the last third of pregnancy.

PROCEDURES AND RESULTS

Pregnant C57BL/6J mice were divided into 3 groups on the 13th day of gestation. Group I received daily injections of phenobarbital (20, 40 or 80 mg/kg in saline) until parturition. Group II received daily injections of an equivalent volume of saline. Group III was untreated.

Injecting pregnant mice with the various doses of phenobarbital (PB) did not significantly alter littler size. Offspring mortality during the first four weeks after birth, however, was higher in the drug groups. Percentage of offspring dying during this period for the various groups were 16, 12, 20, 30, and 43 for the UC, SC, phenobarbital 20 mg/kg (PB20), phenobarbital 40 mg/kg (PB40) and phenobarbital 80 mg/kg (PB80) groups respectively. X_2 analysis established significantly increased mortality for the PB 40 group compared with the UC- or SC- groups and for the PB 80 group compared with the UC-, SC-, or PB20- groups.

The effects of the treatments on body weights of mature (60 day) offspring are summarized in Figure 1. Body weight at this age was decreased for both sexes with increasing doses of phenobarbital. Weights of male animals prenatally exposed to the drug compared to the UC group were reduced by 7, 10, or 12% for the 20, 40, or 80 mg/kg dosages respectively. A similar pattern but increased decrement was noted in females (12, 16, and 19% reductions). Mean body weights for saline-control groups of both sexes are lower than untreated controls; however, these differences are not statistically significant (males, $t = .816$, $df = 24$, p .2; females, $t = 1.106$, $df = 21$, p .1). Since the phenobarbital was administered in a saline solution, effects of the drug on body weights were statistically analyzed by comparing drug groups with SC groups in a 2 x 4 (Sex x Treatments) ANOVA. The results of this analysis established significant sex differences ($F = 176.3$, $df = 1, 93$, p .01) and treatment effects (f $= 5.50$, $df = 3, 93$, p .01) but no Treatment x Sex interaction. Further comparison of individual drug group means with the SC group within each sex via Dunnett's t statistic (Weiner, 1962) established significantly lower body weights for both sexes of the PB80 group and for females of the PB40 group.

The effects of the highest dosage of phenobarbital (80 mg/kg) on brain

TABLE IV
Effects of Phenobarbital (20-, 40-, and 80 mg/kg) during
Pregnancy on Litter Size and Offspring Mortality

Treatment	Number of Litters	Avg. No. Per Litter	% Died or Destroyed by 4 Wks. After birth
Untreated Control	9	7.9	16
Saline Control	8	7.1	12
Phenobarbital (PB)			
20 mg/kg	9	7.1	20
40 mg/kg	9	6.3	30*
80 mg/kg	10	7.3	43**

*PB 40 > SC, UC; Differences significant at .05 or less, x^2 test
**PB 80 > PB 20, SC, UC

macromolecules have been determined. Proteins and nucleic acids were assayed by a modification of the method of Santen and Agranoff (1963).

DNA, RNA and protein contents of individual brains were determined at intervals from the day of birth through 28 days. These data are summarized in Figure 2. The data were analyzed by a 3 (Treatments) x 8 (Days) ANOVA. The relevant variables for this study were Treatment effects and Treatment by Days interactions. Evaluation of group differences within a particular day was made by comparing group means, with least squares differences of .05 or less considered significant.

For brain DNA the Treatment effect was not significant ($F = 1.74$; $df = 2$, 128; p .05); however, there was a significant Treatment by Days interaction (F = 2.864; $df = 14$, 128; p .01). The interaction effect is accounted for by initially lower DNA levels (days 5-14) and then heightened levels (days 21 and 28) for phenobarbital animals compared to controls.

Analysis of RNA data established a significant Treatment effect (F = 8.713; $df = 2$, 133; p .01) but no Treatment by Days interaction (F = 1.527; df 14, 133; p .05). Depressed RNA values for the phenobarbital animals are noted beginning 5 days after birth and continuing throughout the 28-day assessment. On day 28 the phenobarbital mean is significantly lower than either of the control groups.

Analysis of the protein data established a significant Treatment effect (F = 13.726; $df = 1$, 131; p .01) and a Treatment x Days interaction (F = 3.122; df = 14, 131; p .01). As noted for the effect of phenobarbital on brain RNA, the

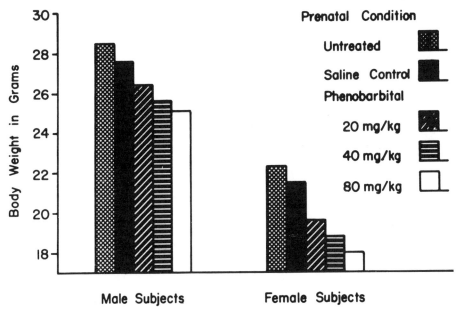

FIG. 1.   Mean body weights for 60-day old offspring of mice uninjected, injected with saline, or injected with phenobarbital for the last third of pregnancy.

depression in protein begins on day 5 and continues through the day 28 assessment. Lower doses of phenobarbital (20, 40 mg/kg) had no measurable effect on brain macromolecules.

Prenatal exposure to 80 mg/kg phenobarbital appears to depress levels of brain macromolecules during the period of rapid brain growth from about the fifth postnatal day until at least 14 days after birth. Although levels of RNA and protein continue to be depressed 21 and 28 days after birth, DNA levels are higher than control values at this time. Since DNA is a reflection of cell number (Winick and Noble, 1965), it is possible that prenatal exposure to phenobarbital retarded or prevented neurogenesis during the early stages of development. The higher levels of DNA noted 21 and 28 days after birth could reflect either recovered development of functionally normal neurons or, perhaps, a compensatory increase in glial cell number. The latter interpretation is compatible with the observed continued reduction in RNA and protein, indicating reduction in cell size, at times when DNA has returned to control levels or above (i.e., although cell number has increased, cell size remains below that of controls).

The mechanism of the phenobarbital-induced changes in macromolecules is unresolved by these data. Whether the effect of phenobarbital is due to a direct action on the fetal brain or a maternally mediated action is not clear. It has been reported that this drug does cross the placenta readily and can be found in the fetus after maternal injections (Villee, 1965). It is also possible that with-

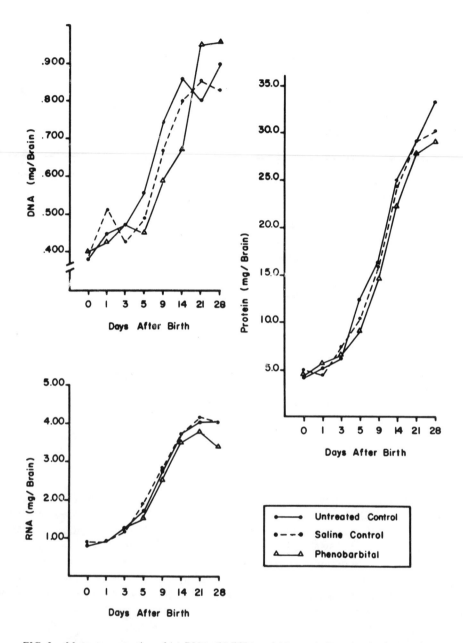

FIG. 2. Mean concentration of (a) DNA, (b) RNA and (c) protein in mouse brain at various intervals after birth. Phenobarbital animals were offspring of dams injected with the drug (80 mg/kg) for the last third of pregnancy. Saline control dams were injected with .9% saline for the same time period. Untreated controls were included to assess possible effects of the injection procedure.

drawal from phenobarbital following delivery has altered maternal care of the neonate, thus producing the developmental alterations.

Chronic phenobarbital administration also induces a mild to severe folate deficiency (Reynolds, 1968). Folate derivatives are required in large quantities in the developing fetus for nucleic acid and protein synthesis. It may be that the effects of phenobarbital are the result of a deficiency in this essential cofactor. Of interest in this regard is that perinatal folate deficiency also reduces brain macromolecules (Shaw, Schreiber, and Zemp, 1973).

One further possibility for the effect of phenobarbital on retarding development could be through an interference with the release of trophic hormones of the anterior pituitary. These have been shown to be secreted under the control of hypothalamic releasing factors which then are influenced by neurotransmitter release. Depression of neural activity in the hypothalamus might therefore block release of trophic hormones in the fetus and therby depress growth. It has been reported that catecholamines are involved in the release of pituitary hormones (van Loon, 1973) and that phenobarbital produces a decreased synthesis of dopamine (Corrodi et al., 1966).

That the brain has not returned to functional normality is suggested by the results of the behavioral observations.

Behavioral studies include effects of phenobarbital on reflex development, open-field activity, passive avoidance, and an operant task requiring increasing response output per unit of reinforcement.

Fox (1965) has reported the development of several reflexes in the C57BL/6J mouse. Eight of these reflexes were chosen to determine whether or not prenatal phenobarbital influenced reflex development. The reflexes chosen for observation were righting, hind-limb placing, accelerated righting, forelimb grasp, straight-line walking, vibrissae placing, barholding and crossed extensor reflex. The offspring of phenobarbital-treated animals were compared with untreated controls. Performance was rated every two days from birth until 20 days of age. Animals were tested on a 0-5 scale, with 0 indicating no response and 5 a maximum response. A comparison of the groups was made on the basis of the day on which 75% of the animals tested received a maximal rating. This comparison is presented in Table V and reveals that the offspring of phenobarbital-treated mothers were significantly slower in the development of 5 of the 8 reflexes tested.

In subsequent work, the effect of prenatal exposure to 40 mg/kg phenobarbital on behavior after maturity was assessed. At 75 days of age, the animals were tested in the open field as described above.

The results of this experiment are summarized in Table VI. An ANOVA on total activity (locomotion, rearing, and grooming) established only a sex difference, with females being more active than males ($F = 6.01$; df 1, 74; p .05). There was no drug effect ($F = 2.54$; df 2, 74; p 0.10) or drug by sex interaction ($F = 0.82$; df 2, 74; p 0.25). The sex difference was determined entirely by the

TABLE V
Effects of Prenatal Phenobarbital Injection on the
Development of Some Motor Reflexes
Day on Which 75% of Animals Received
A Maximal Rating

Test	UC	N	Pheno-barbital	N	x^2	p
Righting	10	24	10	44		n.s.
Hind Limb Placing	10	24	14	44	8.82	0.01
Accelerated Righting	14	32	16	36	12.69	0.0001
Forelimb Grasping	10	24	12	42		n.s.
Straight-Line Walking	12	32	14	44	14.75	0.001
Vibrissae Placing	12	32	14	44		n.s.
Bar holding	12	32	16	44	17.15	0.001
Crossed Extensor	6	33	*	51	18.4	0.001

*The Crossed Extensor develops and then is inhibited during maturation. The variability of the treated animals on this measure was extensive enough that the 75% criterion was never reached.

saline ($t = 2.241$, p 0.035) and untreated ($t = 1.985$, p 0.05) groups with no difference between male and female offspring of dams treated with phenobarbital.

Analysis of the results within sexes revealed no group differences for female offspring. For the male offspring, saline and untreated control animals did not differ on either total activity or on any of three subcategories. These groups were combined for comparison with the phenobarbital-treated group. The phenobarbital-treated group had higher total activity scores (locomotion, rearing, and grooming) than the combined saline and untreated control animals ($t = 2.216$, p 0.05). This difference is due primarily to heightened locomotor activity ($t = 2.700$, p 0.01). It is also noted than the phenobarbital group had a lower frequency of grooming responses. This difference, however, is only marginally significant ($t = 1.812$, p 0.10).

Since male offspring of phenobarbital-treated animals differed from controls on the open-field test and this test may reflect alterations in fear or arousal, male offspring of the three groups were also tested on a passive-avoidance task.

TABLE VI
Effects of Injections of Phenobarbital on
Open-Field Activity at 75 Days of Age

Experi-mental Treat-ment	N^d(Litters)[e]	Total Activity	Squares Entered	Rearing	Grooming
		Male Offspring			
		$\bar{X} \pm$ S.D.	$\bar{X} \pm$ S.D.	$\bar{X} \pm$ S.D.	$\bar{X} \pm$ S.D.
D[a]	11 (5)	182 ± 43^f	145 ± 38^g	33 ± 10	4 ± 4
S[b]	13 (6)	150 ± 32	114 ± 22	28 ± 12	9 ± 9
U[c]	20 (8)	159 ± 27	122 ± 22	27 ± 8	9 ± 7
		Female Offspring			
		$\bar{X} \pm$ S.D.	$\bar{X} \pm$ S.D.	$\bar{X} \pm$ S.D.	$\bar{X} \pm$ S.D.
D	12 (5)	187 ± 23	156 ± 23	27 ± 7	4 ± 6
S	13 (4)	178 ± 25	148 ± 25	27 ± 7	2 ± 1
U	11 (5)	181 ± 31	149 ± 30	28 ± 10	3 ± 3

[a] Offspring of mice injected with phenobarbital for the last third of pregnancy.

[b] Offspring of mice injected with saline for the last third of pregnancy.

[c] Offspring of untreated mice.

[d] Number of animals tested.

[e] Number of litters represented.

[f] D<S,U (p<.05)

[g] D<S,U (p<.05)

Some of the data appearing in this table will be published in Devel. Psychobiol. and is reprinted with permission of John Wiley & Sons, Inc.

This task has also been used as an index of fear or arousal (Weiss et al., 1969). Testing was completed between 1:00 and 5:00 P.M. when the offspring were 90 days of age.

The apparatus was a trough-shaped box divided into two compartments by a guillotine door. The start compartment was constructed of clear Plexiglas with a hardward cloth floor. The compartment was 5 cm wide x 9 cm long x 19 cm high. The shock compartment (5 cm wide x 17.8 cm long x 19 cm high) was constructed of black Plexiglas with a grid floor. A photocell mounted 9 cm from the door and 1.3 cm above the grid floor detected entrance into the compartment. During acquisition, the animal was placed in the start box facing away from the door. The door was immediately raised initiating a latency timer. Entrance into the shock chamber stopped the latency timer and initiated programming equipment to deliver a one sec .6 ma d.c. constant current shock 5 sec later. The door was closed to prevent escape. A retention test following the same procedure with the exception of shock was administered 24 hours later.

Latencies for entering the shock compartment were similar for the saline and untreated control groups during both the acquisition (Xsaline = 22.6 sec vs Xuntreated = 23.3 sec, t = .538, p .3) and the test (Xsaline = 112.5 sec vs Xuntreated = 140.4 sec, t = .606, p .3) phases of this task. These groups were pooled for statistical comparison with the phenobarbital group. During acquisition, the mean latency for entering the shock compartment was lower for offspring of animals treated with phenobarbital; however, this difference was not statistically significant (Xphenobarbital = 15.4 sec vs Xcontrol = 23.5 sec, t = 1.802, p .05). Latencies to enter the shock compartment increased during the test phase for all three groups; however, phenobarbital-treated animals had shorter latencies than controls (Xphenobarbital = 54.0 sec vs Xcontrol = 129.8 sec, t = 2.058, p .05).

Eight female animals from each of the groups tested in the open field were run on a progressive fixed ratio schedule. The schedule required the animal to make an increasing number of responses per reinforcement across days. After one week on a food-deprivation schedule to reduce body weights to 75%-85% of *ad libitum* levels the animals were self-trained to produce food reinforcement. After this, the animals were run 30 min per day for two days on continuous reinforcement, five days on an FR 5 schedule (five responses per reinforcement); five days on an FR 20; and five days on an FR 40 schedule.

To assess whether a noted response decrease during FR 40 in the treated group was due to the length of time on food deprivation or to the schedule of reinforcement, some of the animals were run for an equal length of time on FR 5. Four untreated, six saline, and six phenobarbital-treated animals were used. After two weeks with food available *ad libitum*, the animals were again placed on food deprivation for one week as described above. After three 30-minute sessions with reinforcement available for each response, the animals were tested for 15 consecutive days on FR 5. All testing for assessment of performance under ratio schedules of reinforcement was completed between 1:00 and 5:00 P.M.

There was no noticeable difference among the groups during acquisition of the response to produce food reinforcement. Animals in each group required from one to three 30-minute sessions to acquire the response. During the CRF phase of the experiment, animals typically produced more food pellets than they would eat during a 30-minute session. This was noted in all groups during CRF but did not occur during any of the other schedules of reinforcement.

Mean responses per session per group across days on the various schedules

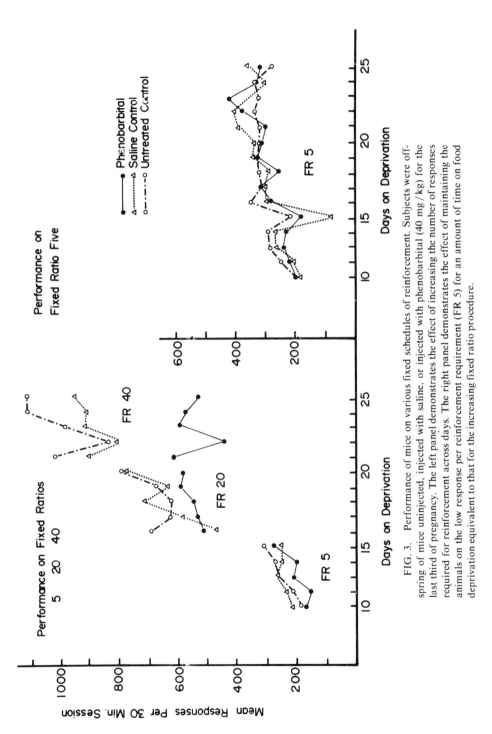

FIG. 3. Performance of mice on various fixed schedules of reinforcement. Subjects were offspring of mice uninjected, injected with saline, or injected with phenobarbital (40 mg / kg) for the last third of pregnancy. The left panel demonstrates the effect of increasing the number of responses required for reinforcement across days. The right panel demonstrates the effect of maintaining the animals on the low response per reinforcement requirement (FR 5) for an amount of time on food deprivation equivalent to that for the increasing fixed ratio procedure.

of reinforcement are shown in Figure 3. As noted in the left panel of the figure, there was no difference among the three groups until FR 20 when the phenobarbital-treated animals tended to respond less than controls. This response decrement became pronounced under the FR 40 schedule of reinforcement. When maintained on FR 5 for an amount of time equivalent to that during the progressive fixed ratio phase, there were no group differences. These data are summarized in the right panel of Figure 3.

Since individual performance across days varied considerably, mean responses per five block sessions on each schedule were calculated to provide an index of an animal's performance on that particular schedule. Mean responses on the fixed ratio 5 and 20 schedules were not different for the three groups. On FR 40, however, offspring of mice exposed to phenobarbital responded much less than either saline (t = 2.78, p   .05) or untreated (t = 2.57,   .05) control mice.

DISCUSSION

The results of these experiments demonstrate that injections of subanesthetic doses of phenobarbital to mice during the last third of pregnancy can alter the behavior of offspring after they have reached maturity. These alterations are noted in the absence of any overtly noticeable morphological abnormalities.

The results of the open-field experiment suggest that prenatal exposure to phenobarbital may have a more severe effect on male offspring. In this experiment prenatally treated male offspring had heightened total activity (locomotion, rearing, and grooming) in an open-field maze, where female offspring appeared to be unaffected. An analysis of the various subcategories of activity revealed that the major factor contributing to heightened activity was the locomotor component. In contrast, the frequency of grooming was somewhat lower for the treated group. Heightened locomotor activity in the open field is commonly interpreted as reflecting a lower level of fear or arousal (Hall, 1936; DeFries et al., 1970). Qualitative differences in the locomotor component, however, could make the reverse interpretation possible. Combined with the results of the passive avoidance and fixed ratio assessments, however, interpretation of the increased locomotion in terms of lowered arousal would seem appropriate.

Animals prenatally exposed to phenobarbital were deficient on a one trial passive-avoidance task. This conditioning procedure has frequently been used as an index of fear with increased latencies of entrance into the compartment previously associated with shock reflecting a higher degree of fear. In these terms, animals prenatally exposed to phenobarbital demonstrated less fear than control animals.

The lower number of responses emitted by treated animals on the high fixed ratio schedule noted in the third experiment suggests lowered responsiveness to stimuli associated with food deprivation. This finding eliminated increased reactivity to food deprivation as a possible cause of the response per-severation noted in mice prenatally exposed to phenobarbital in our earlier studies (Zemp et al., 1974).

A possible interpretation accounting for most of the noted behavioral alter-ations is that prenatal exposure to phenobarbital in some way has altered the animals' reactivity to intero- or extero-ceptively derived stimuli. Treated ani-mals show altered reactivity to fear-provoking stimuli associated with the open field and passive-avoidance task; and to interoceptively derived stimuli associat-ed with food deprivation. The behavioral alterations may be mediated by drug-produced alterations in neural and/or endocrine systems involving ca-techolamines, since these systems have been reported to begin development dur-ing the time of gestation covered by our treatments.

There are two readily apparent mechanisms by which phenobarbital might produce changes in hypothalamic-pituitary-adrenal function. First, phenobarbi-tal may alter monoamine development and through changed monoamine func-tion alter pituitary output of ACTH (van Loon, 1973), which is essential for adrenal development (Jost, 1966). Secondly, it has been reported that phenobar-bital competes with various steroids for hydroxylase enzymes. This would alter plasma concentration of corticosterone which controls release of ACTH in a negative feedback loop. This alteration might in turn alter the hormonal pro-gramming of the brain, as suggested by Levine (1966), thus producing perma-nent changes in behavior.

SUMMARY

Amphetamine. Prenatal intraperitoneal injection of d-amphetamine sulfate (5 mg/kg) produces decreases in the levels of catecholamines in the brain the day of birth and increases on day 30. Open-field activity from days 12 to 31 was higher for the group of animals injected with amphetamine or saline if scores were totaled across all test days. At day 75 the offspring of amphetamine-inject-ed mothers exhibited altered open-field behavior. The effects were not observed with subcutaneous injection regardless of the dose used (2.5, 5.0, and 10.0 mg/kg). The lowest subcutaneous dose decreases neonatal viability.

Phenobarbital. Prenatal intraperitoneal injection of phenobarbital (80 mg/kg) resulted in decreased litter size, increased mortality, and decreased amounts of nucleic acid and protein in the brains of surviving offspring. Beha-vioral deficits associated with response perseveration could be demonstrated at 60 days in the mice prenatally exposed to this dosage. Subcutaneous injections of phenobarbital to pregnant mice at 80 and 40 mg/kg, but not 20 mg/kg, doses increased neonatal mortality. Mature animals prenatally exposed to 40 mg/kg phenobarbital have altered open-field behavior and differ from control animals on a passive avoidance task. Mature offspring prenatally exposed to the 20 or 40 mg/kg dose also responded less than controls on an operant task requiring an increasing number of responses per reinforcement. These studies suggest that prenatal exposure to phenobarbital has in some way altered the animals' reactivity to stimulation.

Notes

This project was supported by USPHS Grant MH-17455 (now DA-00041) and by South Carolina State Appropriation for Research to the Medical University of South Carolina.

References

Anton, A. H., and Sayre, D. F. A study of the factors affecting the aluminum oxide-trihydroxindole procedure for the analysis of catecholamines. *Journal of Pharmacology Experimental Therapeutics,* 1962, *138.* 360-375.

Appel, S. H. Inhibition of brain protein synthesis: An approach to the biochemical basis of neurological dysfunction of amino-acidurias. *Transactions New York Academy of Sciences,* 1966, *29* (1). 63-70.

Axelrod, J. Noradrenalin: Fate and control of its biosynthesis. *Science,* 1971, *173* (3997). 589-606.

Bell, R. W., Drucker, R. R., and Woodruff, A. B. The effects of prenatal injections of adrenalin chloride and d-amphetamine sulfate on subsequent emotionality and ulcer-proneness of offspring. *Psychonomic Science,* 1965, *2. 269-270.*

Bergstrom, R. M. Neurophysiological effects of teratogenic agents in ontogeny. *Acta Neurologica Scandinavica,* 1967, *43* (31). 37-42.

Brown, D. S. Pituitary follicle-stimulating hormone in immature female rats treated with drugs that inhibit the synthesis or antagonize the actions of catecholamines and 5-hydroxytryptamine. *Neuroendocrinology,* 1971, *7.* 183-192.

Clark, C. V. H., Gorman, D., and Vernadakis, A. Effects of prenatal administration of psychotropic drugs on behavior of developing rats. *Developmental Psychobiology,* 1970, *3 (4).* 225-235.

Cohen, R. L. Evaluation of the teratogenicity of drugs. *Clinical Pharmacology and Therapeutics,* 1964, *5* (4). 480-514

Coyle J. T., and Henry, D. Catecholamines in fetal and newborn rat brain. *Journal of Neurochemistry,* 1973, *21.* 61-67.

DeFries, J. C., Wilson, J. R., and McClearn, G. E. Open-field behavior in mice: Selection response and situational generality. *Behavior Genetics,* 1970, *1.* 195-211.

Desmond, M. M., Schwanecke, R. P., Wilson, G. S., Yasunaga, S. and Burgdorff, I. *Journal of Pediatrics,* 1972, *80* (2). 190-197.

Dobbing, J. Vulnerable periods in developing brain. In A. Davison and J. Dobbing (Eds.), *Applied Neurochemistry.* Philadelphia: Davis, 1968. 278-316.

Eiduson, S. 5-Hydroxytryptamine in the developing chickbrain: Its normal and altered development and possible control by end-product repression. *Journal of Neurochemistry, 13.* 923-932.

Fox, W. M. Reflex-otogeny and behavioural development of the mouse. *Animal Behaviour, 1965, 13* (2). 234-241.

Forfar, J. O., and Nelson, M. N. Epidemiology of drugs taken by pregnant women: Drugs that may affect the fetus adversely. *Clinical Pharmacology Therapeutics,* 1973, *14* (4). 632-642.

Haggendal, J., and Lindquist, M. (1963). Behaviour and monoamine levels during long-term administration of reserpine to rabbits. *Acta Physiologica Scandinavica,* 1963, *57.* 431-436.

Hall, C.S. Emotional behavior in the rat. III. The relationship between emotionality and ambulatory behavior. *Journal of Comparative Psychology,* 1936, *22.* 345-352.

Hill, R. M. Drugs ingested by pregnant women. *Clinical Pharmacology and Therapeutics*, 1973, *14* (4) 654-659.

Hoffeld, D. R., McNew, J., and Webster, R. L. Effect of tranquillizing drugs during pregnancy on activity of offspring. *Nature (London)*, 1968, 218 (5139). 357-358.

Hoffeld, D. R., and Webster, R. L. Effect of injection of tranquillizing drugs during pregnancy on offspring. *Nature (London)*, 1965, *205* (4976). 1070-1072.

Hoffeld, D. R., Webster, R. L., and McNew, J. Adverse effects on offspring of tranquillizing drugs during pregnancy. *Nature (London)*, 1967, *215* (5097). 182-183.

Javoy, F., Thierry, A. M., Kety, S. S., and Glowinsky, J. Effect of amphetamine on the turnover of brain norepinephrine in normal and stressed rats. *Communications in Behavioral Biology*, 1968, *1* (1). 43-48.

Joffe, J. M. *Prenatal Determinants of Behavior*. New York. Pergamon. 1969.

Jost, A. Problems of fetal endocrinology: The adrenal glands. *Recent Progress in Hormone Research*, 1966, *22*. 541-574.

Karnofsky, D. A. Drugs as teratogens in animals and man. *Annual Review of Pharmacology, 1965*, *5*. 447-472.

Karavolas, H. J., Gupta, C., and Meyer, R. K. Steroid biosynthesis and metabolism during phenobarbital (PB) block of PMS-Induced ovulation in immature rats. *Endrocrinology*, 1972, *91* (1). 157-167.

Kramer, J. C., Fischman, V. S., and Littlefield, D. C. Amphetamine abuse: Pattern and effects of high doses taken intravenously. *Journal of the American Medical Association*, 1967, *201* (5). 305-309.

Levine, S., and Mullins, R. J., Jr. Hormonal influences on brain organization in infant rats. *Science*, 1966, *152* (3729). 1585-1592.

Lidbrink, P., Corrodi, H., Fuxe, K., and Olson, L. Barbiturates and meprobamate: Decreases in catecholamine turnover of central dopamine and noradrenaline neuronal systems and the influence of immobilization stress. *Brain Research*, 1972, *45*. 507-524.

Markiewcis, L. Biochemical and functional effects of long-term administration of reserpine in mice. *Acta Physiologica Scandinavica*, 1963, *58* (4). 276-380.

McColl, J. D., Globus, M., and Robinson, S. Drug induced skeletal malformations in the rat. *Experientia*, 1963, *19* (4). 183-184.

McIlwain, H., and Bachelard, H.S. (1971). *Biochemistry and the Central Nervous System*, Williams and Wilkins, Baltimore, 1971. 406-444.

Noach, E. L., Joosting Bunk, J., and Wijling, A. Influence of electroshock and phenobarbital on nucleuc acid content of rat brain cortex. *Acta Physiologica et Pharmacologica Neerlandica*, 1962, *11*. 54-69.

Nora J. J., Trasler, D. G., and Fraser, F. C. Malformations in mice induced by dexamphetamine sulfate. *Lancet*, 1965, 2 (7420). 1021-1022.

Reynolds, E. H. Mental effects of anticonvulsants and folic acid metabolism. *Brain*, 1968, *91* (2). 197-214.

Sadusk, J. E., Jr. Symposium on nonnarcotic addiction: Size and extent of the problem. *Journal of the American Medical Association*, 1966, *196* (8). 707-709.

Santen, D. J., and Agranoff, B. W. Studies on the estimation of deoxyribouncleic acid and ribonucleic acid in rat brain. *Biochemica et Biophysica Acta*, 1963, *72*. 251-262.

Seliger, D. L. Effect of prenatal maternal administration of d-amphetamine on rat offspring activity and passive avoidance learning. *Physiological Psychology*, 1973, *1* (3). 273-280.

Shoemaker, W. J., and Wurtman, R. J. Perinatal undernutrition: Accumulation of catecholamines in rat brain. *Science*, 1971, *171* (3975). 1017-1022.

Sparber S. B., and Shideman, F. E. Prenatal administration of reserpine: Effect upon hatching, behavior, and brainstem catecholamines of the young chick. *Developmental Psychobiology*, 1968, *1* (4). 236-244.

Sparber, S. B., and Shideman, F. E. Estimation of catecholamines in the brains of embryonic and newly hatched chickens and the effects of reserpine. *Developmental Psychobiology,* 1969a, *2* (2). 115-119.

Sparber S. B., and Shideman, F. E. Detour learning in the chick: Effect of reserpine administered during embryonic development. *Developmental Pscyhobiology,* 1969b, *2* (2). 56-59.

Sparber, S. B., and Shideman, F. E. Elevated catecholamines in thirty-day-old chicken brain after depletion during development. *Developmental Pscyhobiology,* 1970, *3* (2). 123-129.

van Loon, G. R. Brain catecholamines and ACTH secretion. In W. F. Ganong and L. Martini (Eds.). *Frontiers in Neuroendocrinology.* London, Oxford University Press, 1973, 209-237.

Weiss, J. M., McEwen, B. S., Silva, M. T. A., and Kalkut, M. F. Pituitary-adrenal influences on fear responding. *Science,* 1969, *163* (3863). 197-199.

Werboff, J., and Gottlieb, J. S. Drugs in pregnancy: Behavioral teratology. *Obstetrical and Gynecological Survey,* 1963, *18.* 420-423.

Werboff, J., Gottlieb, J. S., Havlena, J., and Word, T. Behavioral effect of prenatal drug administration in the white rat. *Pediatrics,* 1961, *27* (2). 318-324.

Werboff, J., and Havlena, J. Postnatal behavioral effects of tranquillizers administered to the gravid , rat. *Experimental Neurology,* 1962, *6* (3). 263-269.

Werboff, J., and Kesner, R. Learning deficits of offspring after administration of tranquilizing drugs to the mothers. *Nature (London),* 1963, *197* (4862). 106-107.

Wilson, J. G. Embryological considerations in teratology. *Annals of the New York Academy of Sciences,* 1965, *123* (1). 219-227.

Winer, B. J. *Statistical Principles in Experimental Design.* New York: McGraw-Hill, 1962. 90-91.

Yeung, C. Y., Tam, I. S., Chan, A., and Lee, K. H. Phenobarbitone prophylaxis for neotal hyperbilirubinemia. *Pediatrics,* 1971, *48* (3). 372-376.

DISCUSSION

Q. *Dr. Slotkin:* I have a couple of questions concerning the amphetamine studies. One of the difficulties in trying to correlate a behavioral measure with catecholamine levels alone is that the level does not tell you whether it is decreased because of neuronal hypoactivity, and that synthesis is therefore reduced, or whether it is reduced because of neuronal hyperactivity, and the levels are reduced because of increased release. Now, have you done any studies with radioactive precursors to determine whether or not the neurons are hyperactive or hypoactive as a result of amphetamine administration?

A. *Dr. Zemp: With amphetamine, we have not done these studies as yet. We have been doing them with folic acid deficiency but we hope now to get back to the drug effects and to do these studies just as you suggest. I agree, we have to do the studies.*

Q. *Dr. Slotkin:* My second questions concerns problems using this route of administration, i.e., with I.P. vs Sub-Q. I do not recall whether or not you ran saline-injected controls (I.P.) to see if it was, in fact, only a stress-induced effect.

A. *Dr. Zemp: Saline controls were I.P. saline injections.*

Q. *Dr. Slotkin:* So you could not account for it solely on the basis of stress?

A. *Dr. Zemp: No, it was partially accounted for on the basis of stress because the saline control animals did exhibit increased levels of catecholamines over the untreated controls, and increased activity as compared to untreated.*

Q. *Dr. Slotkin:* The question I have pertaining to the effect of the route of administration is that perhaps the greater activity I.P. might result from the fact that, when you inject I.P., the drug has to go through the liver first, and it might be biotransformed to active products such as parahydroxyamphetamine.

A. *Dr. Zemp: I think that probably is a very reasonable suggestion for what is happening.*

Q. *Dr. Braude:* Most of your studies are on rats. Do you think that species differences could account for some of the differences between Dr. Slotkin's findings and yours? The reason I raised this point is that most of the pre-clinical experiments concerning effects of morphine on enterohormone have been done in mice and I am wondering about conditions between mice and rat data.

A. *Dr. Zemp: I would think that a more important difference is the fact that Dr. Slotkin's data are for adrenal glands and ours are for the central nervous system, not to mention the use of different drugs. We use the same explanation for some of the effects. We are taking a long chance by comparing mice directly to rats. We have done some studies that have indicated that the increase in levels of catecholamines which were found in mice over the first 30 days were similar to the levels found in rats over the first 30 days.*

Addictive Diseases: an International Journal 2 (2): 333-345 (1975)

Somatic Growth Effects
of Perinatal Addiction

GERALDINE S. WILSON
Department of Pediatrics
Baylor College of Medicine
Newborn Nursery and High Risk Clinic
Jefferson Davis Hospital
Maternity and Infant Care Project
City of Houston Health Department
Houston, Texas

INTRODUCTION

Of major concern to me as a clinician is the possibility that perinatal addiction may produce permanent sequelae in involved infants. Our preliminary follow-up study of infants of heroin addicts indicates that long-term effects may exist (Wilson, 1973). The effect most readily assessable is somatic growth impairment. It has been generally accepted that low birth weight in this population results from a variety of adverse factors affecting the addict's pregnancy. Our study demonstrated that postnatal growth disturbance also occurs. Offspring with appropriate measurements at birth may subsequently show evidence of impaired somatic growth. Exploration of this delayed growth effect may be helpful in delineating the effect of narcotic dependence in the developing organism.

The effect of perinatal addiction upon fetal growth is receiving increasing attention as investigators focus on the addict during pregnancy. Early studies reflect a 40-50% incidence of low birth weight in infants born to addicts (Goodfriend, 1956; Cobrinik, 1959; and Rosenthal, 1964). With the exception of Krause (1958) who reported one infant premature by weight but term by gestational age, authors failed to differentiate the small-for-dates term baby from the premature of less than 37 weeks' gestation. Calculation of gestational age was considered unreliable because of poor histories and irregular menses. Standards for assessing gestational age on physical and neurological criteria became available in the late 1960's. Since that time, Zelson (1971) has reported low birth weight in 49% of 384 heroin addicts' infants. Twenty percent of his study were small-for-gestational age. Forty-five percent of Reddy's (1971) 40 patients were small-for-dates, and 27% of our 30 patients were undergrown (Wilson, 1973).

Since the advent of methadone treatment for addiction, the relative merits of methadone use during pregnancy have been extensively discussed. By studying the outcome of the methadone-maintained woman's pregnancy, which theoretically eliminates some of the negative features of the addict's pregnancy, we hope to gain some understanding of factors affecting fetal growth.

METHADONE DURING PREGNANCY— EFFECT ON INTRAUTERINE GROWTH

In offspring of mothers using methadone during pregnancy, Blinick (1973), Rajegowda (1972), Pierson (1972), and Zelson (1973) reported mean birth weights of 2580-2700 grams, comparable to mean birth weights for heroin addicts' infants. Kandall (1974) found a mean birth weight of 3017 grams in a group of 35 infants, and reported a direct linear relationship between methadone dosage and birth weight. Infants small-for-gestational age comprise 20% of Reddy's five patients and 22% of Zelson's 46 patients. Among these studies, the scope of methadone treatment varied widely. Duration of treatment ranged from ten days to several years, dosage varied greatly, and the method of obtaining methadone varied from strict inpatient administration to use of "street" methadone.

At Houston's city-county hospital, we have studied the pregnancies of 39 mothers using methadone during gestation. Twenty-nine of these women participated in federally regulated methadone programs for a period of three months or longer during pregnancy (Table I). Sixteen began maintenance prior to conception, three began during the first trimester of pregnancy, and ten began three to six months prior to delivery. Four women were detoxified prior to delivery. Ten women, designated "methadone-other" in Table II, either had less extensive methadone use, enrolling during the last trimester of pregnancy or discontinuing methadone after a brief period, or obtained their methadone from a source other than a federally regulated program. Ninety-seven per cent of infants delivered to mothers maintained on methadone programs had birth weights appropriate for gestational age. Four infants were premature by dates. These figures contrast sharply with the 50% incidence of small-for-dates infants born to women with limited methadone maintenance or unprescribed use and may explain the difference between our data and that previously cited.

Table II presents the incidence of subnormal birth weight, length, and head

TABLE I
Methadone Experience of 29 Mothers in
Maintenance Program 3 months or longer

Duration of methadone maintenance	– 3 mo.–3 yr. (Average 11.9 mo.)	
Methadone use prior to pregnancy	–	16 patients
Methadone initiated 1st trimester	–	3 patients
Methadone initiated 2nd trimester	–	10 patients
Detoxified prior to delivery	–	4 patients
Methadone dosage during pregnancy	– 30–80 mg/day	

TABLE II
Intrauterine Growth Retardation
Incidence of birth measures below 10th percentile
for gestational age by Lubchenco's criteria

	Number of Patients	Weight	Length	Head Circumference
Maternal Heroin	30	27%	14%	25%
Maternal Methadone Program	29	3%	0	0
Maternal Methadone (Other)	10	50%	20%	30%
Maternal Barbiturate	15	0	0	0

circumference in drug-affected pregnancies. Length at birth was inappropriate for gestational age in 14% of heroin addicts' infants and in 20% of offspring of mothers with unprescribed or brief methadone use. Head circumference was small-for-gestational age in 25 and 30% of these groups, respectively. In three infants, small heads were the only evidence of impaired growth.

We evaluated fifteen babies of mothers abusing barbiturates or using prescribed barbiturates consistently during pregnancy (Desmond, 1972). Intrauterine growth was unimpaired.

ETIOLOGY OF INTRAUTERINE GROWTH RETARDATION

Any number of factors may contribute to impaired fetal growth. The addict's life is characterized by drug-seeking activity, prostitution, and neglect of normal hygiene, health, and nutrition. Several women related that they in-

TABLE III
Complications of Pregnancy

	Heroin	Methadone Program
Total number of cases	30	29
No prenatal care	15 (50%)	3 (10%)
Antepartum hemorrhage		3 (10%)
Hyperemesis gravidarum		4 (14%)
Toxemia	2 (7%)	6 (21%)
Anemia		6 (21%)
Overdose – sedatives		2 (7%)
Infection		
Hepatitis	1 (3%)	1 (3%)
+ VDRL test for syphilis	2 (7%)	5 (24%)
Urinary tract infection	1 (3%)	5 (24%)
Gonorrhea		1 (3%)
Vaginitis		6 (21%)

terpreted symptoms presenting during pregnancy as signs of withdrawal and "treated" them by using heroin. We suspect that infections and other problems were frequently undiagnosed and untreated in the addicted mothers.

COMPLICATIONS OF PREGNANCY

Table III lists complications of pregnancy in heroin addicts and addicts on methadone treatment programs. The number of methadone mothers seeking medical care prenatally actually reflects the altered life-style of this group. Obstetrical and pediatric units and methadone-maintenance programs cooperated in assisting these pregnant women to achieve a stable source of income and maintain optimal health and nutrition during pregnancy. Participation in a "methadone mothers' group" directed their attention to the issues of their health and the future of themselves and their child.

The apparent increased incidence of complications in methadone-maintained mothers may, in some instances, be attributable to more accurate diagnosis through increased contact during pregnancy. Limited contact with heroin mothers, who often have no medical care prior to the onset of active labor, would tend to obscure complications of early pregnancy and limit the opportunity to diagnose and treat infection. The increased incidence of anemia in methadone-maintained mothers has not been explained.

MATERNAL NUTRITION

Improved nutrition in methadone-maintained mothers may explain improved fetal size. Naeye (1973) has investigated the birth weight of addicts' infants and demonstrated that small size of organs in infants exposed to heroin in the third trimester of pregnancy was due mainly to a subnormal number of cells, while undernutrition in non-addicted women restricts the size of individual cells as well as their number.

Naeye assessed pre-pregnancy nutritional status and weight gain during pregnancy of 36 addicts and 500 controls, categorizing them as overweight or underweight prior to pregnancy and as gaining more or less than optimal weight during gestation. Weights of infants, expressed in percent of published "normal" values, were significantly lower in all nutritional categories of heroin addicts' infants as compared to controls, suggesting that maternal nutrition was not the only factor responsible for growth restriction.

HEROIN EFFECT

Naeye suggests that a direct effect of heroin on antenatal growth appears likely. Our clinical data indicate that the issue is complex, and that the presence of heroin during pregnancy does not necessarily disturb growth.

In the series of 29 mothers participating in Houston methadone programs for three months or more during pregnancy, 50% reported continuing heroin abuse, some sporadically and others on a daily basis. Doses of heroin varied from a "pinch" to several papers daily. The low incidence of intrauterine growth retardation in their offspring indicates that factors other than chronic exposure to heroin must be operant in affecting fetal growth. Kandall's data suggest that methadone administration during pregnancy appears to correct in a dose-dependent manner heroin-associated fetal growth retardation (Kandall, 1974). Our data do not corroborate his findings. Birth measures are similar for four infants of mothers receiving 80 mg of methadone daily and all other study infants, whose average maternal methadone dose was 30 mg daily.

MATERNAL INFECTION

As indicated by the rare documentation of infection in the heroin addict's pregnancy, the role of maternal infection in fetal growth retardation has been difficult to evaluate. Addicts are prone to acquire hepatitis, venereal disease, and bacterial infections in pursuit of their addiction. Naeye has studied the size of infants of non-addicted mothers who had hepatitis just prior to or during pregnancy and found that hepatitis had little influence on fetal growth.

Naeye was impressed, however, with the high incidence of acute inflammation identified in a study of 59 addicts at the time of delivery. Three mothers had

TABLE IV

*Incidence of Measurements Below 10th Percentile
(Harvard Growth Grid) at 9-36 Months of Age*

	Heroin During Pregnancy	Methadone Program During Pregnancy
	N - 14	N - 13
Weight	28%	15%
Length	35%	25%
Head Circumference	28%	25%

TABLE V

*Comparison of Subnormal Birth Measurements and Subnormal Measurements
on Follow-Up in Infants of Heroin Addicts*

	X = Birth Measures Below 10th Percentile (Lubchenco)			X = Measurements Below 10th Percentile (Harvard) At 9 – 36 Mos.		
Patient	Weight	Length	FOC	Weight	Length	FOC
1					X	X
2		X	X		X	X
3				X	X	X
4	X			X	X	X
5	X		X			
6				X	X	X

cellulitis or furuncles, while three had significant pyuria. Thirty had unexplained fever and/or inflammation of placental membranes. The mean gestational age of infants born to addicted mothers who had chorioamnionitis or fever was 35 3 weeks, as compared to 39 2 weeks for infants born to mothers with no signs of infection. Infection appears to play a role in the premature onset of labor in addicts.

POSTNATAL GROWTH

To this point, discussion has dealt with factors affecting intrauterine growth. I would like to shift now to the postnatal growth of children chronically exposed to narcotics during gestation.

Table IV presents the incidence of measurements below the 10th percentile at 9-36 months of age of 14 infants of heroin addicts and 13 infants of mothers participating in methadone programs during pregnancy. Sixteen of the original group of heroin infants were not available for study. Four methadone babies could not be located, one died at two months of age, and 11 are currently less than nine months of age.

Comparison of birth and follow-up measurements of children born to heroin addicts demonstrates a fairly consistent rate of low weight and head circumference. The incidence of short stature increases with postnatal growth. Table V presents the relationship between subnormal birth measurements and subnormal measures at nine to 36 months. The decline in growth rate is usually evident by six months.

Although infants of methadone-maintained mothers had normal intrauterine growth, the length and head circumference of 25% of the 13 patients measured after nine months have fallen below the tenth percentile. Ting (1974) has also found short stature in 26% of 25 children aged 6 to 41 months whose mothers were methadone-dependent. Head circumference remained within two standard deviations.

GROWTH—THREE TO SIX YEARS

Studies of three- to six-year-old children of heroin addicts are currently being completed in Houston (McCreary, 1974). The study compares children exposed to narcotics during gestation with children raised by currently addicted parents who did not use drugs during that gestation, and children of similar socioeconomic and cultural backgrounds who have not been exposed to drugs or to the drug culture. Analysis of data is in progress.

Figure 1 depicts the distribution of height in percentiles for the study population and normal controls. It illustrates a high incidence of short stature in the heroin-affected population as compared to controls, who are also shorter than the norm. The head circumference of the study population tends to be below the norm (Figure 2), with almost 30% of the drug patients measuring below the tenth percentile. All controls are above the tenth percentile. Figure 3 illustrates distribution of weight by percentiles.

Interpretation of data concerning the postnatal growth of addicts' children may be difficult because the sample is very small. If the data can be assumed to be valid, explanations for the findings must be sought.

HEIGHT

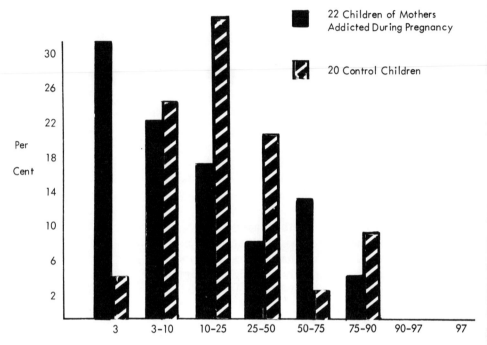

PERCENTILE DISTRIBUTION OF HEIGHT AT 3-6 YEARS
ON HARVARD GROWTH GRID

FIG. 1

NUTRITION

The first explanation to be considered in this population is chronic under-nutrition. In our study population, heroin addicts rarely care for their children personally during the first years and tend to place children with relatives or foster parents. Socioeconomic status of foster families was higher than the mean for our clinic population. Methadone-maintained mothers assumed responsibility for their infants, and were given assistance in obtaining food and milk. These mothers tended to overfeed their infants, offering milk whenever the infant cried. Deprivation of food is suspected to be a factor affecting growth in only one patient.

Most infants tend to develop large appetites, consuming almost twice as much formula as the normal term infant as noted previously by Hill et al. (1963). In spite of high caloric intake beginning within the first week, babies with severe withdrawal tend to lose 10-15% of their birth weight. Birth weight was regained at a median age of 20 days, which exceeds the usual mean.

HEAD   CIRCUMFERENCE

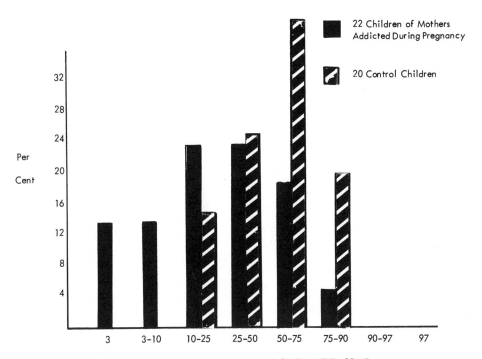

PERCENTILE DISTRIBUTION OF HEAD CIRCUMFERENCE AT
3-6 YEARS ON HARVARD GROWTH GRID

FIG. 2

Abnormally high caloric intake persists, certainly through 9-12 months and perhaps longer. High caloric intakes, ranging from 124 to 272 calories per kilogram, were calculated for 11 drug-study infants aged six weeks to 17 months. These figures do not represent a random sample of addicts' babies, as a nutritionist initially obtained detailed dietary information from mothers complaining of their baby's unusual appetite. Our most extreme patient at five months consumed 64 ounces of formula and four jars of baby food daily.

The excessive quantity of formula ingested may result in high-volume diarrhea.

Three infants developed milk intolerance at 2-3 months of age and required special formulas to control vomiting and diarrhea.

INFECTION

An area which we are just beginning to explore is that of postnatal infection. During the newborn period, infections were frequent. In 30 consecutive in-

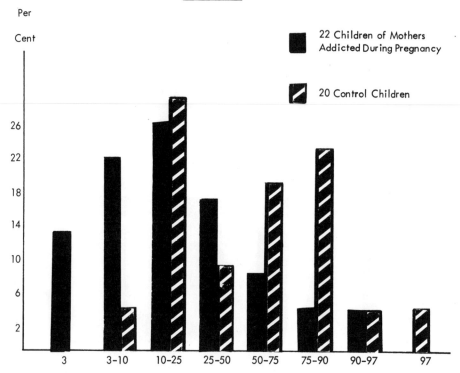

WEIGHT

FIG. 3

fants of heroin or methadone mothers, they included oral and perineal monilia-sis (six cases), cellulitis secondary to abrasions of knees (three patients), and asymptomatic salmonella infection in one infant. Five infants with a positive VDRL test for syphilis had no clinical signs of congenital syphilis.

One infant with neonatal moniliasis had persistent mild infection in spite of extensive therapy. At ten months, he developed generalized oral-cutaneous monilial infection. Immunologic studies were normal. His somatic growth was not disturbed.

Australia antigen hepatitis has been identified in two babies who had no symptoms suggestive of hepatitis. One had multiple minor malformations, growth disturbance and psychomotor retardation. The second had poor weight gain, short stature and abnormal liver function. Weight gain improved when liver function reverted to normal. Short stature persists.

Three babies hospitalized at six to nine months for evaluation of persistent excessive irritability or abnormal sleep patterns were found to have unsuspected infections, including urinary tract infection, chronic otitis media, and mild broncho-pneumonia. It is possible that these infections may have affected the somatic growth of these children. Further study will be necessary to establish this point. To date, we have identified definite problems in each of seven babies admitted for observation and evaluation; symptomatology of patients was not classic for the disease in any case.

HYPOTHALAMIC EFFECT

A hypothalamic-pituitary disturbance has been suggested by several investigators based on their findings in animals and adult addicts. Friedler and Cochin (1972) found transient postnatal growth retardation in rats whose mothers were habituated to morphine prior to but not during pregnancy. This they related to possible disturbance of hypothalamic-pituitary mechanisms. Cushman (1972) measured growth hormone, the most sensitive index of pituitary function, in adult heroin addicts. He demonstrated a mild reduction of growth hormone secretion in response to insulin-induced hypoglycemia in heroin addicts and methadone users. Resting levels of growth hormones were unaffected and clinical significance is uncertain.

Corssen (1974) demonstrated that human epithelial cells in tissue culture develop tolerance to morphine and become dependent upon its presence. Growth arrest and even cell death occurred in response to sudden withdrawal of morphine. Whether such a direct cellular action has bearing on the neonate withdrawn from opiates requires investigation.

SLEEP DISTURBANCE

Preliminary investigations of sleep in drug-dependent infants raise the question of possible significance of sleep disturbance as a factor affecting growth. Schulman (1974) studied eight full-term infants whose mothers used heroin until delivery. These infants had mild withdrawal but did not require therapy. She reported absence of quiet sleep and significant decrease in REM sleep as compared to normal controls. Sisson (1969) studied ten infants of heroin or methadone users. Infants were treated with chlorpromazine for management of withdrawal. He reports that methadone and heroin obliterated REM sleep and allowed rare periods of quiet sleep prior to treatment. Although periods of REM sleep increased with therapy, abnormality persisted. Clinically we see sleep disturbance continuing beyond a year of age. Since it is postulated that neuronal protein synthesis is most active during REM sleep, disturbance of this sleep period may be of significance.

SUMMARY

Intrauterine growth retardation occurs in a large percentage of infants born to mothers addicted to heroin during pregnancy. This is seen less often in infants of mothers who faithfully attend methadone programs.

Postnatally, a decline in linear growth and head circumference is seen during the first year in both heroin- and methadone-exposed infants. The basis for this postnatal growth retardation requires further investigation.

The birth weights, lengths and head circumferences were appropriate for gestational age in 28 of 29 infants delivered to mothers participating in methadone-maintenance programs three months or longer during pregnancy. Absence of intrauterine growth retardation seems to reflect the addict's improved lifestyle.

Postnatally, growth disturbance occurred in 35% of infants exposed to heroin and 25% of infants exposed to methadone during gestation.

Several cases of chronic unsuspected infections in addicts' infants are reported, raising the question of the significance of undiagnosed infection as it affects growth.

Notes

Supported by the Maternity and Infant Care Project No. 06H-000-016-09, American Legion Erna and Albert Siegmund Child Welfare and Rehabilitation Foundation, United States Public Health Service Grant No. RR-00188, United States Public Health Service Grant No. MCT-000436-18-0, and Department of Health, Education and Welfare Grant No. 1-660-00-53.

Requests for reprints should be addressed to Geraldine S. Wilson, M.D., Baylor College of Medicine, Department of Pediatrics, 1200 Moursund Avenue, Houston, Texas 77025.

References

Blinick, G., Wallach, R.C., and Jerez, E. Pregnancy in narcotics addicts treated by medical withdrawal. *American Journal of Obstetrics and Gynecology*, 1969, *105*(7). 997-1003.

Cobrinik, R. W., Hood, R. T., and Chusid, E. The effect of maternal narcotic addiction on the newborn infant. *Pediatrics*, 1959, *August*, 288-304.

Corssen, G., and Skora, I. A. "Addiction" reactions in cultured human cells. *Journal of the American Medical Association*, 1964, *187*(5). 92-96

Cushman, P. Growth hormone in narcotic addiction. *Journal of Clinical Endocrinology and Metabolism*, 1972, *35*(3). 532-358.

Desmond, M.M., Schwanecke, R. P., Wilson, G. S., Yasunaga, S., and Burgdorff, I. Maternal barbiturate utilization and neonatal withdrawal symptomatology. *Journal of Pediatrics*, 1972, *February, 80*. 190-197.

Friedler, G., and Cochin, J. Growth retardation in offspring of female rats treated with morphine prior to conception. *Science*, 1972, *175*. 654-656.

Goodfriend, M.J., Shey, I.A., and Klein, M.D. The effects of maternal narcotic addiction on the newborn. *American Journal of Obstetrics and Gynecology*, 1956, *71*. 29-36.

Hill, R. M., and Desmond, M. M. Management of the narcotic withdrawal syndrome in the neonate. *The Pediatric Clinics of North America*, 1963, *February*, 67-85.

Kandall, S. R., Gartner, L. M., and Berle, B. B. Birth weights and maternal narcotic use. *Pediatric Research,* 1974, *8*(4), 364/90 (abstract).

Krause, S. O., Holmes, J. B., and Burch, R. Heroin addiction among pregnant women and their newborn babies. *American Journal of Obstetrics and Gynecology,* 1958, *April,* 754-756.

McCreary, R., Wilson, G. S., and Kean, J. Unpublished data.

Naeye, R. L., Blanc, W., Leblanc, W., and Khatamee, M.A. Fetal complications of maternal heroin addiction: Abnormal growth, infections, and episodes of stress. *Journal of Pediatrics,* 1973, *83*(6). 1055-1066.

Pierson, P.S., Howard, P., and Kleber, H.D. Sudden deaths in Infants born to methadone-maintained addicts. *Journal of the American Medical Association,* 1972, *220*(13). 1733-1744.

Rajegowda, B. K., Hugh, E. ., Maso, G., Swartz, D. P., and LeBlanc, W. Methadone withdrawal in newborn infants. *Journal of Pediatrics,* 1972, *81*(3). 532-533.

Reddy, A. M., Harper, R. G., and Stern, G. Observations on heroin and methadone withdrawal in the newborn. *Pediatrics.* 1971, *48*(3). 353-357.

Rosenthal, T., Patrick, W. S., and Krug, D. C. Congenital neonatal narcotics addiction: A natural history. *American Journal of Public Health,* 1964, *54*(8). 1252-1262.

Schulman, C. A. Alterations of the sleep cycle in heroin-addicted and "suspect" newborns. *Neuropadiatrie,* 1969, *1*(1). 89-100.

Sisson, T. R. C., Wickler, M., Tsai, P., and Rao, I. P. Effect of narcotic withdrawal on neonatal sleep patterns. *Pediatric Research,* 1974, *8*(4), 451-177 (abstract).

Ting, R., Keller, A., Berman, P., Finnegan, L. P., and Delivoria-Papadopoulous, M. Followup studies of infants born to methadone-department mothers. *Pediatric Research,* 1974, *8*(4), 346-72 (abstract).

Wilson, G. S., Desmond, M. M., and Verniaud, W. M. Early development of infants of heroin-addicted mothers. *American Journal of Diseases of Children,* 1973, *126.* 457-462.

Zelson, C., Rubio, E., and Wasserman, E. Neonatal narcotic addiction: 10 year observation. *Pediatrics, 1971, 48*(2). 178-189.

Zelson, C., Sook, J. L., and Casalino, M. Neonatal narcotic addiction: Comparative effects of maternal intake of heroin and methadone. *New England Journal of Medicine,* 1973, *289*(23). 1216-1220.

Addictive Diseases: an International Journal 2 (2): 347-355 (1975)

Differential Effects of Heroin and Methadone on Birth Weights

STEPHEN R. KANDALL
SUSAN ALBIN
EVAN DREYER
MARCIA COMSTOCK
JOYCE LOWINSON
Division of Neonatology
Department of Pediatrics
Albert Eistein College of Medicine
and Rose F. Kennedy Center for Research
in Mental Retardation
and Human Development
and Department of Psychiatry
Albert Einsetein College of Medicine
Bronx, New York.

INTRODUCTION

An analysis of birth weight of 207 neonates in relation to history of maternal narcotic usage was undertaken. Mean birth weight of infants born to mothers abusing heroin during the pregnancy was low; this was felt to be primarily an effect of intrauterine growth retardation. The same low mean birth weight was seen in infants born to mothers who had abused heroin in the past, but not by history during the current pregnancy. Infants born to mothers on methadone maintenance during the pregnancy had higher mean birth weights. A dose-related effect between maternal methadone dosage in the first trimester and birth weight was observed, i.e. the higher the dosage, the larger the infant.

Heroin abuse during pregnancy has been known for some time to be associated with a population of neonates who are of low birth weight (Krause,

1958; Cobrinik, 1959; Sussman, 1963; Rosenthal, 1964; Perlmutter, 1967; Stone, 1971; Statzer, 1972; and Glass, 1973). This has been reported to be a combination of intrauterine growth retardation and true prematurity. It was first reported that birth weights of infants born to mothers taking heroin or methadone, were not different (Rajegowda, 1972), but subsequent reports (Zelson, 1973, Naeye, 1973), have suggested that methadone usage during pregnancy was associated with higher birth weights in the newborns. Recently Newman (1974) observed these higher birth weights and tentatively suggested that a dose-related effect between maternal methadone dose and birth weight might exist.

Because of this controversy, a systematic review of our records was undertaken to determine birth weight patterns in populations of women with varying drug histories.

PATIENTS AND METHODS

Review of all births at the Albert Einstein College of Medicine—Bronx Municipal Hospital Center from January 1, 1971, to December 31, 1973, was undertaken to identify all infants born to mothers with histories of past or present narcotic usage. This review included records from the Divisions of Obstetrics, Neonatology, and Social Service.

All of these babies were cared for in the term or intensive care nursery of the Bronx Municipal ospital Center. There were 194 such patients identified during the three-year study period. In addition, 13 patients within Group IV (see below) born to mothers followed at the Albert Einstein College of Medicine—Bronx State Hospital Methadone Maintenance Treatment Program, born at other local hospitals were included in the study.

This total of 207 neonates were divided into four study groups.

(a) Group I consisted of 58 neonates born to mothers who admitted to heroin abuse of significant degree during the current pregnancy. There were two stillbirths and 7 early deaths. Of the 53 babies who lived for at least 4 days, 44 showed withdrawal symptoms; 25 of the 44 required specific treatment for withdrawal symptoms.

(b) Group II consisted of 27 neonates born to mothers with a past history of significant heroin usage, but who claimed to be drug-free during the current pregnancy. All such mothers were interviewed carefully by the Social Service or Drug Abuse Divisions of the hospital before such histories were accepted. There were no withdrawal symptoms in the infants and no neonatal deaths.

(c) Group III consisted of 46 newborns of mothers who admitted to use of both heroin and methadone in large amounts during the pregnancy. All such mothers were interviewed in the same way as those mothers in Group II. One infant was stillborn. Of the remaining 45, 43 showed withdrawal symptoms within our period of observation, 33 of whom were treated.

(d) Group IV consisted of 63 infants born to mothers who had taken methadone as their sole or major drug throughout the entire pregnancy. All had prior histories of heroin addiction before entry into Methadone Maintenance Treatment Programs. Fifty-seven of the 63 had withdrawal symptoms; 55 received specific treatment for withdrawal.

A subgroup of 30 infants born to mothers who were registered in the Albert Einstein College of Medicine—Bronx State Hospital Methadone Maintenance Treatment Program throughout their entire pregnancy was identified (Group V). Since complete dosage schedules and urine analyses for drugs were available on each of these patients, this group was analyzed separately after their inclusion in Group IV.

A control group of 40 neonates (Group VI) was generated randomly by choosing the next baby born following one of the methadone group. This group was free of history of maternal narcotic usage, but was not controlled in any other way.

RESULTS

The results were as follows (Table I):

TABLE I
Birth Weight

GROUP	NO.	MEAN AND S.E.	GESTATIONAL AGE
I. HEROIN	58	2481G $\pm$ 82	38.4 WKS $\pm$ 0.4
II. PAST HEROIN	27	2540G $\pm$ 75	38.1 WKS $\pm$ 0.5
III. HEROIN AND METHADONE	46	2530G $\pm$ 101	38.2 WKS $\pm$ 0.6
IV. METHADONE	63	2963G $\pm$ 77	39.2 WKS $\pm$ 0.3
V. BRONX STATE MMTP	30	3065G $\pm$ 103	39.5 WKS $\pm$ 0.2
VI. CONTROL	40	3282G $\pm$ 66	39.9 WKS $\pm$ 0.1

Legend: Table showing means of birth weights and gestational age in the six groups.

Newborns in Group I had a mean birth weight of 2481G ± 82, in Group II 2540G ± 75, and in Group III 2530G ± 101, with gestational ages noted in the table. Two-tailed t-test analysis revealed no statistically significant differences between these three groups. Mean birth weight of the methadone group (IV) was 2963G ± 77; when compared to the Groups I, II, III combined, the difference was highly significant (p< 0.001). The difference in gestational age approached significance (p < .10).

The infants in the control group had significantly higher birth weights (p<0.01)and gestational ages (p<0.05)than the infants in the methadone group.

The subpopulation of Bronx State MMTP patients (Group V) was analyzed separately. There were no significant differences in birth weight between this group and the total methadone group (IV). Since methadone dosages were available in all patients for the entire pregnancy, the relationship between birth weight and maternal dosage during each trimester was examined. In this analysis a highly significant relationship was found between first trimester dosage and eventual birth weight, i.e., the higher the methadone dosage in one first trimester, the higher the birth weight. The generated regression line had an R value of 0.524 (p<0.005).

DISCUSSION

The effects of maternal drug use on the developing fetus are incompletely understood. Although birth weight is a biologic endpoint subject to many influences, it was hoped that an analysis of birth weight in relation to maternal drug history would provide clues into some of these effects.

First, this study confirms the observation that babies born to mothers abusing heroin during pregnancy tended to be of low birth weight. Since in our study the large majority of these babies were at or near term, this effect was mainly one of intrauterine growth retardation, rather than shortened gestation. This population of mothers tended to be black, of low maternal age and lacking in prenatal care, all factors suspected of being contributory to the production of low birth weight infants. Despite these factors, the remarkably consistent association of heroin abuse and low birth weight in the literature, confirmed in our data, suggests that heroin use itself may be extremely important in this regard, as suggested by Naeye et al. (1973).

Birth weights in Group II, babies born to past heroin users, are identical with those in Group I. This suggests for the first time that heroin abuse in the past, despite abstinence during the current pregnancy, may still contribute to fetal growth retardation. Although consideration of the ex-addict's life-style is of obvious importance, it is quite possible that heroin may induce physiologic or biochemical changes which extend beyond the period of addiction. An example of such a delayed effect is the reported postnatal growth retardation in young rats born to mothers who had exposure to morphine in the past, but not during the current pregnancy (Friedler, 1972).

The higher birth weights noted in the methadone group confirm recent studies in the literature. This group was compared to the other groups combined with respect to several variables that might influence birth weight. A significantly higher proportion of mothers taking methadone attended prenatal clinic greater than six times during the pregnancy than in the other combined group (p< 0.001). An analysis of the mothers' pre-pregnancy weights showed no statistically significant differences between the methadone group and the other combined groups. In terms of racial distribution, there were significantly fewer black women in the methadone group (p< 0.05). In the breakdown of maternal ages, there were fewer teenage mothers in the methadone group (p< 0.02). Although males made up 66% of the methadone group and 50% of the other drug group, this difference was not statistically significant. Since it had been observed that males generally weigh more than females at birth, the birth-weight figures were sex-adjusted, and the comparisons repeated, with no change in significance.

In spite of these confounding variables, a direct effect of methadone dose on fetal growth is still suggested by the relationship of birth weight to first trimester methadone dosage. The relationship between birth weight and dose in the last two trimesters was not significant. This suggests that an early drug effect may be operative. The mechanism of this effect is not known, but speculation involves three major possibilities. The first is that methadone alters fetal carbohydrate metabolism. It has been known for many years that infants of diabetic women are frequently overgrown, and it has been suggested that hyperglycemia and hyperinsulinism are responsible for this increased weight gain. The hyperglycemic effect of morphine has been known for many years (Vassalle, 1961), and there is suspicion that methadone, acting through the hypothalamus, may have similar properties.

A second possibility is that methadone acts on maternal hormones involved in part in the regulation of carbohydrate homeostasis. Glass (1973), reported a lower level of circulating corticosteroids in pregnant heroin addicts at term. It is possible that methadone corrects this relative adrenal hypofunction, restoring carbohydrate homeostasis to normal. It is also possible that large amounts of methadone in the first trimester may establish a pattern of adrenal hyperfunction with subsequent fetal overgrowth.

A third postulate is that methadone corrects in a specific but unknown manner the reduction in organ cell number in the infants of heroin-addicted mothers (Naeye, 1973). These authors reported normal cell size, and concluded that fetal growth retardation could not be explained by the state of maternal nutrition alone.

These findings have wide-ranging implications. First, they are of direct importance in the management of the addict's pregnancy, since effects on fetal growth must be taken into consideration in the manipulation of drug dosage. Second, they raise questions about the differential effects on fetal organ development and maturation in relation to the mother's methadone dose. The effect on the developing brain would be a critical issue to consider. Third, it opens for close inspection the basic mechanisms which affect and determine fetal growth in general. The development of a suitable laboratory animal model would be of great benefit in seeking these answers.

Notes

Requests for reprints should be addressed to Stephen R. Kandall, M.D.: Dept. of Pediatrics, Albert Einstein College of Medicine, 1300 Morris Park Avenue, Bronx, New York 10461.

References

Cobrinik, R. W., Hood, T. R., Chusid, E. The effect of maternal addiction on the newborn infant. Review of the literature and report of 22 cases. *Pediatrics*, 1959, *24*. 288-304.

Friedler, G., and Cochin, J. Growth retardation in offspring of female rats treated with morphine prior to conception. *Science*, 1972, *175*. 654-655.

Glass, L., Rajegowda, B. K., and Mukherjee, T. K. Effect of heroin on corticosteroid production in pregnant addicts and their fetuses. *American Journal of Obstetrics and Gynecology*, 1973, *117*. 416-418.

Krause, S., Murray, P. M., Holmes, J. B., et al. Heroin addiction among pregnant women and their newborn babies. *American Journal of Obstetrics and Gynecology*, 1958, *75*. 754-758.

Naeye, R. L., Blanc, W., Leblanc, W., et al. Fetal complications of maternal heroin addiction: Abnormal growth, infections, and episodes of stress. *Journal of Pediatrics*, 1973, *83*. 1055-1061.

Newman, R. G. Pregnancies of methadone patients. *New York State Journal of Medicine*, 1974, *74*. 52-54.

Perlmutter, J. Drug addiction in pregnant women. *American Journal of Obstetrics and Gynecology*, 1967, *99*. 569-572.

Rajegowda, B. K., Glass, L., Evans, H. E., et al. Methadone withdrawal in newborn infants. *Journal of Pediatrics*, 1972, *81*. 532-534.

Rosenthal, T., Patrick, S. W., and Krug, D. C. Congenital neonatal narcotics addiction: A natural history. *American Journal of Public Health*, 1964, *54*. 1252-1262.

Statzer, D. E., and Wardell, J. N. Heroin addiction during pregnancy. *American Journal of Obstetrics and Gynecology*, 1972, *113*. 273-278.

Stone, M. L., Salerno, L. J., Green, M., et al. Narcotic addiction in pregnancy. *American Journal of Obstetrics and Gynecology*, 1971, *109*. 716-720.

Sussman, S. Narcotic and methamphetamine use during pregnancy. *American Journal of Diseases of Children*, 1963, *106*. 325-330.

Vassalle, M. Role of catecholamine release in morphine hyperglycemia. *American Journal of Physiology*, 1961, *200*. 530-534.

Zelson, C., Lee, S. J., and Casalino, M. Neonatal narcotic addiction. *New England Journal of Medicine*, 1973, *289*. 1216-1220.

DISCUSSION

Q. *Dr. Kron:* In Philadelphia, we have had some experience with comparing groups of infants born to mothers attending methadone clinics, and those who have not been attending methadone clinics. I think that one problem is in what we call these people. I do not think that we can really call them heroin addicts, but just people who are not attending our clinic. Even the so-called methadone clinic attenders are not methadone addicts necessarily; they may be taking a variety of other drugs as well. But we have had similar findings to your own, namely, something like 300 gram differential between the groups we have studied, and there are very similar numbers too. These range from a mean of about 2500 grams, for the babies being born to people coming off the street, and about 2800 or 2850 for those coming through the clinic, at least in the study I am referring to now.

A. *Dr. Kandall: The regression line was generated only from the 30 babies from the Bronx State Hospital program on whom we had urines weekly throughout the pregnancy, and knew their dosages. This should not be one confounding factor, although the point has been raised that you do not know whether they are "topping off" on the street. We obviously do not, but this was a relatively clean group that was studied.*

Dr. Kron: I am not contradicting the data; I am simply adding a question, because we have data that run exactly contrary to that. Mainly, in groups of women attending the methadone clinic, the weight of the infants, again in the particular population I am referring to, was inversely related to the length of time that they were in the clinic. In other words, those who were in the clinic for nine months or longer, up to three years, had smaller babies (still within the normal range). The prematurity rate in that group was slightly less than 20 percent vs the 50 percent of the street addicts. However, our regression line ran in the opposite direction to your own, and I think that it may have to do with differences in things other than methadone, that is a multifactorial issue, and that there may be other characteristics of your program, as contrasted to ours, or the difference in the population separate from the methadone dose, which might explain the differences between our data.

Dr. Kandall: I have no quarrel with that. Birth weight is a very complex biologic endpoint, obviously. It has always been amazing to me that birth weights of babies born to heroin-using mothers cluster around 2500 grams, whether they are black, white, or Puerto Rican; whether they have had prenatal care or have not had prenatal care. This is very striking evidence that there is a direct drug effect, and it is not a long jump to say that methadone should have some effect on the birth weight. We feel very secure that this is what we are seeing, although there are obviously many variables that have to be considered.

Dr. Roloff: I still do not quite see why you look for a growth-stimulating explanation for this effect, if they did not reach the control weights.

A. *Dr. Kandall: There was a definite effect on growth. Weights were increased to 3065 grams in the Bronx State group, and, as you can see from the regression line, the ones born to mothers taking more than 80 mg a day in the first trimester weighed over 3200 grams, which is the control weight.*

Q. *Dr. Remeteria:* Have you had a chance to follow these babies postnatally as far as what happens to their weights?

A. *Dr. Kandall: I have no follow-up data to report. It is much too sketchy.*

Q. *Dr. Abrams:* I would just like to ask Dr. Wilson whether or not she has any information on growth hormone levels or thyroid function studies in the children who are showing growth failure in the first year?

A. *Dr. Wilson: Not at this point.*

Dr. Kandall: I suspect that insulin levels might be more helpful than growth hormone levels, but we do not have that data yet.

Q. *Dr. Finnegan:* When we discussed our data with the Veterans Administration program in Philadelphia, Dr. Chuck O'Brien, who is in charge of that program, and Dr. George Woody were interested in our increase in birth weights in the methadone group. They also had observed with their veteran male patients that, after going on methadone, there was an increase in weight. I wonder if anyone here has observed that in nonpregnant individuals, and if there is any correlation between this increase of body weight in the adult and this increase here in the babies?

A. *Dr. Kandall: I can give you some information on that. We did check with the Bronx State program. Dr. Lowienson, who heads that program, says that it is commonly known that when patients in the adult nonpregnant population go on methadone they gain weight.*

Q. *Dr. Abrams:* Is there water retention?

A. *Dr. Kandall: I do not think that was ever really studied in the adult. Apparently, when you lower the methadone dose in the adult population, the weight gain starts to subside.*

Q. *Dr. Kron:* That brings up the question of whether it is indeed methadone which is bringing about the changes, or the ancillary, helpful effects of prenatal care or, in the case of the methadone addict, association with the clinic. Is there a variety of methadone-addict population who is not attending clinics and in whom this can be compared?

A. *Dr. Kandall: Not that I know of, because that puts them into the uncontrolled group, where we do not have the urines. And then, one is never sure what one is dealing with in terms of groups. We tried to isolate a relatively pure group on whom we had all the data, and could be relatively sure that they were not taking other drugs of abuse as well. That is why we are looking for an animal model, but the rat does not appear to be a suitable model, as Dr. Rosen has told me. The rats, when they are on high methadone dosage, die during pregnancy. And in the low doses, there was no effect on the birth weight.*

Dr. Abrams: I have heard it said that those on methadone treatment have ex-

cessive cravings for carbohydrates, and that may play a part as well.

A. *Dr. Kandall: Yes, it all may be related.*

Dr. Ostrea: It is true that we also see less of these small for gestational age babies if the mothers are on methadone. However, there is a significant difference; but we do not classify these methadone babies as large for gestational age. As an answer to the previous question, the postnatal weight loss of the babies whose mothers are on methadone tend to be much greater compared to the postnatal weight loss of the babies whose mothers are on heroin. This probably speaks more for the fact that the babies whose mothers are on heroin are small for gestational age.

Dr. Hug: This may relate to the rat data and it may not. You say that the rats which were given the high dose of methadone simply died. One of the things which we routinely did for years was to put a rat on a maintenance schedule. This is to induce tolerance and physical dependence, and to follow body weight. Of course, if you start with a high dose to begin with, they do not thrive and they do die. If you start with a low dose of morphine and build it up, then what you find is the differential between the saline-injected and the morphine-injected rats. Now this may be disruptive.

A. *Dr. Kandall: These were all rats that were morphinized first, and then converted to low-dose methadone, and slowly built up; and then they all died.*

Q. *Dr. Hug:* Did you get viable offspring from those who did survive?

A. *Dr. Kandall: We were pushing up to 100 mg per kilo per day, which was higher than the literature said we could go, but we did get them up there.*

Dr. Nuite: If I could just make a couple of comments. The National Institute on Drug Abuse did some contract work, both on chronic studies of methadone, and on LAAM, a similar long-acting compound. We also did reproductive studies (the standard three-phase reproductive studies). We found that we could bring animals to high levels of methadone, as long as we started with a 0.5 mg per kilogram dose, and then brought them up very slowly. We did find that, with methadone, one has to be very careful and watch the development of tolerance. But if you were careful, and adjusted the dose to the level of tolerance that developed in the animal, you could bring rats and rabbits up to 20 mg per kilogram and maintain them at that level.

Dr. Hug: I think that one of the things that you have to keep in mind in this situation is the pharmokinetics of the drug you are dealing with. Because if you try to inject animals—and I only know about morphine—one dose a day, and build up the dose by making that one dose larger and larger, you are going to be, I think, relatively unsuccessful. If you do it on a three-dose basis and maintain them at their continual weight gain, even though it is lower than controls, you can get them up to enormous doses of morphine. The question that comes to mind is that if you have them morphinized and you switch to methadone, and if you follow the same dosage regimen, you may either be giving them inadequate doses, or you may be getting an accumulation of methadone.

Addictive Diseases: an International Journal 2 (2): 357-368 (1975)
© 1975 by Spectrum Publications, Inc.

Effect of Heroin on Perinatal Respiration

LEONARD GLASS
Jewish Hospital and Medical Center of Brooklyn
Brooklyn, New York

HUGH E. EVANS
Jewish Hospital and Medical Center of Brooklyn
Brooklyn, New York

B.K. RAJEGOWDA
Lincoln Hospital Center
Bronx, N.Y.

ERIC J. KAHN
Harlem Hospital Center
New York, N.Y.

INTRODUCTION

Antenatal exposure of the fetus to heroin has a profound effect on neonatal respiratory performance. It was apparent from our clinical observations at Harlem Hospital Center, during the late 1960s, that there was a marked decrease in the incidence of the respiratory distress syndrome (RDS) among low birth weight infants of heroin users, and that those infants with postnatal signs of narcotic withdrawal had unusually rapid respiratory rates. We therefore undertook a retrospective comparison of the prevalence of RDS in infants of addicted and nonaddicted mothers (Glass et al., 1971). This was followed by a prospective study correlating respiratory rates with acid-base status of neonates undergoing heroin withdrawal (Glass et al., 1972).

Since administration of 17 hydroxycorticosteroids (17-OH CS) is associated with increased production of pulmonary surfactant (Kotas et al., 1971), we carried out a prospective study in order to determine if increased 17-OH CS production by fetuses of heroin-addicted mothers is responsible for the apparent decrease in RDS noted in this group (Glass et al., 1973).

The results of these three studies are presented in this paper.

METHODS AND MATERIALS

Because of the high incidence of intrauterine growth retardation among infants of addicted mothers, only those of gestational age of 32 to 37 weeks, inclusive, were included in the study.

Charts were reviewed for 33 consecutively born infants in this gestational age group who exhibited signs of heroin withdrawal and for 123 consecutive nonaddicted infants of comparable gestational age. Infants were grouped within a 2-week range, e.g., 32-33, 34-35, and 36-37 weeks. The characteristics of these infants are shown in Table I.

The diagnosis of RDS was based on the presence of chest retractions, expiratory grunt, cyanosis in room air, blood gas studies, and the absence of any other recognized causes of respiratory distress, such as pneumonia or pneumothorax. Chest X-rays were diagnostic of RDS in 12 of the 26 infants who developed the disorder and equivocal in another three. In the four fatal cases, post mortem examination confirmed the diagnosis.

The diagnosis of heroin withdrawal was made on the basis of a positive maternal history, together with typical signs, such as coarse flapping tremors, irritability, and shrill, high-pitched cry.

TACHYPNEA AND RESPIRATORY ALKALOSIS

Twenty-two infants of heroin-addicted mothers were selected for the study when major signs of withdrawal (irritability and coarse flapping tremors) were first observed. The mothers of these infants used from 3 to 40 bags of heroin daily; none of them used methadone. Twenty of the mothers were cigarette smokers, nine were moderate to heavy consumers of alcohol, and there was sporadic use of barbiturates and marijuana.

The birth weights of these infants ranged from 1,220 to 3,370 grams, with a median of 2,070 grams; the gestational age ranged from 32 to 40 weeks with a median of 37 weeks. Aside from signs of heroin withdrawal, none had evidence of obvious illness. In 16 of these infants, withdrawal signs were severe enough to necessitate treatment with 7 mg of phenobarbital/kg/day, administered in three divided oral doses.

Nineteen control infants, also free of illness, and closely matched with the study infants for birth weight and gestational age, were randomly selected.

While none of their mothers used narcotics or consumed appreciable amounts of alcohol, eight were cigarette smokers. The birth weights of these infants ranged from 1,250 to 4,400 grams, with a median of 1,980 grams, and gestational age from 32 to 40 weeks, with a median of 36 weeks. All infants were raised under conditions of thermoneutrality.

Respiratory rates were counted four times a day, and the average of the four readings tabulated as the daily mean. Tidal volumes were not measured.

Measurements of blood pH and PCO_2 were performed on arterilized capillary blood, obtained by heel prick, after warming the extremity for about 15 minutes. Blood samples were obtained on 11 study and 8 control infants on the first day of life, 21 study and 16 control infants on the second day, all infants on the third day, and 15 study and 16 control infants on the fourth day. Additional analyses were made on 10 study and 10 control infants between the fifth and seventh days of life, and on five members of each group during the second week of life.

CORTICOSTEROID PRODUCTION

Concentrations of 17-OH CS were determined, using a modification of the Mattingly method (1971) on cord sera of 18 infants of heroin-addicted mothers (including one set of twins), and 15 infants of nonaddicted mothers. All infants were delivered vaginally and none were asphyxiated. The infants of the addicted mothers had birth weights of 720 to 3,400 grams, with a median of 3,290 grams, and gestational ages of 26 to 40 weeks, with a median of 38 weeks.

Control infants had birth weights ranging from 1,020 to 3,800 grams with a median of 40 weeks. With the exception of the pair of twins whose gestational age was 26 weeks, all of the infants survived and had uneventful postnatal courses.

In addition, 17-OH CS concentrations were measured in all 17 addicted mothers and 12 of the 15 control mothers immediately after delivery. Similar analgesic and anesthetic agents were used for both groups of women during labor and delivery.

RESULTS

Absence of RDS

None of the infants exhibiting signs of heroin withdrawal developed RDS. Fourteen of 26 non-addicted infants in the 32-33 week category, 8 of 39 in the 34-35 week category, and 4 of 53 infants in the 36-37 week category developed RDS (Table I). In general, the illness tended to be less severe with advancing gestational age.

TABLE I
Incidence of RDS in Premature Infants of Addicted and Nonaddicted Mothers

Gestational Age	Number	Median Birth Weight (gm)	Number of Cases Of RDS
32-33 Weeks:			
Addicted	6	1,600	0
Nonaddicted	26	1,530	14
34-35 Weeks:			
Addicted	9	1,780	0
Nonaddicted	39	1,870	8
36-37 Weeks:			
Addicted	18	1,980	0
Nonaddicted	58	1,990	4

TABLE II
Effect of Heroin on Corticosteroid Concentrations, Median and Ranges
(ug/100 ml)

	Maternal	Cord Blood
Addicted	22. 7 (12. 0- 71. 0)	12. 3 (8. 3- 20. 6)
Nonaddicted	38. 5 (23. 2- 75. 5)	13. 0 (4. 8- 21. 0)

Tachypnea and Respiratory Alkalosis

Infants in the heroin-withdrawal group had significantly higher respiratory rates than the controls during the first week of life (Figure 1); their PCO_2 levels were significantly lower (Figure 2) and blood pH was elevated significantly on the second, third, and fourth days (Figure 3). In a small number of patients investigated during the second week of life, these differences were less apparent. Calculated base excess values were approximately the same in both groups throughout the study period.

All findings were independent of birth weight, gestational age, and, as far as could be determined, the severity of withdrawal. Respiratory rates did not appear to be influenced by the use of phenobarbital.

Corticosteroid Production

Comparable concentrations of 17-OH CS were observed in the cord bloods of both infants (Table II), with a median value of 12.3 ug/100 ml for the heroin

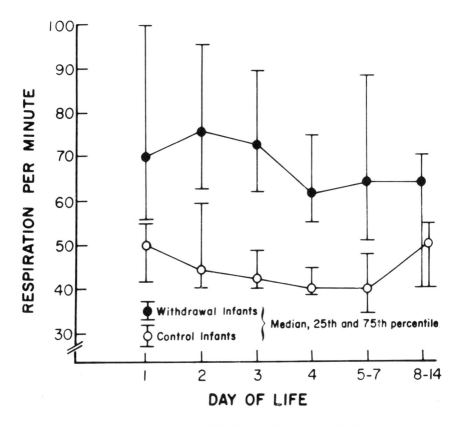

FIG. 1.   Respiratory Rates in Infants With Heroin Withdrawal and in Normal Controls

group, and 13.0 *ug* / 100 ml for the control group. In contrast, the levels found in addicted mothers (median value 21.0 *ug*/100 ml) were significantly lower than those found in nonaddicts (median value 38.5 *ug*/100 ml, Table II). These differences were statistically significant ($p < 0.01$).

DISCUSSION

Our retrospective study confirmed our impression that RDS was extremely rare in premature infants who were exposed to heroin in utero. The reasons for this finding, however, could not be readily explained.

Premature delivery in heroin-addicted women has been associated with a high incidence of intrauterine infection (Naeye et al., 1973). It has also been observed that prolonged rupture of membranes (Bauer et al., 1974) and intrauterine infection (Naeye et al., 1971) are associated with a decreased incidence of RDS, presumably due to the effect of increased cortisol secretion on pulmonary

362

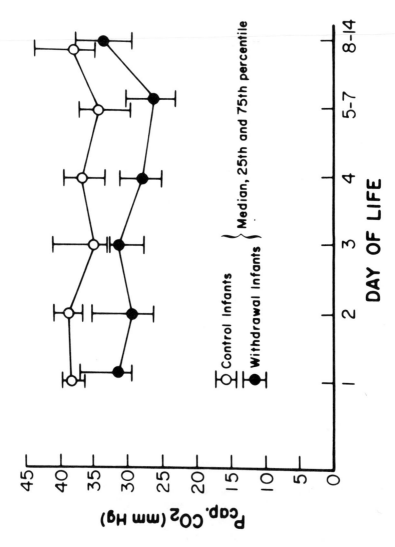

FIG. 2. Capillary Blood PCO2 Values in Infants With Heroin Withdrawal and Normal Controls

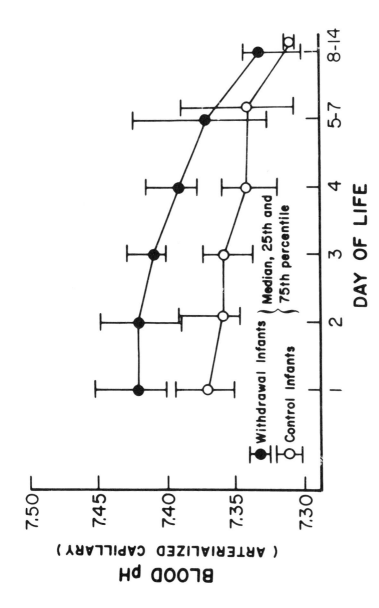

FIG. 3. Capillary Blood pH Values in Infants With Heroin Withdrawal and Normal Controls

363

surfactant production. However, our finding that 17-OH CS concentrations are not elevated in infants of addicted mothers would point to another mechanism responsible for the decreased incidence of RDS in these infants. The low 17-OH CS levels noted in addicted mothers is consistent with previous observations in nonpregnant adults that opiates suppress the hypothalamic anterior pituitary axis (Goodman et al., 1970).

We may speculate that heroin acts as an enzyme inducer, resulting in accelerated production of pulmonary surfactant. However, further studies are necessary to clarify this point.

Finnegan et al. (1974) observed that the P$_{50}$ of cord blood erythrocytes is higher in infants of heroin-addicted mothers than in normal controls. This shift to the right of the oxyhemoglobin dissociation curve is associated with increased delivery of oxygen to tissues, a factor which may be at least in part associated with the decreased incidence of RDS.

The cause of the observed tachypnea was not determined, although in adult addicts it is believed to be attributable to an increased sensitivity of the respiratory center to carbon dioxide (Martin, 1966). In our patients a metabolic acidosis could be excluded as the cause of the hyperventilation beause there were no significant differences in calculated base excess values between patients and controls.

The relationship between the observed respiratory alkalosis and absence of RDS is not completely clear. While it is unlikely that there is a causal relationship, one may conjecture that the normal or elevated blood pH observed in these infants affords protection against pulmonary hypoperfusion, which is often observed in RDS in association with low blood pH (Chu et al., 1967).

Notes

This work was supported in part by USPHS grant 5PO 1-HD-03993 and by the Tuberculosis and Respiratory Disease Association of New York.

Requests for reprints should be addressed to Leonard Glass, M.D., Jewish Hospital and Medical Center of Brooklyn, 555 Prospect Place, Brooklyn, New York 11238.

The three figures are reprinted by permission from the *New England Journal of Medicine*, 286:746, 1972.

References

Glass, L., Rajegowda, B. K., Evans, H. E. Absence of respiratory distress syndrome in premature infants of heroin-addicted mothers. *Lancet* 1971, *2*, 685-686.
Glass, L., Rajegowda, B., Kahn, E., Floyd, M. Effects of heroin withdrawal on respiratory rate and acid-base status in the newborn. *New England Journal of Medicine*, 1972, *186*, 746-748.
Kotas, R. V., and Avery, M. E. Accelerated appearance of pulmonary surfactant in the fetal rabbit. *Journal of Applied Physiology*, 30:358, 1971.

Glass, L., Rajegowda, B. K., Mukherjee, T. K., Roth, M. M., and Evans, H. E. Effect of heroin on corticosteroid production in pregnant addicts and their fetuses. *American Journal of Obstetrics and Gynecology,* 1973, *117*, 416-418.

Mattingly, R., Method for the determination of plasma corticosteroids, *British Medical Journal,* 1971, *25*, 310-315.

Naeye, R. L., Blanc, W., Leblanc W., Khatamee, M. A. Fetal complications of maternal heroin addiction: Abnormal growth, infections, and episodes of stress. *Journal of Pediatrics,* 1973, *83*, 1055-1061.

Bauer, C. R., Stern, L., and Colle, E. Prolonged rupture of membranes associated with a decreased incidence of respiratory distress syndrome. *Pediatrics,* 1974, *53*, 7-12.

Naeye, R. L., Harcke, H. T., Jr., and Blanc, W. A. Adrenal gland structure and the development of hyaline membrane disease. *Pediatrics,* 1971, *47*, 650-657.

Goodman, L. S., and Gilman, A. *The Pharmacologicl Basis of Therapeutics,* London, Macmillan Publishing Co., Inc., 1970, p. 242.

Finnegan, L. P., Shouraie, Z., Emich, J. P., Connaughton, J. F., Schut, J., and Delivoria Papadopoulos, M. Alteration of the oxygen hemoglobin dissociation curve and red cell 2, 3—Diphosphoglycerate (2, d-DPG) in cord blood of infants born to opiate dependent women. *Pediatric Research,* 1974, *8*, 363 (abstract).

Martin, W. R. A homeostatic and redundancy theory of tolerance to and dependence on narcotic analgesics, *The Addictive States: Proceedings of the Association for Research in Nervous and Mental Disease, 1966.* Edited by A. Wikler. Baltimore, Williams and Wilkins Company. 1968.

Chu, J., Clements, J. A., Cotton, E. K., Klaus, M. H., Sweet, A. Y., Tooley, W. H., Bradley, B. L., and Brandorff, L. C. Neonatal pulmonary ishcemia. Part I. Clinical and Physiological Studies. *Pediatrics,* 1967, *40* (Suppl.), 709-782.

DISCUSSION

Q. *Dr. Nathenson:* Your clinical data referred to babies who were heroin-addicted. There has been some suggestion made that methadone may not have the same effect in the prevention of hyaline membrane disease. Do you have any data on this?

A. *Dr. Glass: We see so few premature infants with maternal use of methadone that I just cannot really give you any data. Some people have observed RDS in premature infants of mothers using methadone. Our experience with preemies of methadone-addicted mothers is so scanty.*

Q. *Dr. Nathenson:* Ours has been also; that is why I ask. I wondered if anyone in the audience could comment on that?

A. *Dr. Harper: We have seen four such babies that were premature, whose mothers were on methadone, and who had hyaline membrane disease and were posted with their hyaline membrane.*

Q. *Dr. Merritt:* Your initial observations were very important in the initiation of a number of studies in pulmonary enzymology. However, Dr. Gluck has noted an abnormal elevation of the LS ratios in a variety of conditions at gestational ages in which it is normally much less than one. *You mentioned premature ruptured membranes, non-hypertensive glomerulonephritis, placental infarcts, and* *mid-trimester bleeding. Did you control these variables when you looked at perinatal addiction?*

A. *Dr. Glass: This was not a controlled study, it was a retrospective study.*

Q. *Dr. Merritt:* In the study where you reported the similarity between cord blood and corticosteroids, was the duration of labor between the addicted and nonaddicted mothers similar?

A. Dr. Glass: They were similar. May I comment about the LS ratios. *In one recent report, published in July in the* American Journal of OB-GYN *(1974), in which we correlated the Bubble-Stability test, the LS ratios, and the antinatal detection of RDS, interestingly the one negative Bubble-Stability test, in which the infant did not develop RDS, was in a mother who used heroin and also had prolonged rupture of membranes. The LS ratio was quite low and the Shake test was negative. This is one infant who did not develop RDS, whatever that means.*

Dr. Neumann: I just wanted to introduce a cautionary note about administering a narcotic antagonist to a depressed neonate with a history of drug intake over a period of time. I have not done it myself, so I cannot speak of it, but I understand others have and, similar to adult experience, have precipitated very severe and difficult-to-treat withdrawal.

Q. *Dr. Abrams:* I was interested in your cortisol data; on what day of life did you get these blood samples from the infants?

A. *Dr. Glass: These were cord bloods. The maternal bloods were taken right after delivery on the table.*

Dr. Abrams: We did a study at Roosevelt Hospital a few years ago on 50 normal newborn infants looking for the effect of stress on infants. We found high levels, relatively speaking, of plasma cortisol on the first day of life. And the curve came down by day three or four and this is in keeping with what is published in the literature. Just coincidentally, we were not doing any studies on the addicted infants, the three or four heroin babies were the ones that seemed to have even higher levels than the average, on the first day of life as well.

Q. *Dr. Glass:* Were these cord bloods before they developed withdrawal?

A. *Dr. Abrams: Yes, they were cord bloods.*

Q. *Dr. Desmond:* I was wondering whether anyone had seen idiopathic respiratory distress and withdrawal occurring at the same time. One of the first findings in idiopathic respiratory distress is hypotonicity and inactivity, as shown by the data of Rudolph, et al. A hypotonic baby cannot tremor and I was wondering if these are not really two mutually exclusive syndromes?

A. *Dr. Glass: I really cannot answer that question. It is a very good point and I wonder if anyone has any experience.*

Dr. Finnegan: As I mentioned to you, we have seen four babies, two of which are heroin-addicted, and two of which are methadone-addicted, who have developed clinical signs of respiratory distress syndrome and who died, and whose pathological specimens are consistent.

Q. *Dr. Glass:* Did they have withdrawal signs?

A. *Dr. Finnegan: Two of these babies were treated for respiratory distress and were treated with phenobarbital.*

Q. *Dr. Glass:* Did they have the classic withdrawal signs?

A. *Dr. Finnegan: They had tremors.*

Q. *Dr. Glass:* What were the gestational ages?

A. *Dr. Finnegan: One was a 1400 gram baby, with a gestational age of 32 weeks, and I cannot remember the other one.*

Q. *Dr. Kandall:* Could you speculate on the role of the effect of the drugs on the respiratory system, and the subsequent development of the sudden death syndrome, as mentioned very briefly by Dr. Desmond yesterday? We now have about nine cases of sudden death syndrome, and we are trying to relate it to the effect on the respiratory system.

A. *Dr. Glass: It is an interesting hypothesis. I think we have discussed it with Dr. William Martin at Lexington, who originally showed the effects of withdrawal in adult abstinence. It is a very good possibility that there may be some aberrations of the response of the respiratory center to CO_2. I do not know the answer. We have been asking that question for a half a dozen years now.*

Dr. Roloff: I would like to offer some speculation regarding the hyperventilation. If indeed the P50 is increased, this might have the same effect as raising oxygen which, in premature infants, is a respiratory stimulant.

A. *Dr. Glass: Well, we know that exchange transfusions with fresh blood having a high P50 is one of the treatments of respiratory distress syndrome.*

Dr. Nathenson: I might make a comment that peripherally touches upon one previous question regarding the concomitant occurrence of hyaline membrane disease and withdrawal symptomatology. We have not seen this, but I have been impressed by the fact that addicted infants who are otherwise ill—one, for instance, with severe meconium aspiration and another with congenital pneumonia demonstrated no withdrawal during the period of respiratory illness, but, on recovery from the acute illness, they began to have delayed withdrawal manifestations. I wondered whether or not other insults to the newborn who is addicted may, in fact, suppress the onset of withdrawal until these effects are over. Perhaps then the central nervous system operates otherwise to demonstrate withdrawal.

A. *Dr. Glass: I cannot answer that either. It is a good question; I think we have to look specifically for that. We just are not seeing very much pure heroin withdrawal these days, but once the new Turkish crop comes in, I suppose we will be getting our share of heroin-addicted infants again.*

Q. *Dr. Garrettson:* Have you measured simple respiratory rate as you followed the babies or have you done any tidal-volume measurements?

A. *Dr. Glass: We did not at that time measure tidal volume; it was simply respiratory rate measured by the same observer.*

Q. *Dr. Garrettson:* Are you now measuring the tidal volume?
A. *Dr. Glass: Not at the present time.*

Dr. Garrettson: The reason I ask this is that in the adult, the two classic drugs, morphine and Demerol, are respiratory depressants, one depressing rate more than volume, and the other depressing volume more than rate. In the infant, it is clear that when one looks at the tidal volume at different ambient CO_2's, morphine is distinctly a more depressing drug, even at ambient CO_2, than is Demerol. This is with drugs given to the nonaddicted infants receiving a single dose. One wonders what the response then is.

Q. *Dr. Glass:* Did you say that morphine was distinctly more depressive on rate?
A. *Dr. Garrettson: No, on tidal volume. This is a study that was done in human neonates and published in* Clinical Pharmacology and Therapeutics *about four or five years ago. The question then is, How does methadone behave in the newborn in this regard? As I say, one must get at a minute volume; and I think it will have very important implications for us, possibly, as we discussed whether or not we should be switching to low doses of methadone for treating withdrawal syndrome, or whether we should stay with the opium preparations, such as morphine. And it is a quesiton of which is more depressive and this may be of importance in some infants.*

Q. *Dr. Hug:* Just to amplify that last point a little bit more in terms of the importance of the minute volume as opposed to either rate or tidal volume, we are doing studies on adults, anesthetized adults, and it is quite dramatic when we give an intravenous dose of morphine, to see what happens; both tidal volume and rate fall very quickly. Tidal volumes were recovered and actually go to greater than controlled stable levels, and the rate and minute volume are what parallel each other as the drug is essentially eliminated. But the point is that even within that, there is considerable variability in the thing that shows the smoothness, presumably parallels the drug most closely in minute volumes. Another comment about the naloxone, have people here seen withdrawal in the neonate—that is the newborn given naloxone? My question is, Did you see withdrawal before you saw antagonism to the respiratory depression? Were you able to distinguish? Years ago, Wickler reported that adult human addicts, as they are exposed longer and longer to morphine, become more and more sensitive to the antagonist. Of course, he was using nalorphine, and even to the point where you might precipitate an acute withdrawal syndrome without fully reversing the respiratory depressant factor.

Q. *Dr. Remeteria:* I was wondering; instead of an effect on the respiratory center, or directly on the lungs, we also might consider another possibility, i.e., when an infant is going into withdrawal, the increased muscular activity is going to increase his metabolic rate, his need for oxygen, and, therefore, his respiratory rate. Could this be a respiratory compensation for the increased oxygen needs?

A. *Dr. Glass: I do not think that anyone has ever demonstrated an increased oxygen consumption.*

Addictive Diseases: an International Journal 2 (2): 369-379 (1975)

Morphine Administration to Pregnant Rabbits: Effect on Fetal Growth and Lung Development

DIETRICH W. ROLOFF
WILLIAM F. HOWATT
WILLIAM P. KANTO, JR.
ROBERT C. BORER, JR.
Department of Pediatrics and Communicable Diseases
University of Michigan
Ann Arbor, Michigan

INTRODUCTION

The observation by Glass, Rajegowda, and Evans (1971) that premature infants of heroin-addicted mothers have a lower prevalence of idiopathic respiratory distress syndrome (RDS) than those of non-addicted mothers suggested that opiates are among the agents which may enhance pulmonary organ maturation when given prenatally. Because pressure/volume curves from lungs of prematurely delivered rabbits correlate well with histochemical, histological, and physical characteristics of developing lung maturity (Kotas and Avery, 1971), we used this model to test the hypothesis that the administration of morphine to rabbits during most of their pregnancy might accelerate fetal lung maturation.

MATERIALS AND METHODS

Morphine injections

Time-bred New Zealand rabbits whose normal length of gestation is 31 days were admitted to the animal care facility between the 3rd and 10th day of

369

gestation. They were in the laboratory for three days for acclimatization. Subcutaneous injections of morphine sulfate began three days later from the 6th to 14th gestational day. Injections were given in 6-hour intervals in doses of 10, 5 or 2.5 mg/kg up to sacrifice time. Equal volumes of 0.9% NaCl solution were given to control animals. The solutions were coded as to their identity and the code was not broken until after the conclusion of the experiment and the computation of the results. Intravenous administration of naloxone to 3 test animals produced withdrawal symptoms.

Delivery

On the 27th, 28th, or 29th day of gestation the pregnant rabbits were anesthetized and a laparotomy was performed. In order to prevent spontaneous air-breathing the uterus was left unopened until fetal movements had ceased following interruption of the uterine blood flow by a mass ligature. The fetuses were then removed in their fetal sacs and the amniotic fluid was collected. The position within the uterus was noted and the weight was recorded. Each fetal weight was also expressed as a percentile value relative to the entire litter (Barr and Brent, 1970).

Pressure/volume curves

In order to obtain pressure/volume curves we inserted a plastic catheter into the trachea of the rabbit fetus through a tracheotomy. The chest walls were left intact. Air was injected into the lungs from a syringe attached to a Harvard infusion pump at a rate of 0.15 ml/minute. Corrections were made in the volume measurements for the compression in the system of 0.01 ml/cm H_2O pressure. By means of a transducer connected to the system, airway pressures were recorded. The lungs were inflated to an airway pressure of 35 cm H_2O. After an equilibration period of 5 minutes, more air was injected if the pressure had fallen below 35 cm H_2O in the interval. The direction of the infusion pump was then reversed until atmospheric airway pressures were observed. The amount of air remaining in the lungs when the deflation pressure had fallen to 10 cm H_2O (V_{10}) was then determined and was expressed as the proportion of the volume which had been injected during the inflation to 35 cm H_2O. Kotas, Fletcher, Torday, and Avery (1971) have shown that V_{10} is an adequate measurement of characteristics of the entire deflation limb of the pressure/volume curve. Normal saline was then instilled through the catheter and withdrawn. This lung washing was preserved frozen.

Lecithin/sphingomyelin ratio

Amniotic fluid was aspirated from the amniotic sacs and was stored at -20°C until determination of the lecithin/sphingomyelin (L/S) ratio. A cold

TABLE I
Pregnancy Outcome

	CONTROLS	MORPHINE SULFATE (mg/kg/dose)		
		10	5	2.5
NUMBER OF RABBITS:	31	11	13	23
ABORTED (%):	2 (7)	5 (46)	6 (46)	5 (22)
NOT PREGNANT (%):	10 (32)	4 (36)	5 (39)	7 (30)
PREGNANT (%):	19 (61)	2 (18)	2 (15)	11 (48)

acetone precipitate of a chloroform extract was subjected to thin-layer chromatography, and the spot areas were analyzed for phospholipids (Gluck, Kulovich, Borer, 1974). Saline lung washings were processed similarly. For the human fetus the L/S ratio in the amniotic fluid is a clinically useful indicator of the biochemical maturation of the pulmonary surfactant system; low values are associated with postnatal occurrence of RDS (Gluck and Kulovich, 1973).

RESULTS

Outcome of pregnancies

Almost half of the pregnant rabbits receiving morphine in doses of 10 and 5mg/kg had spontaneous abortions (Table I), most of them on the 25th day. This incidence fell to 22% when the dose was lowered to 2.5 mg/kg. The abortion rate in the control animals was only 7.0%. The number of animals found not to be pregnant upon hysterotomy represent the sum of fertilization failures and early fetal loss with complete resorptions; there were no differences between the treatment and control groups in this regard.

In pregnancies carried to the date of hysterotomy there were no differences in regard to litter size, number of dead fetuses per litter (i.e., intrauterine death before delivery) or percentage of pregnancies with dead fetuses. Thus, the morphine-related pregnancy losses in rabbits appear to be caused by abortions rather than individual intrauterine deaths.

Of the control animals, 84% gained weight during the observed part of their pregnancy, while 70% of the morphine-treated animals lost weight. Of the does losing more than 10% weight, 89% aborted; none aborted if they had gained weight or lost less than 10%.

TABLE II
Comparison of Weight, Lung Volume, and Amniotic Fluid Lecithin/Sphingomyelin (L/S) Ration of Fetuses from Morphine-Injected and Control Rabbits

Gestational Age:	27 days		28 days		29 days	
	morphine	controls	morphine	controls	morphine	controls
Mean fetal weight(g)	17.0	25.2	25.3	30.0	29.7	38.0
(N)	(31)	(59)	(59)	(54)	(40)	(28)
P	< 0.001		< 0.005		< 0.001	
Mean V_{10} (%)	45.2	48.0	49.4	55.5	64.6	65.9
(N)	(10)	(8)	(11)	(22)	(13)	(11)
P	NS		NS		NS	
Mean L/S ratio	0.59	0.66	0.55	0.61	0.63	0.73
(N)	(22)	(16)	(18)	(25)	(10)	(3)
P	NS		NS		NS	

V_{10} = lung volume at 10 cm H_2O pressure in percent of the volume at 35 cm H_2O pressure

NS = no significant difference (t-test)

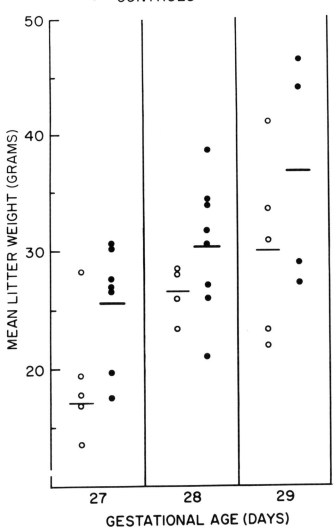

FIG. 1   The effect of morphine given to pregnant rabbits on the mean litter weight of their off-spring. Horizontal lines denote mean values.

FETAL POSITION AND FETAL WEIGHT

○ MORPHINE

● CONTROLS

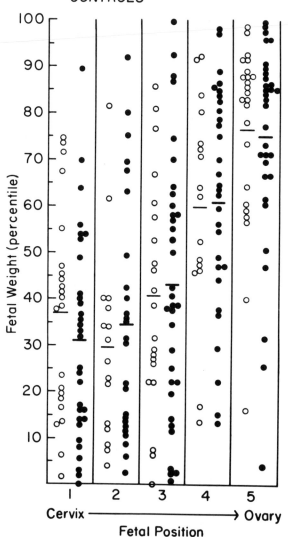

FIG. 2. The effect of intrauterine position on the fetal weight expressed in percentile values Horizontal lines denote mean values.

Fetal weight

As expected, the fetal weight increased with gestational age, but showed considerable intra-litter and inter-litter variance. At all gestational ages examined fetuses from morphine-treated rabbits weighed less (p 0.005) than those from control animals (Figure 1; TableII).

Fetal weight and intrauterine position

It has been noted earlier (Roloff and Howatt, 1973; Rosahn and Green, 1936) that in rabbits one factor influencing fetal growth is the implantation site in the uterine horn whereby the average fetal weight is higher toward the ovarian end of a uterine horn and the lowest toward the cervix. Figure 2 demonstrates this effect by plotting the percentile ranking for the weight of each fetus against its intrauterine location. This effect is not altered by maternal morphine administration.

Pressure/volume curves

Values for V_{10} were calculated from the deflation limb of the pressure/volume curves, and the mean values for each gestational day were compared. There was the expected increase with gestational age (Figure 3). The mean V_{10} values are somewhat lower for fetuses of morphine-treated rabbits, but this is not statistically significant (Table II). In neither sample is there a correlation between the percentile weight and the V_{10} indicating the presence of different regulators for body growth and for the maturation of specific organ systems (Figure 4).

L/S ratio

Determination of the L/S ratio in the amniotic fluid failed to show a rise commensurate with the rise in V_{10} or with the progression of gestation and the groups did not differ (Table II). The phospholipid content in the tracheal washings was too low to be assayed.

DISCUSSION

We conclude that the effect of the administration of morphine to pregnant rabbits resembles the outcome of pregnancies of human narcotic addicts in that it produces underweight offspring. It cannot be stated whether this is a direct effect of the drug on fetal growth at the cellular level or whether the growth failure is a consequence of poor maternal nutrition as suggested by our weight data.

GESTATIONAL AGE AND RESIDUAL LUNG VOLUME

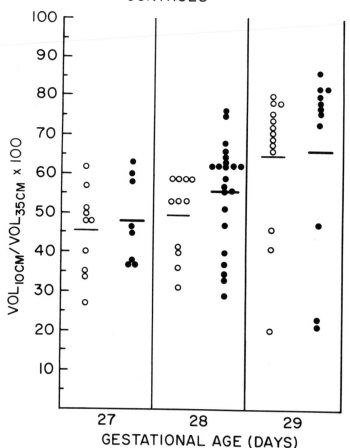

FIG. 3. Comparison of deflation lung volumes (V₁₀) between fetuses of rabbits receiving morphine injections during pregnancy and controls. Horizontal lines denote mean values.

However, Taeusch, Carson, Wang, and Avery (1973) found growth retardation in fetal rabbits whose mothers had received 0.8 to 3.3 mg/kg heroin intravenously twice daily for 3 consecutive days from the 24th day of gestation, but they noted that these does had not lost weight. The failure of maternally administered morphine to induce pulmonary surfactant activity in our more prolonged administration study extends these authors' results from a more acute experiment. They found no difference in the deflation pressure/volume curves of fetuses whose mothers had been injected with heroin, but reported increased

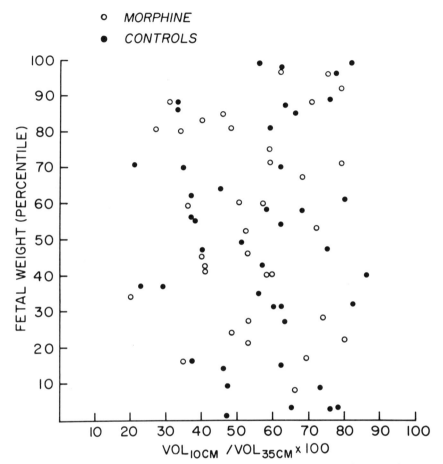

RESIDUAL LUNG VOLUME AND FETAL WEIGHT

o   *MORPHINE*

•   *CONTROLS*

FIG. 4.   Lack of correlation between lung maturation and relative fetal growth.

lung distensibility when 10-20 mg/kg heroin was injected directly into the fetus once on the 24th day. They postulated a dose-related effect. We could not achieve this effect, even by giving the highest doses compatible with the preservation of pregnancies.

A similar difference between the maternal and fetal administration of a drug to rabbits was established for cortisol by Motoyama, Orzalesi, Kikkawa, Kaibara, Wu, Zigas, and Cook (1971). There was also no demonstrable effect on lung maturation by the maternal administration of chlorpromazine in an experiment by Krauer, Rosegger, Salloch, and Scopes (1973) Placental factors have not been investigated. Glass, Rajegowda, Mukherjee, Roth, and Evans (1973) reported that infants of addicted mothers have cord blood cortisol levels equal to those of normal infants. The possible action of a postnatal factor was discussed by Glass, Rajegowda, Kahn, and Floyd (1972), who postulated that the postnatally observed alkalosis of these infants may help prevent RDS.

The fact that the amniotic fluid L/S ratio in rabbits does not correlate with gestational age has been corroborated by Olson (1973). We believe that the discrepancy to human data is due to quantitative rather than qualitative differences in the metabolism of surface-active phospholipids. Gluck and Kulovich (1973) observed earlier than expected rises in the amniotic fluid L/S ratio of 10 infants of mothers addicted to narcotics.

Beyond the obvious species difference, important differences exist between the animal experiment and the human pathophysiology: 1) a chemically pure substance is given to the animals, while a poorly defined mixture of ingredients is used by narcotic addicts; 2) the drug regimen was begun after the onset of pregnancy, whereas human mothers are addicted before they become pregnant; 3) the animals were not regulating the drug intake by self-administration as a human addict would, and thus they might have been periodically in a state of withdrawal. All these factors might result in a different intrauterine environment. The actual mode of action in those situations in which accelerated pulmonary maturation does occur awaits further clarification.

SUMMARY

Morphine was injected subcutaneously in doses of 2.5 to 10 mg/kg every 6 hours into pregnant rabbits from early pregnancy until delivery by hysterotomy on the 27th, 28th, or 29th day. Pregnant control animals received 0.9% NaCl injections. Abortions occurred in 34% of the morphine-treated does as a dose-related effect and in 6.5% of the controls. In preserved pregnancies the prevalence of intrauterine death was identical in both samples. Fetuses of treated animals weighed significantly less than those of the controls. However, the normally present effect of intrauterine position on fetal growth was not altered in fetuses of treated animals, so that growth-retarded as well as normal fetuses weighed more when located in the ovarium rather than the cervical portion of the uterus.

The fetal lungs were inflated to 35 cm H_2O and the remaining air at a deflation pressure of 10 cm H_2O (V_{10}) was determined as a measure of lung stability. There were no differences in this indicator of fetal lung maturity between fetuses of treated and control animals. It was found that the lecithin/sphingomyelin (L/S) ratio in the amniotic fluid of rabbits does not correlate with lung maturity; there were no differences between fetuses of treated and control animals.

Morphine, when administered to pregnant rabbits does not accelerate fetal lung development. Therefore, the observed reduction in the incidence of respiratory distress syndrome in infants of heroin-addicted women has no direct equivalent in this animal model.

References

Barr, M., and Brent, R.L. The relation of the uterine vasculature to fetal growth and the intrauterine position effect on rats. *Teratology*, 1970, *3*. 251-260.

Glass, L., Rajegowda, B.K., and Evans, H.E. Absence of respiratory distress syndrome in premature infants of heroin-addicted mothers. *Lancet*, 1971, *2*. 685-686.

Glass, L., Rajegowda, B.K., Kahn, E.J., and Floyd, M.V. Effect of heroin withdrawal on respiratory rate and acid-base status in the newborn. *New England Journal of Medicine*, 1972, *286*. 746-748.

Glass, L., Rajegowda, B.K., Mukherjee, T.K., Roth, M.M., and Evans, H.E. Effect of heroin on corticosteroid production in pregnant addicts and their fetuses. *American Journal of Obstetrics and Gynecology*, 1973, *117*. 416-418.

Gluck, L., and Kulovich, M.V. Lecithin/sphingomyelin ratios in amniotic fluid in normal and abnormal pregnancy. *American Journal of Obstetrics and Gynecology*, 1973, *115*. 539-546.

Gluck, L., Kulovich, M.V., and Borer, R.C. Estimates of fetal lung maturity. *Clinics in Perinatology*, 1974, *1*. 125-139.

Kotas, R.V., and Avery, M.E. Accelerated appearance of pulmonary surfactant in the fetal rabbit. *Journal of Applied Physiology*, 1971, *30*. 358-361.

Kotas, R.V., Fletcher, B.D., Torday, J., and Avery, M.E. Evidence for independent regulators of organ maturation in fetal rabbits. *Pediatrics*, 1971, *47*. 57-64.

Krauer, B., Rosegger, H., Salloch, R., and Scopes, J. Pretreatment of pregnant rabbits with chlorpromazine—assessment of any enzyme-inducing effect on the fetus. *Biology of the Neonate*, 1973, *23*. 8-10.

Motoyama, E.K., Orzalesi, M.M., Kikkawa, Y., Kaibara, M., Wu, B., Zigas, C.J., and Cook, C.D. Effect of cortisol on the maturation of fetal rabbit lungs. *Pediatrics*, 1971, *48*. 547-555.

Olson, E.B. Personal Communication, 1973.

Roloff, D.W., and Howatt, W.F. Lung maturation and variations in fetal growth. *Journal of Pediatrics*, 1973, *83*. 151-152.

Rosahn, P.D., and Greene, H.S.N. The influence of intrauterine factors on the fetal weight of Rabbits. *Journal of Experimental Medicine*, 1936, *63*. 901-921.

Taeusch, H.W., Carson, S.H., Wang, N.S., and Avery, M.E. Heroin induction of lung maturation and growth retardation in fetal rabbits. *Journal of Pediatrics*, 1973, *82*. 869-875.

DISCUSSION

Q. *Dr. Merritt:* We also have found a notable discrepancy between the gestational age and LS ratio in the rabbit, and, in fact, found our peak total at 28 days, 18 hours, although the LS ratio was less than 1. Also, for Dr. Glass, we noted that although acidosis had profound effects upon the choline incorporation pathways, in both rats and rabbits, the alkalosis was just as bad, and, in fact, we demonstrated this. I have one slide that I will show you. This particular slide is on rats, but the one for rabbits is similar. This is using C 14 choline, with an in vitro incubation over a 30-minute period. We find peak incorporation at 7.4; however, incorporation of C 14 choline precursor was diminished at pH's that we find to be clinically severe in RDS. Why we have that transient elevation at 6.8, I do not know, but I certainly would not recommend it as the optimal pH. But alkalosis is just as bad as acidosis.

Addictive Diseases: an International Journal 2 (2): 381-384 (1975)
© 1975 by Spectrum Publications, Inc.

GENERAL DISCUSSION

Dr. Nathenson: Phenobarbital seems to be ideally suited for preventing seizures, and I wonder what the difference is in the two series, or three series, that we heard about. Was it due to the fact that one group uses phenobarbital, or Valium perhaps, and the other one does not? So, I would like to suggest that the drug that suppresses all symptoms is the wrong type of drug to use in the management of these infants. These infants should be symptomatic. Phenobarbital, as I said before, sedates the infant sufficiently to make him sleep. The symptoms that the infant has, tremors particularly, and the stiffness, the rigidity, are like Parkinsonism. These disappear, or certainly subside tremendously, during treatment with phenobarbital; and the infant is manageable after three to five days. Before I close I would like to appeal to people who experiment with drugs, to use double-blind trials, rather than any other type of approach. Dr. Neuman, who is here, and myself have used it in studying the relative efficacy of phenobarbital and chlorpromazine. Using the double-blind approach is a very sobering experience to anyone.

Dr. Kron: We, in Philadelphia, are very interested in the variety of drugs that are being used currently in the treatment of the neonatal, narcotic abstinence syndrome. Probably our group had the usual prejudices of pediatricians regarding what were the appropriate drugs used, namely, the drugs that have been used over the years, and proven "safe" for the neonate. However, we, too, have had some sobering experiences when we have applied the newer methods for evaluating the behavior of the newborn. We have discovered that the drugs which have been found to be safe and effective over the years are indeed effective in alleviating symptoms, but seem, when we measure the behaviour of the infant using fine-grain techniques, also to suppress what would be considered normal adaptive functioning in the newborn. Now our concern—my being a psychiatrist, Dr. Finnegan, a neonatologist, Dr. Connaughton, an obstetrician—with special interest in these patients, is the effect that this may have upon the developing mother-infant relationship, which to begin with, is sorely stressed in the addict. The addict herself, as pointed out by Dr. Coppolillo, is a person who has very little in the way of resources to invest in this new object; and indeed, in the populations we have studied, we found that often the mothers will deliver their baby, and in spite of the efforts on the part of a social work team to involve the mothers in the attention and care of their infants, they will be surprised to be notified some days or weeks later that there is a baby at the hospital for them to come in and retrieve, to take home. Dr. Finnegan, in her knowledge through contact with these mothers, has, if I can speak for her, indicated that in many cases in the subculture which our addicts come from, there is a concern about investing in the baby too early, before it's a proven product—if it is a preemie, before it comes up to normal weight; or if it is a baby undergoing the throes of withdrawal, before it has overcome this disorder. To begin with, the population in which it is difficult to stimulate the normal mother-infant relationship, and by introducing a variety of the iatrogenic complications, such as medications which may suppress the responsitivity of the infant and make it less interactive with the mother or the mothering object, we may be doing a disservice, in spite of the fact that the drug itself is very effective in alleviating the symptoms or preventing convulsions. The two most effective drugs, in terms of quieting the infants, in our experiment were indeed barbiturates and Valium—Valium, the most potent of all. However, the nurses could, by looking at the babies in the nursery, tell which babies were on barbiturates, which were on Valium, and which were on paregoric. Paregoric babies were lively and responsive. The opiate did not suppress the type of responsivity which, in its exaggerated form, is probably considered a portion of the abstinence syndrome. But in its normal amounts, it is probably an important evoker of maternal responses, an evoker of involvement on the part of the environment. So, I think that besides the efficacy of the drug, we also have to consider in what way the drug may have effects on the social functioning, and interfere with the setting up of the relationship between the mothering figure and the infant, such as has been discussed earlier. So it is a complex issue, not one simply related to the pharmacology of the agent, but also its psychology, the manner in which it is going to influence the very beginnings of what, hopefully, is a normal nurturing and receptive interaction between the child and the mother. But in the case of the addicts it is usually not, and may be further confounded by our interventions. Another point is in terms of a misunderstanding regarding the pharmacology of depressants or sedatives, vis-a-vis the opiates. Opiates, in gradually decreasing amounts, have been found over the years (in work at the Lexington and other centers) to suppress the abstinence syndrome without creating undue central nervous system depression. In order to achieve similar results with other medication, sedatives, for example, it is necessary to give doses to adults which are obtunding. You have to anesthetize the adult in withdrawal, and it is effective if you put an adult addict asleep with a barbiturate; he is free of the symptoms. As soon as he wakes, however, he is once more in the throes of his discomfort, and small amounts of opiates do not create this problem. So that if we are to learn from what is available from animal experiments as well as from adult experience, we would tend to use opiates unless there is some specific contraindication. And, I think that the major contraindication is the feeling that it is wrong, or bad, or inappropriate to be giving it to an infant. You may be creating or potentiating a problem—making an addict out of him. As Dr. Zelson suggests, there are two problems; mainly the psychological addiction or dependence, as well as the biological, biochemical, metabolic need for the drug. But the infant only has the latter. We may probably safely utilize opiates without concern for creating some future potential for addiction. In any case, the baby has been addicted *in utero* for many, many months and we are only probably adding a small, additional risk to whatever is there. This is not a plea for opiates because I would rather that we keep our minds open and look at the data. As I gather, there are many different viewpoints, from today alone there are three different, very strong viewpoints regarding the treatment (pharmacologic). I wonder whether that does not indicate something to us already, that the answer has not yet been achieved, and we still have to do plenty of comparative studies on both the pharmacology and behavioral effect of these drugs before coming to any definite conclusion. May I suggest that, in one of our studies, a single dose of phenobarbital given to a mother within three hours of delivery suppressed the adaptive functioning of the baby throughout the first week of life? I think what has been shown to us is the pharmacologic evidence indicating that such doses of drugs, which are supposed to be benign and short-acting, have, indeed, very profound and prolonged effects, and I am not sure whether we are really just giving a single dose or three doses. But, we are giving a dose, such as when we give an injection of one of the long-acting phenothiazines. It is staying there and it is going to have its effect over a month or two months. Are we willing to, or is it safe? Do we have evidence about it, something that we should do with the baby when we know that there are other drugs that have half-lives of just a few hours, and may at least be excreted by the baby's metabolism in a much shorter period of time? I do not know the answers, but it appears to me that we should not have too strong feelings about it at this point, when we have so little information or data to back up our point of view, other than our clinical sense, which is valuable for generating hypotheses but not adequate to come to conclusions on. It is a way to ask a question but it is not the answer yet.

Dr. Rolloff: In our studies, the Demerol has an effect of about 10 percent of that in the average dosage given to mothers, 10 percent of that of the barbiturate. But it is a real effect.

Dr. Davis: The last comment was that often, phenobarbital or general anesthesia, and other methods of analgesia, cause the same depression of adaptive behavior. We do not have to touch the phenobarbital at this point. I think the concept that I would like to see discussed more is, When is treatment indicated and when is it not, and what are the goals of treatment? Dr. Kron really put emphasis, I think, in the right direction. Whether treatment is required or not depends upon who is looking at the child. What are the criteria for calling a certain kind of behavior a symptom? It is very arbitrary. I have found in my city, from analyzing data from the various hospitals, that the criteria are terribly arbitrary. For example, nurseries where pacifiers were forbidden because of lack of nursing and fear of infection, have a high rate of babies being treated. Nobody could stand a baby crying constantly. Nurseries where pacifiers and other methods were used had a lower rate of treatment indication. And further, by the application of other observations of the behavior, treatment could be handled in such a way that they could be pacified without pharmacological agents. As far as pharmacological agents are concerned, I have not used any narcotics in the last 100 babies. Of course, I am not a neonatalogist. Only because of my research and involvement as a consultant, a neonatalogist would follow my recommendations; and it has been my observation that it is Valium which reduces the time for hospitalization, which I think is crucial. With paregoric, hospitalization has been longer, as with methadone babies. There is a great difference between methadone and heroin babies. They are much more responsive and faster on the heroin. Therefore, paregoric, even if it may be a better medication, can damage and further alienate the mother from the child by prolonging the separation and, therefore, perhaps, we should pay the price of working with the mother and putting more investment in the handling of the treatment only in a different direction.

Subject Index

A

Abortion, 26, 72, 106-108, 371, 378
Abscesses, 259
Abstinence syndrome, 113-121, 141-158, 257-275, 381-382
  manifestations, 116-118, 143, 198, 258
  norepinephrine production, 304-305
  score sheet, 31, 145-147, 159-168
  seizures, 209
Acetophenetidin, 54
Acetylcholine, 277
Acetylcholinesterase, 277, 278
Acetylcycloheximide, 291
Acidosis, 364, 379
Adenine nucleotides, 293
  ATP, 293, 296, 301
Adrenal function,
  fetal, 40, 41
  phenobarbital effects, 327
  rats, 293-305
Adrenaline, 305
Adrenergic neurons, 293
Adrenocorticotropin (ACTH), 327
Alcohol,
  control of alcoholism, 162-163
  dehydrogenase, 40
  fetal syndrome, 79-88
  in combination with other drugs, 1, 2, 9-16, 102, 107, 109, 209, 232, 358, 359
  placental transfer of, 55
  statistics of use, 16-18
Alkaline phosphatase (HSAP), 89-99
Alkaloids, 55
Alkalosis, 117, 358-359, 364, 378, 379
Amnionitis, 28, 29
Aminopyrine, 38, 51
Amitriptyline, 11
Amniocentesis, 99
Amniotic fluid,
  drug detection, 114, 175
  L/S ratio, 370-372, 378
Amobarbital, 8, 131, 132, 133
Amphetamine,
  analysis of, 26

catecholamine levels, 309, 312-316, 330, 331
chromosomal damage, 66
drug screen for, 91, 93, 173, 178
in mice, 279, 287
placental transfer of, 55
prenatal exposure, 307-316, 327
statistics of use, 1, 8, 11, 12-15, 17
teratogenic effects, 46, 48
Amytal (Amobarbital), 8, 131, 132, 133
Analgesics
  effect on adaptive behavior, 383
  in combination with other drugs, 13
  narcotic, 27
  statistics of use, 8, 15-16, 18
Anemia, 29, 30, 336
Anesthetics, 54, 55, 383
Aniline, 38, 51
Anotia, 58
Anoxia, 118
Anti-depressants, 8, 11, 12, 17
Antihistamines, 55
Apgar,
  effects of obstetrical sedation, 263, 266
  heroin addict mothers, 115
  methadone-maintained mothers, 172, 190, 192, 197, 215, 228, 238, 239, 258
  study parameter, 194, 195, 237, 238
Apnea, 163
Asphyxia, 31, 33, 172, 199
Asthma, 29
Ataxia telangiectasia, 73
Atelectasis, 33

B

Barbiturates,
  analysis of, 26
  chromosomal effects, 66, 69
  effects on sucking behavior, 265, 267, 273
  in combination with other drugs, 69, 91, 93, 107, 109, 114, 165, 173, 178, 209, 232, 358
  placental transfer, 54, 55
  seizures, 291
  statistics of use, 7-10, 17

teratogenic effects, 46, 48, 316
treatment for neonatal withdrawal, 167, 236, 260, 382, 383
Bayley Scales (of Infant Development), 215, 217, 218, 230, 231, 239, 240, 242
Benzedrine, 13
3, 4-Benzpyrene, 38, 43, 51
Bilirubin, 163, 195-197, 228, 229, 232
Biotransformation, 37-43, 51
Birth order, 237, 239
Blood,
    chromosomal abberations in, 66-68, 73, 77
    gas, 161, 358-360, 362, 364
    3HSAP detection, 92-94
    pH, 359, 360, 363, 364
Bloom's syndrome, 73
Bradycardia, 163
Brazelton Neonatal Assessment Scale, 166, 167, 204, 215, 217, 226, 230, 231, 239, 240, 242-245, 261, 262, 268-271, 274
Breech, 259
Bubble-Stability test, 366
Butabarbital, 8, 132
Butisol (Butabarbital), 8

C

Caffeine, 49, 55
Caesarian section, 228, 239
Calcium, 31, 181, 192, 196, 228, 229
Camphor, 156, 157, 167, 168
Cannabis, 46, 134, 135, 185
Carbamazepine, 132, 133
Carcinogen, 38, 39, 43
Cardiac disease, 29
Catechol products, 42, 305
Catecholamines (see also dopamine),
    effects of drugs on, 220, 295-303, 305, 309, 311-316, 321, 327, 331
    effects of stress, 330
    running response in mice, 289
    synthesis of, 293, 294, 308
Cellulitis, 29, 30, 338, 342
Cerebral palsy, 230
Clastogen, 63
Child abuse, 205, 230
Chloral Hydrate, 54
Chlordiazepoxide, 10, 49
Chlorpromazine,
    gas chromatography, 124, 125

lung maturation, 377
metabolism, 38
neonate withdrawal treatment, 31, 67, 69, 143, 162, 163, 165, 167, 178, 236, 260, 343, 381
placental transfer, 54, 55
teratogenic effects, 46
Chlorothiazide, 54
Cholelithiosis, 51
Choline acetyltransferase, 277
Chorioamnionitis, 338
Chromosome damage, 63-77
Cirrhosis, 87
Cleft palate, 46, 48, 57
Cocaine,
    analysis of, 26
    chromosomal damage, 66, 67, 69
    in combination with other drugs, 91, 92, 173
    in mice, 279, 287
    statistics of use, 18
Codeine, 135
Coma, 260
Constipation, 162
Convulsions, 118, 119, 190, 197, 199, 258, 263
Coombs test, 229
Corticosteroids, 351, 360, 366
Corticosterone, 327
Cortisol, 361, 366, 377
Cyclazocine, 135
Cycloheximide, 277, 279, 286, 288, 289
Cytochrome P-450, 38
Cytogenic effects,
    pharmacological, 63-77
    viral, 63
Cytomegalic-inclusion disease, 111

D

Darvon (Propoxyphene), 15
DDT, 124
Dehydration, 163, 164, 259
Delirium tremens, 87
Demerol (Meperidine), 211, 260, 368, 383
Deserpidine, 46
Desipramine, 52
Desmethylimipramine, 38
Dexedrine, 13
Dextro amphetamine (Dexedrine), 54, 55
Dextrorphan bitartrate, 279, 284
Diabetes, 29, 90, 351

Diaphoresis, 215
Diarrhea, 117, 120, 164, 173, 190, 191, 196, 197,
    215, 216, 220, 236, 258, 341
Diazepam (see also Valium), 38, 49, 143, 149,
    152, 156, 209
Diethylstilbesterol, 41
DNA, 318, 319, 320, 321
Diphenylhydantoin, 46, 48, 55, 57
Donnatal, 229, 233, 236, 239
Dopamine,
    assay of, 311
    effects of drugs on, 220, 295, 296, 305, 312,
        313, 315, 321
    in mice, 291
    in rats, 299, 300, 302, 303
    synthesis of, 293, 294
Doriden (Glutethimide), 9, 93
Doxepin, 11
Dysmorphogenesis, 80

E

Elavil (Amitriptyline), 11
Electroencephalograph, 214, 219, 224, 231, 240,
    247-249, 251, 252, 255, 259, 287
Electrophysiological studies, 236, 240-255
Embryo, 3, 45, 57, 307
Encephalitis, 119
Epilepsy, 163, 316
Epinephrine, 296-299, 301
Epoxide, 38, 39, 43
Equanil (Meprobamate), 10
Ethambutol, 69
Ethchlorvynol, 9
Ethinamate, 9, 46
Ethylmorphine, 38
Exocytosis, 296, 305
Extrapyramidal symptoms, 165

F

Fanconi's anemia, 73
Fetal alcohol syndrome, 79-88
Fever, 116, 173, 258, 338
Fiorinal (Butabarbital), 8
Folate deficiency, 29, 321, 330
Furuncles, 338

G

Gas chromatography,
    biomedical application, 123, 137
    methadone analysis, 169-178
Gastrointestinal Distress, 113, 115, 117, 118,
    120, 190, 191, 195, 197, 229, 236, 239, 258,
    275
Gastroschisis, 33
Glomerulonephritis, 365
Gonorrhea, 29, 30, 336
Glucuronide, 39, 40, 41
Glutathione, 38, 39, 43
Glutethimide, 9, 93
Gravidity, 193, 194, 195

H

Hallucinogenic drugs, 13, 63
Haloperidol, 46
Hemorrhage, 28, 29, 33, 119, 336
Hepatitis (serum), 29, 30, 259, 336, 337, 342
Hernia, 111, 210
Heroin,
    child abuse, 230
    chromosome damage, 65-69, 71-77
    effect on autonomic system, 163
    in combination with other drugs, 13
    mycolonic jerks, 217
    neonatal complications, 118, 119
    pregnant addict, 21-35, 89, 91, 92, 94, 104,
        105, 108, 109, 112, 114, 115, 119, 159, 160,
        165, 169, 187, 188, 192, 193, 196-199, 213,
        224, 225, 227, 229, 232, 233, 235-239, 241-
        255, 258, 259, 265, 273, 274, 333-344, 347-
        355, 357-368, 369, 384
    rabbits, 376, 377
    seizures, 211
    statistics of use, 18
    sweating, 168
    teratogenic effects, 53-55
Herpes, 67
Hexobarbital, 38, 51
Hyaline membrane disease, 365, 367
Hydrocarbons, 38, 39, 41, 52
Hydroceles, 210
Hydrocephalus, 210
Hydronephrosis, 57
Hydrops fetalis, 33
Hydroxycorticosteroids, 357-361, 364

Hyperactivity, 216, 219, 241, 258
Hyperacusis, 115, 120
Hyperbilirubinemia, 163, 179, 182, 195, 255, 316
Hyperemesis gravidarum, 336
Hyperglycemia, 351
Hyperinsulinism, 351
Hyperphagia, 117, 120
Hyperserotoninemia syndrome, 220
Hypertension, 29
Hyperthermia, 215
Hyperthyroidism, 119, 305
Hypertonus, 116, 172, 190, 196, 197, 215, 219, 236, 241, 258, 366
Hypnotics, 1, 102
Hypocalcemia, 118, 119, 161, 181
Hypoglycemia, 118, 119, 160, 161, 301, 343, 351
Hypomagnesia, 119
Hypothalamus, 305, 321, 327, 343, 351, 364
Hypotension, 163

I

Imipramine, 11, 46, 55
Inanition, 259
Insulin, 301, 302, 343, 354
Ion Monitoring (selected), 131-136
Isoniazide, 69
Irritability, 119, 173, 196, 197, 215-217, 225, 229, 230, 233, 245, 247, 253, 258-260, 265, 267-271, 343, 358

J

Jaundice, 33, 40, 118, 163, 232, 255

K

Kernicterus, 255
Klinefelters, 75

L

Landavreflexes, 216
Laryngospasm, 162

Lecithin, 364, 365, 370-372, 375, 378, 379
Leukemia, 73
Levorphanol, 279, 284
Librium (Chlordiazepoxide), 10
Lumbar puncture, 31
Lung, rabbit, 369-381
LSD (Lysergic Acid Diethylamide), 18, 47, 49, 54, 55, 64, 65, 210

M

Marijuana, 14, 18, 185, 358
Mass spectroscopy, 125-139
Meconium, 33, 99, 103, 115, 118, 228, 367
Meningitis, 111, 119, 158, 160, 199, 258
Meningomyelocoele, 210
Meperidine, 211, 260, 368, 383
Mepivacaine (carbocaine), 54
Meprobamate, 10, 55
Mescaline, 47
Metaraminol, 296-298, 300, 301
Methadone,
    chromosome damage, 65-69, 71, 74-76
    disposition, 52-56, 169-178
    induced toxicity, 2
    jaundice, 118
    maintenance for pregnant addicts, 21-35, 89-99, 101-112, 114, 115, 119, 150, 159, 160, 163, 165, 167, 187, 192-195, 197-199, 209, 210, 213-226, 227-233, 235-239, 241-255, 258, 259, 265, 267-270, 274, 334-344, 347-355, 358, 365, 366
    treatment for withdrawal, 156, 157, 168, 260, 273, 275, 368, 384
    urinalysis for, 161, 166, 173-175
Methaqualone, 9, 47, 91, 92, 133, 134
N-methylaniline, 38
Methyclothiazide, 54
Methylphenidate, 47
Methyprylon, 9
Miltown (Meprobamate), 10
Moniliasis, 342
Monoamine oxidase, 309, 327
Morbidity, 22, 32, 34, 72, 106, 109, 142, 169, 210, 226, 259
Moro response, 216
Morphine,
    chromosome damage, 65
    effect on catecholamines, 295-305
    mice, 255, 277-291

rabbits 369-379
rats, 343, 350, 351, 355
seizures, 209, 211
sulfurylation by fetus, 41
teratogenic effects, 47, 54
tidal volume, 368
urinalysis for, 91, 93, 160, 163, 165, 178, 187, 188, 192, 193, 195, 198, 229, 230
vapor phase analysis, 133, 135
Mortality, 22, 32, 34, 54, 72, 79, 85, 101, 102, 105, 107, 109, 111, 142, 199, 210, 260, 315, 317, 318, 327, 348
Mother-child relationship, 3, 201-208, 214, 219, 316, 381, 382, 384
Mouse,
    effects of amphetamine on, 309-316, 327
    effects of phenobarbital on, 316-328
    perinatal addiction, 277-291
Mutagenic effects,
    drug induced, 48, 49, 72
    radiation, 73
Myoclonic jerks, 198, 199, 217, 220

N

Nalorphine, 368
Naloxone, 279, 284, 287, 289, 291, 368, 370
Narcosis, 261
Nasal stuffiness, 196, 197, 258
Nembutal (Pentobarbital), 8
Neoplasia, 43
Neurotube defects, 210
Neurotransmitters, 308, 309, 315
Nialamide, 47
Nicotine (smokers), 54, 358, 359
Noludar (Methyprylon), 9
Norepinephrine, 304, 305, 311, 312, 315
Normetanephrine, 131
Normeparadinic acid, 211
Nutrition, 29, 84, 213, 232, 255, 259, 299, 308, 335, 337, 340, 341, 351, 375

O

Obesity, 29
Opisthotonos, 220
Organogenesis, 49, 57, 58, 307
Otitis media, 343
Oxyhemoglobin, 364

P

Pain, 119
Pallor, 258
Parachloraphenylalanine, 291
Paregoric,
    camphor in, 156, 157, 167, 168
    dosage, 143, 148, 162
    effects on sucking, 151-154, 263, 265, 273, 274
    treatment of withdrawal, 31, 67, 144, 149, 150, 229, 233, 236, 260, 274, 275, 382, 384
Parity, 238, 239
Pemoline (Pentazocine), 47
Pentazocine, 15, 47, 135
Pentobarbital, 8, 130
Pharmacokinetics, 2, 3, 52, 169, 185, 355
Phenelzine, 47
Phenobarbital,
    disposition in neonate, 179-185
    dosage, 143, 148, 158, 162
    effect on sucking, 150-154, 263, 272, 273
    in mice, 52-54
    neonatal withdrawal, 31, 143, 144, 148, 149-154, 156, 209, 239, 265, 275, 360, 367, 381
    prenatal exposure, 166, 307, 308, 316-328, 383
    statistics of use, 1, 3, 8
    vapor phase analysis, 132
Phenothiazines (see also Chlorpromazine), 55, 67, 69, 165, 178, 383
Phocomelia, 48, 58
Phototherapy, 229
Placenta,
    Abruptio, 28, 29, 34, 228, 230, 236, 265
    enzymes in, 38, 42, 90, 97
    inflamation of, 338
    transfer of drugs, 4, 39, 41, 51-56, 58, 67, 84, 89, 169, 174, 176, 219, 299, 315, 319
    weight, 94
Placidyl (Ethchlorvynol), 9
Pneumonia, 33, 163, 343, 358
Pneumothorax, 358
Polycythemia, 119
Pre-eclampsia, 22, 23, 24, 28, 29, 34, 90, 91, 111
Premature births, 101, 102, 232, 237, 255, 259, 333, 334, 338, 348, 353, 361, 365, 367, 369
Prochlorperazine, 47
Propoxyphene, 15
Prostitution, 29

Protein,
  determination, 318
  effects of drugs on synthesis, 277, 308, 319,
    320, 323, 343
Psychedelics, 66
Pyridoxine dependence, 119
Pyuria, 338

Q

Quaalude (Methaqualone), 9, 92
Quinine, 26, 54, 65, 91, 93, 160, 161, 165, 199

R

Rabbit, 369-379
Rat,
  acidosis in, 379
  adrenal development, 293-305, 331
  affect of amphetamines on, 309, 315
    methadone on, 354, 355
    morphine on, 343, 351
    tranquilizers on, 308
Reserpine, 47, 54, 309, 315
Respiratory distress, 33, 89, 99, 117, 118, 158,
    162, 163, 173, 255, 258, 357-368, 369, 371,
    378, 379
RNA, 316, 318-321

S

Salicylate, 47, 54, 55
Salmonella, 342
Scopolamine, 49
Secobarbital, 8, 130, 184, 263, 267
Seconal (Secobarbital), 8
Seizures,
  audiogenic in mice, 255, 287-290
  neonatal, 3, 119, 143, 173, 198, 199, 291
  treatment of, 162, 163, 381
Sedatives,
  barbiturates, 144, 153, 162, 163, 178, 316, 382
  in combination with other drugs, 9, 11-13, 16,
    17, 102
Sepsis, 161
Septicemia, 119
Serotonin, 220, 289, 291
Shock, 260

Sinequan (Doxepin), 11
Sleep studies, 214, 240, 247-252
  REM, 165, 216, 219, 220, 247, 343
SKF 525A, 52, 53
Sneezing, 190, 196, 197, 236, 258, 263
Sopor, 9
Sphingomyelin, 364-366, 370-372, 375, 378, 379
Spinal tap, 259
Splanchnic nerve, 295, 298, 301
Stillbirths, 107, 108, 348
Sucking behavior,
  effects of drugs on, 150-154, 166, 184, 185
  in neonatal withdrawal, 2, 117, 167, 190, 196,
    197, 214-216, 219, 236, 246, 258, 261-274
  measurement of, 261-274
Sudden death, 210, 367
Sulfurylation, 41
Suprapubic tap, 31
Surfactant, 357, 364, 376
Swaddling, 31, 116, 121, 143, 158, 216, 219,
    229, 236, 246
Sweating, 115, 117, 120, 168, 190, 196, 197, 258
Syphilis, 25, 29, 30, 336, 342

T

Tachypnea, 33, 158, 191, 215, 360, 364
Talipes equinovarus, 210
Talwin (Pentazocine), 15
Tegretol (Carbamazepine), 132, 133
Teratology, teratogenic effects,
  dietary deficiency, 45
  drug induced, 46, 47, 48, 49, 52, 57, 58
  radiation, 45
  rubella, 45
Tetany, 160, 194
Tetrahydrocannabinol, 134, 135
Thalidomide, 1, 48-50, 57, 58
Thiazides, 54
Thiopental, 185
Thrombophlebitis, 163, 259
Thorazine (Chlorpromazine), 67, 69, 178
Thyrotoxicosis, 305
Tidal volume, 359, 367, 368
Tofranil (Imipramine), 11
Toxemia, 23, 259, 336
Tranquilizers,
  in combination with other drugs, 9, 12, 16
  in pregnant rats, 308
  maternal use, 48, 111, 204

neonatal withdrawal, 157, 162, 167, 214
statistics of use, 1, 8, 10, 11, 17, 18
Transsynaptic inductions, 293, 296, 303
Tremors, 3, 115, 119, 143, 157, 158, 163, 173,
    190, 191, 196, 197, 198, 207, 215, 219, 258,
    358, 366, 367, 381
Trophic hormones, 321
Tuberculosis, 69
Tumor, 39, 277, 278
Tyrosine, 293-296, 299, 300, 302, 303, 305

V

Vaginitis, 336
Valium (Diazepam),
    effect on sucking, 263
    maternal abuse, 178
    neonatal withdrawal, 31, 67, 162, 163, 168,
        209, 229, 233, 236, 239, 260, 381, 382, 384
    statistics of use, 10, 11
Valmid (Ethinamate), 9
Vapor Phase Analysis, 123-139
Venereal disease, 259, 337
    VDRL, 228, 229, 336
Vesicles (storage), 293, 296-304
Vomiting, 117, 162-164, 173, 190, 191, 196, 197,
    215, 216, 236, 258, 341

W

Weight
    gain, 197, 229, 230
    heat stable alkaline phosphatase, 94
    induced low birth, 2, 46, 47, 89
        by alcohol, 80, 81, 85
        by heroin/methadone, 22-25, 27, 29, 32,
            34, 101, 102, 106-109, 115, 119, 149, 151,
            172, 189, 190, 195, 197, 214, 215, 228,
            231, 232, 237-239, 255, 259, 333, 334,
            337-340, 347-355, 357-360
    loss, 191, 194, 196, 258
    rabbits, 370-377
    rats, 299
Withdrawal,
    assessment scales, 2, 143-155, 157, 161, 166,
        167, 191, 204, 215-218, 220, 226, 230, 231,
        238-253, 261-271, 274
    effects on mothering behavior, 205, 206, 208,
        209, 214, 246, 340, 382

maternal, 25-27, 29, 103
neonatal, 22, 24, 31-34, 55, 67, 69, 89, 102,
    107, 108, 111-121, 141-158, 159-168, 169-
    178, 179, 180, 187, 199, 209, 215, 216, 219,
    220, 257-275, 336, 343, 348, 349, 357, 358-
    363, 366, 368
rats, 295, 297
subacute, 120
tyrosine levels, 305

X

Xenobiotics, 51

Y

Yawning, 116, 190, 196, 197, 236, 258, 263